New Concepts in Neoplasia as Applied to Diagnostic Pathology

INTERNATIONAL ACADEMY OF PATHOLOGY
MONOGRAPHS IN PATHOLOGY

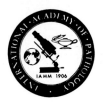

SERIES EDITOR, Nathan Kaufman, M.D.
Secretary-Treasurer
US-Canadian Division
International Academy of Pathology

No. 1. **The Lymphocyte and Lymphocytic Tissue**
JOHN W. REBUCK *and* ROBERT E. STOWELL, *Editors*
No. 2. **The Adrenal Cortex**
HENRY D. MOONE *and* ROBERT E. STOWELL, *Editors*
No. 3. **The Ovary**
HUGH G. GRADY *and* DAVID E. SMITH, *Editors*
No. 4. **The Peripheral Blood Vessels**
J. LOWELL ORBISON *and* DAVID E. SMITH, *Editors*
No. 5. **The Thyroid**
J. BEACH HAZARD *and* DAVID E. SMITH, *Editors*
No. 6. **The Kidney**
F. K. MOSTOFI *and* DAVID E. SMITH, *Editors*
No. 7. **The Connective Tissue**
BERNARD M. WAGNER *and* DAVID E. SMITH, *Editors*
No. 8. **The Lung**
AVERILL A. LIEBOW *and* DAVID E. SMITH, *Editors*
No. 9. **The Brain**
ORVILLE T. BAILEY *and* DAVID E. SMITH, *Editors*
No. 10. **The Skin**
ELSON B. HELWIG *and* F. K. MOSTOFI, *Editors*
No. 11. **The Platelet**
K. M. BRINKHOUS, R. W. SHERMER, *and* F. K. MOSTOFI, *Editors*
No. 12. **The Striated Muscle**
CARL M. PEARSON *and* F. K. MOSTOFI, *Editors*
No. 13. **The Liver**
EDWARD A. GALL *and* F. K. MOSTOFI, *Editors*
No. 14. **The Uterus**
HENRY J. NORRIS, ARTHUR T. HERTIG, *and* MURRAY R. ABELL, *Editors*
No. 15. **The Heart**
JESSE E. EDWARDS, MAURICE LEV, *and* MURRAY R. ABELL, *Editors*
No. 16. **The Reticuloendothelial System**
JOHN W. REBUCK, COSTAN W. BERARD, *and* MURRAY R. ABELL, *Editors*
No. 17. **Bones and Joints**
LAUREN V. ACKERMAN, HARLAN J. SPJUT, *and* MURRAY R. ABELL, *Editors*
No. 18. **The Gastrointestinal Tract**
JOHN H. YARDLEY, BASIL C. MORSON, *and* MURRAY R. ABELL, *Editors*
No. 19. **The Lung**
Structure, Function, and Disease
WILLIAM M. THURLBECK *and* MURRAY R. ABELL, *Editors*
No. 20. **Kidney Disease: Present Status**
JACOB CHURG, BENJAMIN H. SPARGO, F. K. MOSTOFI, *and* MURRAY R. ABELL, *Editors*
No. 21. **The Pancreas**
PATRICK J. FITZGERALD *and* ASHTON B. MORRISON, *Editors*
No. 22. **Perinatal Diseases**
RICHARD L. NAEYE, JOHN M. KISSANE, *and* NATHAN KAUFMAN, *Editors*
No. 23. **Current Topics in**
Inflammation and Infection
GUIDO MAJNO, RAMZI S. COTRAN, *and* NATHAN KAUFMAN, *Editors*
No. 24. **Connective Tissue Diseases**
BERNARD M. WAGNER, RAUL FLEISCHMAJER, *and* NATHAN KAUFMAN, *Editors*
No. 25. **The Breast**
ROBERT W. McDIVITT, HAROLD A. OBERMAN, LUCIANO OZZELLO, *and*
NATHAN KAUFMAN, *Editors*
No. 26. **The Pathologist and The Environment**
DANTE G. SCARPELLI, JOHN E. CRAIGHEAD, *and* NATHAN KAUFMAN, *Editors*
No. 27. New Concepts in Neoplasia as Applied to Diagnostic Pathology
CECILIA M. FENOGLIO-PREISER, RONALD S. WEINSTEIN, *and* NATHAN KAUFMAN, *Editors*

INTERNATIONAL ACADEMY OF PATHOLOGY MONOGRAPH

New Concepts in Neoplasia as Applied to Diagnostic Pathology

EDITED BY

CECILIA M. FENOGLIO-PREISER, M.D.

Chief, Laboratory Services
Veterans Administration Medical Center
Albuquerque, New Mexico
and
Professor, Department of Pathology
University of New Mexico School of Medicine
Albuquerque, New Mexico

RONALD S. WEINSTEIN, M.D.

Harriet Blair Borland Professor and Chairman
Department of Pathology
Rush Medical College
Rush-Presbyterian-St. Luke's Medical Center
Chicago, Illinois

NATHAN KAUFMAN, M.D.

Secretary-Treasurer
United States-Canadian Division
International Academy of Pathology
Augusta, Georgia

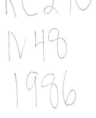
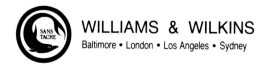

WILLIAMS & WILKINS
Baltimore • London • Los Angeles • Sydney

Editor: George Stamathis
Associate Editor: Carol Eckhart
Copy Editor: Stephen Siegforth
Design: Bob Och
Illustration Planning: Joseph P. Cummings
Production: Anne Seitz

Copyright © 1986
The United States-Canadian Division of
THE INTERNATIONAL ACADEMY OF PATHOLOGY

Printed in the United States of America

Library of Congress Cataloging-in-Publication Data

Main entry under title:

New concepts in neoplasia as applied to diagnostic pathology.

   (International Academy of Pathology monograph; no. 27)
   Based on presentations for a long course entitled "New concepts in neoplasia as applied to diagnostic pathology" held during the 15th International Congress of the International Academy of Pathology, Sept. 1984, in Miami Beach, Fla.
   Includes index.
   1. Cancer—Diagnosis—Congresses. I. Fenoglio-Preiser, Cecilia M., 1943–   .
II. Weinstein, Ronald S. III. Kaufman, Nathan, 1915–   . IV. International Academy of Pathology. International Congress (15th: 1984: Miami Beach, Fla.) V. Series: Monographs in pathology; no. 27. [DNLM: 1. Neoplasms—diagnosis—congresses. 2. Neoplasms—pathology—congresses. W1 M0568H no. 27/ QZ 241 N5287 1984]
RC270.N48   1986   616.99′2075   85-91274
ISBN 0-683-03151-1

Printed at the
Waverly Press, Inc.

86   87   88   89   90   10 9 8 7 6 5 4 3 2 1

Foreword

This 27th monograph in the series *Monographs in Pathology* is the first in the series to be based on a course given at an International Congress, rather than at our annual meeting. Since this congress was hosted by this Division and the Long Course organized along the same lines as our previous Long Courses, it was felt appropriate to include this particular material in this series.

The Long Course presented at the XV International Congress of the International Academy of Pathology in September 1984 entitled "New Concepts in Neoplasia as Applied to Diagnostic Pathology" was considered to be timely because of the recent developments of these concepts. It was very ably organized and directed by Drs. Cecilia M. Fenoglio-Preiser and Ronald Weinstein. This publication gives us an opportunity to present up-to-date material by experts on the various topics in a manner which is more detailed, more extensive, and more documented than the oral presentations.

The Academy wishes to express its appreciation to Drs. Fenoglio-Preiser and Weinstein, to the other distinguished contributors to this monograph, and to the publisher, Williams & Wilkins, for valuable support and cooperation.

NATHAN KAUFMAN, M.D.
Series Editor

Contributors

ROBERTO BUFFA, M.D.
   Department of Human Pathology and Histopathology, Histochemistry and Ultrastructure Center, University of Pavia, Pavia, Italy

CARLO CAPELLA, M.D.
   Department of Human Pathology and Histopathology, Histochemistry and Ultrastructure Center, University of Pavia, Pavia, Italy

MARIA I. COLNAGHI, PH.D.
   Director of the Division of Experimental Oncology E, Istituto Nazionale per lo Studio e la Cura dei Tumori, Milano, Italy

R. C. COOMBES, M.D.
   Ludwig Institute for Cancer Research (London Branch), Royal Marsden Hospital, Sutton, Surrey, England

JOHN S. COON, M.D., PH.D.
   Department of Pathology, Rush Medical College and Rush-Presbyterian-St. Luke's Medical Center, Chicago, Illinois

MATTEO CORNAGGIA, M.D.
   Department of Human Pathology and Histopathology, Histochemistry and Ultrastructure Center, University of Pavia, Pavia, Italy

LUIS FELIPE FAJARDO, L-G, M.D.
   Professor of Pathology, Stanford University School of Medicine and Chief, Laboratory Service, Veterans Administration Medical Center, Palo Alto, California

CECILIA M. FENOGLIO-PREISER, M.D.
   Chief, Laboratory Services, Veterans Administration Medical Center and Professor, Department of Pathology, University of New Mexico School of Medicine, Albuquerque, New Mexico

B. GUSTERSON, M.D.
   Ludwig Institute for Cancer Research (London Branch), Royal Marsden Hospital, Sutton, Surrey, England

KLAUS E. KUETTNER, PH.D.
   Departments of Biochemistry and Pathology, Rush-Presbyterian-St. Luke's Medical Center, Chicago, Illinois

LANCE A. LIOTTA, M. D., PH.D.
   Chief, Laboratory of Pathology, Chief, Tumor Invasion and Metastasis Section, National Cancer Institute, National Institutes of Health, Bethesda, Maryland

MARGARET B. LISTROM, M.D.
   Attending Pathologist, Veterans Administration Medical Center, Albuquerque, New Mexico

MARVIN A. LUTZNER, M.D.
*National Cancer Institute, National Institutes of Health, Bethesda,
Maryland, and Unite des Papillomavirus, Institut Pasteur, Paris,
France*

RENATO MARIANI-COSTANTINI, M.D.
*Research Assistant of the Division of Anatomical Pathology and
Cytology, Istituto Nazional eper lo Studio e la Cura dei Tumori, Milano,
Italy*

R. A. J. MCILHINNEY, M.D.
*Ludwig Institute for Cancer Research (London Branch), Royal Marsden
Hospital, Sutton, Surrey, England.*

SYLVIE MENARD, PH.D.
*Research Associate of the Division of Experimental Oncology E, Istituto
Nazionale per lo Studio e la Cura dei Tumori, Milano, Italy*

P. MONAGHAN, M.D.
*Ludwig Institute for Cancer Research (London Branch), Royal Marsden
Hospital, Sutton, Surrey, England*

A. MUNRO NEVILLE, M.D., PH.D.
*F.R.C. Path., Director, Ludwig Institute for Cancer Research (London
Branch), Royal Marsden Hospital, Sutton, Surrey, England*

BENDICHT U. PAULI, D.V.M.
*Departments of Biochemistry and Pathology, Rush-Presbyterian-St.
Luke's Medical Center, Chicago, Illinois*

FRANCO RILKE, M.D.
*Director of the Division of Anatomical Pathology and Cytology, Istituto
Nazionale per lo Studio e la Cura dei Tumori, Milano, Italy*

GUIDO RINDI, M.D.
*Department of Human Pathology and Histopathology, Histochemistry
and Ultrastructure Center, University of Pavia, Pavia, Italy*

DANIEL SCHWARTZ, M.D.
*Department of Pathology, Rush Medical College and Rush-Presbyterian-
St. Luke's Medical Center, Chicago, Illinois*

ENRICO SOLCIA, M.D.
*Professor, Department of Human Pathology and Histopathology, Histo-
chemistry and Ultrastructure Center, University of Pavia, Pavia, Italy*

ELDA TAGLIABUE, PH.D.
*Research Assistant of the Division of Experimental Oncology E, Istituto
Nazionale per lo Studio e la Cura dei Tumori, Milano, Italy*

PATRIZIA TENTI, M.D.
*Department of Human Pathology and Histopathology, Histochemistry
and Ultrastructure Center, University of Pavia, Pavia, Italy*

THOMAS B. TOMASI, M.D., PH.D.
*Distinguished University Professor, Director of the Cancer Center, Chair-
man, Department of Cell Biology, University of New Mexico, Albuquerque, New Mexico.*

GABRIELLA DELLA TORRE, PH.D.

Research Assistant of the Division of Experimental Oncology A, Istituto Nazionale per lo Studio e la Cura dei Tumori, Milano, Italy

TIMOTHY J. TRICHE, M.D., PH.D.

Chief, Ultrastructural Pathology Section, Laboratory of Pathology, National Cancer Institute, National Institutes of Health, Bethesda, Maryland

RONALD S. WEINSTEIN, M.D.

Harriet Blair Borland Professor and Chairman, Department of Pathology, Rush Medical College, Rush-Presbyterian-St. Luke's Medical Center, Chicago, Illinois

JORGE J. YUNIS, M.D.

Professor of Pathology, Department of Laboratory Medicine and Pathology, University of Minnesota Medical School, Minneapolis, Minnesota

Contents

Chapter 1

Introduction

CECILIA M. FENOGLIO-PREISER AND RONALD S. WEINSTEIN

Benign and malignant neoplastic proliferations occur in a population of cells which were previously normal and in some way have lost their usual regulatory mechanisms such that unrestricted growth occurs and tumors develop. Not all cells have the same potential to undergo neoplastic proliferations and, further, even a cell which may be rendered neoplastic relatively easily may not become transformed in every individual exposed to an oncogenic agent. In this volume, some specific oncogenic agents will be discussed. After considering current ideas on how cells become neoplastic, several chapters discuss the biology of the hallmarks of malignant growth, namely, tumor invasion and metastases. Then, tumor cell phenotype is considered from the standpoint of diagnostic pathology. The usefulness of several markers in identifying the progenitor cells of specific human malignancies is considered, as well as the use of cytoplasmic and cell surface markers in predicting the clinical course of the malignant dyscrasia in individual patients.

Cancer is clearly a multifactorial disease. Operationally, oncogenic agents can be subclassified into genetic, physical, chemical, infectious, and immunologic categories. There are specific associations between certain cancers and their presumed etiologic agents. Several examples exist of genetic disorders associated with an increased incidence of cancer. Specific chemicals are known to cause tumors both in experimental animals and in humans. Physical agents such as irradiation can irreversibly transform cells. Infectious agents such as certain viruses, both endogenous and exogenous, are oncogenic in experimental systems and are associated with some human malignancies.

Since the interaction of cells with dissimilar oncogenic agents can result in the production of a pathologically identical tumor, such as a squamous cell carcinoma, it is plausible that each of these agents may act through a common pathway, possibly the activation of an endogenous virus or an oncogene. Various aspects of this subject are explored in the chapters by Drs. Tomasi, Yunis, and Fajardo. This is followed by a presentation of the spectrum of lesions caused by one class of viruses, the papillomaviruses, by Dr. Lutzner.

Whatever the etiologic agent for a particular tumor in an experimental system or in man, tumors evolve over a period of time, and the individual cell populations comprising them apparently pass through various stages of abnormal growth control regulation. It is also clear that even though a specific agent is oncogenic in some settings, most agents are unable to cause malignant proliferations in many cells lines or in all individuals, either due to unique interactions required of the agent with the progenitor cells, differences in host responses, or other factors. It is well established that some families are more prone to develop cancer than others. Some may have a definable genetic syndrome or karyotype abnormality as discussed by Listrom and Fenoglio-Preiser. Others may not have morphologically recognizable karyotypic abnormalities but may have chromosomes which are unusually susceptible or resistant to the mutagenic effects of a particular agent. This subject is explored by Dr. Yunis, especially with regard to fragile sites on chromosomes.

Mere exposure to potential carcinogens in the foods we eat or the air we breathe may be insufficient to cause cancer, until they are activated by enzymes to create an alkyl or aryl derivative, which then binds preferentially to DNA, RNA, or cell proteins. Radiation can interact with cells to cause lipid peroxidation of cell membranes, either the plasma membrane or membranes of individual organelles. Of greater importance to the cancer problem, radiation is known to induce chromosomal damage which may be manifested as deletions, gaps, or translocations within individual chromosomes which might directly activate oncogenes. The relationship of one type of physical injury, *i.e.*, ionizing radiation, to the subsequent development of neoplasia is discussed in detail in the chapter by Dr. Fajardo.

Tumors, once established, are influenced by growth factors, growth inhibitors, hormones, and biogenic amines. There are numerous growth promoters and modifiers. One which has generated a large literature and captured the imagination of the scientific community is so-called tumor angiogenesis factor. This is produced by successful neoplasms which have the capacity to induce the proliferation of endothelial cells to form new blood vessels, thereby allowing them to maintain sufficient access to oxygen and nutrients required for a sustained increase in tumor mass. It has been hypothesized that inhibition of tumor angiogenesis factor would stunt tumor growth and thus render malignant cell proliferations innocuous. In recent years, it has been suggested that angiogenesis factor is nonspecific, possibly restricting its potential clinical value. In a chapter on alternative approaches to restricting tumor dissemination, Drs. Kuettner and Pauli characterize endogenous stromal proteinase inhibitors that may partially explain differences in host susceptibilities to tumor invasion. It remains to be seen whether proteinase inhibitors are of therapeutic value. This is followed by a chapter by Drs. Liotta and Ras on the biology of tumor invasion, stressing the interactions of tumor cell surface receptors with extracellular matrix components.

A broad spectrum of nuclear, cytoplasmic and cell surface changes have been detected in neoplasms. Some, such as the laminin receptors described by Drs. Liotta and Ras may be mechanistically related to the invasive process whereas the expression of others may represent epiphenomena unrelated to tumor behavior but, nevertheless, of value for tumor diagnosis, classification, or as prognostic factors. The chapters by Dr. Neville and his associates and Dr. Rilke and associates describe the use of monoclonal antibodies to breast carcinomas in detecting micrometastases in bone marrow. This provides an important approach to the identification of patients with "dormant" carcinoma, undetectable by conventional histopathology. Drs. Weinstein, Schwartz, and Coon describe the prognostic significance of the deletion of normal epithelial cell surface components, the tissue blood group antigens, in patients who present with low grade, low stage urinary bladder transitional cell carcinoma, as well as the use of marker profiles for establishing the risk of recurrences and invasion. The chapter by Dr. Solcia and his associates outlines the use of antigenic markers in analyzing various neuroendocrine tumors. Finally, Dr. Triche summarizes the current state of the art in working up the ultimate challenge in tumor classification, the anaplastic tumor.

Chapter 2

Cellular Aspects of Neoplasia

MARGARET B. LISTROM AND CECILIA M. FENOGLIO-PREISER

Pathologists are characteristically able to distinguish between the neoplastic and nonneoplastic phenotype of a given cell population based on specific morphologic features. These features may be visualized using standard histological techniques (Fig. 2.1), ultrastructural analysis, chromosome preparations, or special staining techniques such as immunohistochemistry. In this chapter the morphologic, histologic, and cytologic features of neoplastic cells will be discussed organelle by organelle. No new cellular organelles are seen in neoplastic cells but quantitative and qualitative alterations may be present.[133]

NUCLEUS

GENERAL MORPHOLOGIC FEATURES

Often it is the nuclear characteristics that allow one to recognize the neoplastic phenotype (Fig. 2.1) and to distinquish benign from malignant cells. Criteria that are commonly present in neoplastic cells are an increased nuclear size, producing an increased nuclear cytoplasmic ratio (often with nuclear gigantism), and nuclear pleomorphism, correlating with an abnormal chromosomal number and an altered DNA content, prominent nucleoli, and peripheral chromatin clumping (Fig. 2.1). Abnormalities in nuclear size result from endoreduplication, true endomitosis, and a type of polytenization.[249] In addition, increased mitoses are often present, indicative of an actively proliferating cell population, even though the reproducibility of counting mitosis may be variable.[130, 222, 234]

Ultrastructurally, these nuclear abnormalities are even more prominent, with irregular distribution of the heterochromatin, prominent nucleoli, peripheral chromatin clumping, active mitoses, bizarre shapes (Fig. 2.2), and the presence of nuclear inclusions ranging from viruses to structures known as nuclear bodies (Fig. 2.3).[100, 233, 240, 243]

Many of the nuclear bodies have structures resembling nucleoli.[243] Some are similar to small nucleoli with a filamentous cortex. Others resemble ring-shaped nucleoli (Fig. 2.4) or nucleoli with separation of their components.[240] Others merely represent cytoplasmic inclusions.

In most cells the nucleolus disappears during mitoses; it is thought to disintegrate concomitant with dissolution of the nuclear membrane.[34] Those which

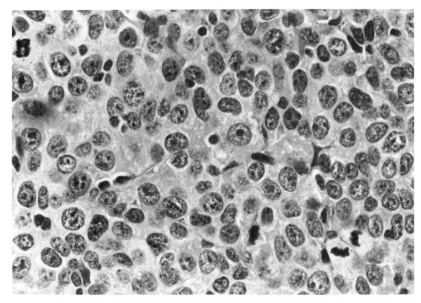

FIG. 2.1. Light micrograph of a malignant islet cell tumor. The cells are pleomorphic with many mitoses evident. In addition, peripheral nuclear clumping and prominent nuclei are noticeable. One would not have difficulty making a diagnosis of neoplasia on such a lesion.

TABLE 2.1. TUMORS CONTAINING INTRANUCLEAR RODLETS

Gliomas
Ependymomas
Pancreatic islet cell tumors
Parathyroid adenomas
Mycosis fungoides
Sarcomas
Neuroepithelial tumors

are retained and persist during metaphase and anaphase are referred to as persistent nucleoli. These may be seen in neoplastic cells,[148, 225] and their number often reflects histological differentiation.[225]

Intranuclear rodlets are composed of proteinaceous material of uncertain origin and function[233] and are found in various tumors,[17, 100, 117, 189, 201, 227, 238, 247] (Table 2.1). The rodlets are composed of individual filaments that measure up to 7–9 nm in width and are not restricted to neoplastic cells.[117] Intranuclear crystalline inclusions with a leaf-like, striated appearance ("zebra bodies") are inducible in tumor cells by viruses.[268] Intranuclear annulate lamellae may also be present.[96, 133]

NUCLEAR MEMBRANE

By definition, human cells are compartmentalized into the nucleus (Fig. 2.1 and 2), which contains the genetic material and structures involved in transcription and processing of transcription products, and into the cytoplasm, which contains the translational apparatus, cellular organelles, and other

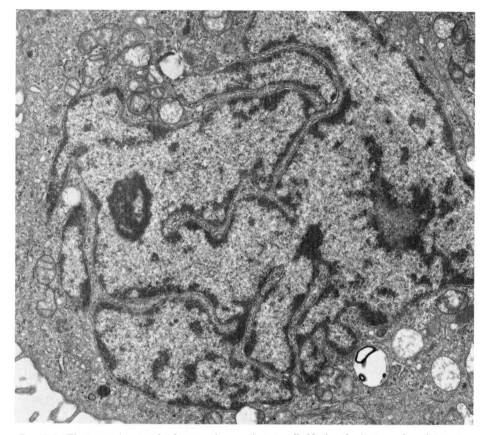

FIG. 2.2. Electron micrograph of an ovarian carcinoma cell. Notice the increased nuclear cytoplasmic ratio with the marked nuclear pleomorphism, cytoplasmic invaginations, peripheral nuclear clumping, and prominent nucleolus.

structures. This compartmentalization is maintained by the nuclear envelope, which is always present except during mitoses[86] (Fig. 2.1–2.5).

One important part of the nuclear membrane is the nuclear pore complex, which functions in nuclear-cytoplasmic exchanges. In some tumors nuclear pore complexes are significantly reduced. This observation has been used to explain the discrepancy that exists between active-appearing nuclei and an indolent-looking cytoplasm. The hypothesis is that there may be a disturbance of nuclear-cytoplasmic transport of proteins. It is further postulated that morphologic signs of nuclear hyperactivity may represent compensation for the nuclear membrane defect.[123]

In neoplastic cells the nuclear membrane may also show blebbing, pockets, and projections, particularly in lymphoma cells.[133] The fibrous lamina may also become quite prominent. This structure appears to be associated with some oncogenes.[75]

As noted above, neoplastic cells are often mitotically quite active. The nucleus undergoes profound alterations when cells enter mitosis: the nuclear envelope breaks down and chromatin condenses into individual chromosomes

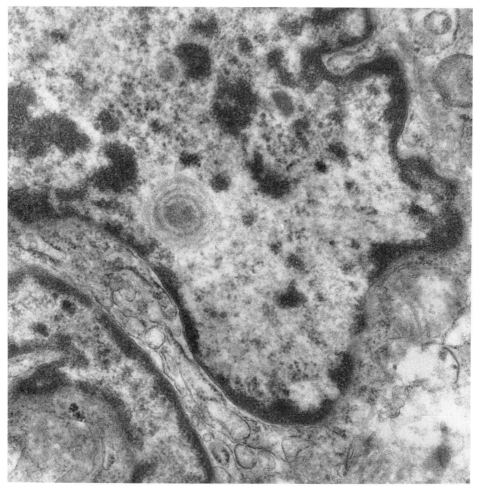

Fɪɢ. 2.3. Electron micrograph of an ovarian cancer. A prominent nuclear body is seen in the nucleus of the cell just left of the center of the illustration.

(Fig. 2.5). Certain proteins become associated with the condensed chromosomes.[196] There is (are) a specific protein(s) (phosphoproteins) that is (are) mitosis-associated.[62] It (they) may phosphorylate the nonhistone proteins necessary to initiate mitosis.[85]

Nuclear Sex Chromatin (Barr Bodies)

Barr bodies are frequently absent in the neoplastic cells of females; this may be due to: (1) the loss of the inactivated X chromosome; (2) the possibility that a previously inactive X chromosome may become activated by the malignant process; or (3) the presence of more than two X chromosomes. There is a direct relationship between ploidy and the incidence of normal single Barr bodies. Atkin[7] showed that approximately 8% of near diploid cervical cancers contain a normal single Barr body, whereas 20% of the aneuploid tumors had a low percentage of these structures. This contrasted with a low frequency of Barr

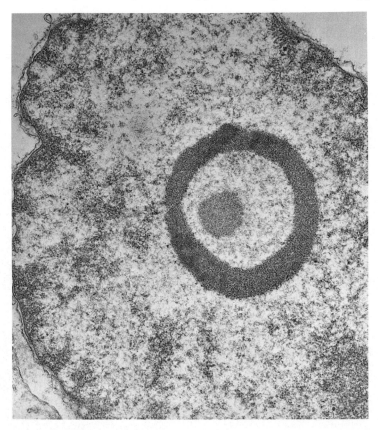

FIG. 2.4. Electron micrograph of a poorly differentiated carcinoma of the endometrium. Notice the prominent ring-shaped nucleolus.

bodies in tumors that had a near triploid pattern. This observation was also confirmed for breast cancer.[7] The relationship of the Barr bodies to the ploidy status has led investigators to suggest that the identification of the Barr body could be used as a prognostic factor in evaluating patients with cancer.[7, 8, 15, 126]

The concept that Barr body analysis could be useful diagnostically is not new and was first introduced in 1954 by Hunter and Lennox.[120] However, the usefulness of detecting these structures may be hampered by physiologic variations pertaining to sex chromatin frequency. For example, estrogen administration is capable of activating the X chromosome, thereby reducing the frequency of finding Barr bodies.[6, 16, 107, 202]

It now appears that in breast cancer patients, tumor grade is not directly related to the presence of these structures, although tumor cells with small, uniform nuclei, as in infiltrating lobular carcinomas, are more likely to have a higher Barr body frequency than cells with large atypical nuclei as seen in medullary carcinoma.[26, 29, 106, 132, 134] There is also a relationship between the age of the patient, the presence of metastatic disease, and the presence of sex chromatin. Finally, large numbers of Barr bodies are usually associated with high levels of estrogen receptors and other receptors in primary breast can-

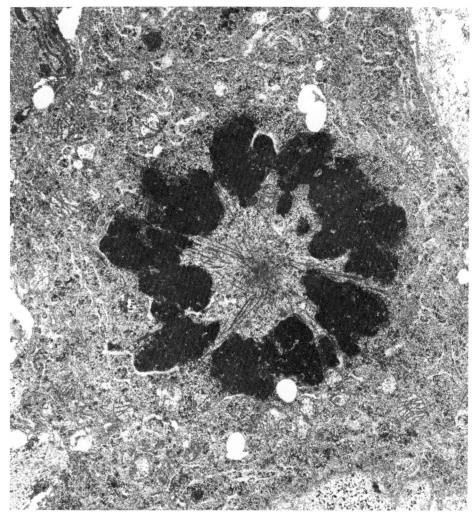

Fɪɢ. 2.5. Electron micrograph of a cell in mitoses. The prominent microtubular network is present in the middle of the condensed chromosomes getting ready to spread these into the mitotic spindle.

cers.[236, 239] Epidermoid cancers of the cervix and endometrial adenocarcinomas in patients with sex chromatin-negative tumors do more poorly over a 5-year period than do those with sex chromatin positive tumors.[41]

Occasionally, one finds the presence of a Barr body, and therefore a female karyotypic pattern, in males with tumors. A sex chromatin-positive melanoma and choriocarcinoma of the testis have been reported, as have male patients with lung cancers containing Barr bodies.[7, 111]

Neoplastic cells may contain more than one Barr body and some have as many as three. Tumors containing more than one Barr body are usually near tetraploid or hyperdiploid. Most near tetraploid tumors in females are sex chromatin-negative, either through the loss of an inactive X chromosome dur-

TABLE 2.2. APPLICATION OF CHROMOSOMAL ANALYSIS TO NEOPLASIA

1. Etiology and causation
2. Diagnosis and classification (Ph in AML)
3. Prognosis and response to therapy
4. Disease characterization
5. Genetic disease and neoplasia
6. Carcinogenesis, prevention, and public health aspects
   a. Monitor chromosomal change and sister chromatid exchanges
   b. Establish specific karyotypic changes for environmental carcinogens

TABLE 2.3. CELLULAR AND VIRAL ONCOGENES

Virus	Viral Gene Abbreviation	Cellular Gene Abbreviation
Rous sarcoma	v-src	c-src
Myelocytomatosis	v-myc	c-myc
Fujinami sarcoma	v-fps	c-fps
Y 73	v-yes	c-yes
VR2 Avian sarcoma	v-ros	c-ros
Carcinoma MH2	v-mht/myc	c-mht//my
Avian erythroblastosis	verb^A/verb^B	c-verb^A/verb^B
Myeloblastosis and erthroblastosis E 26	v-myb or v-ets	c-myb or c-ets
Reticuloendotheliosis	v-rel	c-rel
Abelson murine leukemia	v-abl	c-abl
Harvey and Kirsten rat sarcoma	v-ras$^{HA \text{ or } KI}$	c-ras$^{HA \text{ or } KI}$
Maloney murine sarcoma	v-mos	c-mos
FBJ murine osteosarcoma	v-fos	c-fos
ST and GA feline sarcoma	v-fes	c-fes
SM feline sarcoma	v-fms	c-fms
Simian sarcoma	v-sis	c-sis

ing cytogenetic changes in the tumor or through activation of the inactive X chromosome.[213]

The presence of more than one Barr body occurs exclusively in females, usually in those patients with metastatic disease. This can be helpful in diagnosing effusion cytology, in which the presence of double Barr bodies is strong evidence for the presence of malignancy.[2, 13]

GENETIC FEATURES OF NEOPLASIA

Among others, the genetic study of human cancer mainly involves two aspects: genetic abnormalities in cancer cells and genetic predispositions to develop cancer (Table 2.2).

Perhaps the most exciting development in our understanding of neoplasia comes from the demonstration that the genetic change that probably underlies all cancers involves critical viral genes known as viral oncogenes and their homologues in normal cells (host or cellular oncogenes). We have known for decades that the causes of cancer are manifold and include chemicals, viruses, physical agents, and other agents that fall under the umbrella of "environmental agents." Highly oncogenic retroviruses, papova, and adenoviruses add dominant oncogenes to cells, thereby transforming them. This observation has changed our perception that there are different carcinogenic routes since all agents may act by adding (or activating) an oncogene.[248] These are derived from the normal cellular genome[152] and may become the common denominator between the carcinogenic action of viral and nonviral agents.[152] Because the common pathway in oncogenesis may involve the activation of an oncogene, this area will be covered before considering other nuclear and genetic aspects of the neoplastic cell.

Oncogenes

As discussed in the chapters by Yunis and Tomasi, oncogenes (or transforming sequences) are present in many neoplastic cells and are thought to be the genes whose activation plays a role in the induction of the neoplastic phenotype. In general, the transforming sequences from different cancers are different.[168] However, exceptions exist, for example, similar transforming sequences have been identified in human colon and lung cancer cell lines.[190] Many of the transforming sequences are similar to *c-onc* genes, the cellular homologue of retrovirus *onc* genes (Table 2.3).[66] *C-onc* genes are normal components of the human genome containing genetic sequences homologous to those of the corresponding *v-onc* genes carried by retroviruses.[50]

V-onc genes are responsible for the neoplastic phenotype. The functional significance of *c-onc* genes in nonneoplastic cells is not known, but they are thought to play a role in cellular differentiation. Evidence for this comes from the demonstration of differences in the level of transcription of individual *c-onc* genes during development[167] or regeneration.[102] Other suggested roles for oncogenes (or their products) are listed in Table 2.4.[33, 53, 79, 95, 219, 224, 228–230, 232, 244]

The human equivalents of several oncogenes have been mapped to specific chromosomes by hybridization techniques. These regions (Table 2.5) are sites that often are involved in translocations in human hematologic malignancies (see below).[57, 105, 115, 145, 171, 190, 273]

Point mutations, multiple mutations, inversions, deletions, insertions, and

TABLE 2.4. Postulated Oncogene or Oncogene Product Activity

Guanine nucleotide binding[56]
Kinase for actin microtubular protein[57–60]
Phosphoprotein kinase (cAMP-dependent kinase)[57–59]
Nuclear neoantigens[61]
Adenylate cyclase[62]
ATP synthetase[63]
Specific protein secretion[64]
Altered adhesion plaques, junctions[65]
DNA binding proteins[62]
Platelet-derived growth factor[62]
Transposons[62]
Transferrins[62]

TABLE 2.5. Chromosomal Location of Oncogenes

c-myb	Chromosome 6
c-myc	Chromosome 8
c-mos	Chromosome 8
c-abl	Chromosome 9
c-fes	Chromosome 15
c-sis	Chromosome 22

other structural differences have been identified on *v-onc* and *c-onc* genes.[36] Single-base changes in the oncogene of a human bladder cancer cell line suggests a partial mutational role in some carcinogenic events.[197, 246] A point mutation in *c-ras H* has also been found in leukocytes and normal bladder cells in patients with bladder cancer, suggesting that a mutation in *c-ras H* oncogenes confers predisposition to neoplasia.[169]

More Than One Oncogene(?)

From studying hereditary human cancers, a second class of human cancer genes has been identified. They are known not by their activity but from the lack thereof. The normal form of these genes is believed to suppress the activity of oncogenes, and therefore, they can be thought of as "anti-oncogenes." This class of genes may be responsible for the dominantly inherited predispositions to cancer that account for most "cancer families."[137]

Thus, it appears as if there are at least two genes (not including anti-oncogenes) involved in the already well recognized multistep process that results in the generation of malignant cells. This is not a new concept but one that was introduced in 1941 by Berenblum.[19] It is currently envisioned that at least two genes function in the development of neoplasms, one of which is related to division; the other affects cytoplasmic or cell membrane functions.[142] It is not clear how these specific genes induce nuclear stimulatory machinery, nor is it clear what the effect of altering plasma membrane proteins is.[33] However, the cellular oncogenes constitute a functionally heterogeneous group of genes, members of which can cooperate with one another to achieve neoplastic transformation, probably through a multistep process.[143]

Stanbridge *et al.*[242] proposed a chromosomal hypothesis of oncogenesis which is as follows: each cell contains within its genome genetic material that is associated with a specific chromosomal segment which is necessary for the proliferative activity of that cell. In differentiated cells this proliferative factor is normally suppressed by a contiguous chromosomal segment which is associated with a specific inhibitory factor. These two genetic loci must be adjacent to one another for the interaction to occur. The chromosomal and intrachromosomal location of each of these factors is unique for each cell type. Any chromosomal rearrangement (such as in translocations, deletions, or insertions) that leads to a loss of continuity between these segments may remove the inhibition of the proliferative factor by the inhibitory factor and may result in the expression of the proliferative functions which become manifest as a result of the neoplastic transformation. Conceptually, the proliferative factor in its dormant state could be classified as a proto-oncogene and, when active, could be considered to be oncogenic.

The present unifying concept of carcinogenesis presupposes that neoplastic transformation involves a mutation or translocation of cellular oncogenes, or a nearby regulatory gene, that normally represses the oncogene.[207, 214, 275] However, at present there is no conclusive evidence that an unaltered proto-oncogene can function as a cancer gene simply through enhanced transcription or gene amplification.[69]

CHROMOSOMAL ABERRATIONS

It is clear that the process of malignant transformation is a complicated one with many steps intervening between the initial cellular alteration and final unrestrained growth within the malignant cell. In this section we will examine what role chromosomal alterations may play in tumor development. These genetic abnormalities may be grossly visible chromosomal alterations, or non-visible point mutations, chromosomal rearrangements, or changes in gene dosage.

Constitutive chromosomal abnormalities fall into two classes: numerical abnormalities (aneuploidy) and structural abnormalities.[256] Numerical abnormalities result from an error in division (nondisjunction). Nondisjunction can involve sex chromosomes or autosomes. If the nondisjunctional event involves sex chromosomes, Klinefelter's syndrome (47 XXY), Turner's syndrome (45 X), the XYY state, and triple X female (47, XXX) genotypes result.

When chromosomal analysis is performed on neoplastic cells, gross abnormalities such as abnormal karyotypes, chromosomal breaks, or ring structures are often seen. These are usually random, but nonrandom specific chromosomal abnormalities have been described in numerous conditions[212] (Table 2.6). The classical example is the Philadelphia chromosome seen in 90% of patients with chronic myelogenous leukemia[182] which represents a translocation from chromosome 22 to chromosome 9.[274] Unfortunately, the chromosomes of many tumors have a fuzzy, ill-defined appearance which can make it difficult to interpret banding patterns,[212] and thus, it may be impossible to determine the exact tumor karyotype.

Three basic classes of chromosomal abnormalities have been described in cancers. These include: (1) reciprocal translocations; (2) deletions or nonreciprocal rearrangements that result in the loss of structural material; and (3) duplications of whole chromosomes or chromosomal segments.

TABLE 2.6. NONRANDOM MORPHOLOGICAL CHROMOSOME CHANGES IN HUMAN CANCER[a]

Chromosome Involved	Disease
1p −	Malignant melanoma
1p − (p34)	Neuroblastoma
1q +	Breast cancer
3p −	Small cell cancer (lung)
5q −	Refractory anemia, AML
6q −	Lymphoma, ALL
7q −	AML
11q −	AMOL, AMMOL
12q −	Acute Leukemia
14q +	Lymphoma, ALL, CLL
14q + (q32)	Adult T cell leukemia
i(17q)	CML
20q −	Polycythemia vera
21q −	Thrombocythemia
22q −	CML, meningioma
1p − i(1q)	Endometrial cancer
3p −, 3q −, 5q −, 7q −	Leukemia

[a]Modified from Sandberg, A. A.[212]

In *reciprocal translocations* there is no significant loss of structural material. Classic examples of this kind of abnormality are marker rearrangements associated with particular lymphomas and leukemias, including Burkitt's lymphoma[20, 153, 210] and chronic myelogenous leukemia (Philadelphia chromosome). These translocations are reciprocal in nature without loss of genetic information.[206] This, in combination with the fact that the break points occur in specific locations, suggests that it is the activation of genes carried on the rearranged segments that contribute to cellular transformation.

The structural rearrangements that characterize chronic myelogenous leukemia and Burkitt's lymphoma (as the result of the translocation) involve the movement of at least two *c-onc* genes from their normal position to new positions adjacent to an identifiable gene coding for immunoglobulin synthesis. In chronic myelogenous leukemia, the *onc* gene *c-abl* moves from chromosome 9 to chromosome 22 near the lambda chain locus.[63] In Burkitt's lymphoma the *onc* gene *c-myc* moves from its position on chromosome 8 to chromosome 14 adjacent to the immunoglobulin heavy chain gene complex.[171] It has been suggested that these rearrangements combining oncogenes with an actively transcribing gene (immunoglobulin gene) may result in altered cell proliferation, enhancing oncogene expression, thereby leading to transformation.[114]

Chromosomal exchanges can theoretically activate *c-onc* genes by moving them away from an adjacent suppressor of transcription or next to an endogenous active promoter of transcription.[98] The particular chromosomal segments participating in these genetic rearrangements may or may not be randomly selected. One mechanism for the nonrandomness may be the identification of fragile sites in the karyotype.[277] (Also see the Yunis chapter for further discussion of this subject.)

The second major class of chromosomal abnormalities consists of *deletions* or *nonreciprocal rearrangements* that result in the loss of structural material at specific chromosomal sites. Examples include chromosomal deletions involving chromosomes 11 and 13 in Wilms' tumor and retinoblastoma, respectively. Retinoblastomas, Wilms' tumors, and neuroblastomas all occur in familial, as well as sporadic forms.[136] In familial cases the predisposition to develop cancer is transmitted as a dominant trait from the parent to the child. Not every child who receives the gene develops cancer and not every cell carrying the gene becomes neoplastic. In an effort to explain this, Knudson[136] proposed a two-hit hypothesis in which at least two gene changes are required for the expression of the malignant phenotype (Table 2.7). In the first hit, one inherits the predisposing germ line gene, and a second gene change occurs (second hit) in the susceptible cells (such as the neuroectoderm) that later become transformed. Sporadic cases are explained, also, by the two-hit theory in that it is assumed that the two hits occur as chance events in the same target cell.[30] Consistent chromosomal abnormalities have now been identified in tumor cell karyotypes from these types of cancers. However, not every example of each tumor type contains the deleted marker chromosome.[98]

Single gene changes associated with particular deletions in cancers of specific differentiated cell types suggest that the deleted genes normally control differentiated cell functions. Alteration in the activity of the differentiation

TABLE 2.7. KNUDSON'S "TWO-HIT" MODEL OF CARCINOGENESIS[a]

Prezygotic First Hit	Second Hit
Familial polyposis coli	Colon cancer
Neurofibromatosis	
Neurofibromas	Neurogenic sarcomas, leukemia
Adrenal medullary hyperplasia	Pheochromocytoma
Multiple mucosal neuroma syndrome	
Thyroid C-cell hyperplasia	Medullary carcinoma
Basal cell nevus syndrome	Basal cell carcinoma
Treated retinoblastoma	Osteogenic sarcoma
Nodular renal blastema	Bilateral Wilms' tumor
Trisomy 21	Leukemia, retinoblastoma
Trisomy 18 with nodular renal blastema	Wilms' tumor
Sporadic antiridia 11p−	Bilateral Wilms' tumor
13q− deletion syndrome	Retinoblastoma
Dysgenetic gonads	Seminoma-dysgerminoma
Ataxia telangiectasia	Lymphoma, leukemia
Bloom's syndrome	Leukemia-gastrointestinal carcinoma
Fanconi's anemia	Leukemia, hepatoma, and gastrointestinal carcinoma
Xeroderma pigmentosum	UV-induced skin cancers

[a]Modified from Bolande, R. P., and Vekemans, M. J-J. [30]

associated genes, or an inappropriate time for their expression during development, could lead to the continued proliferation of cell populations producing the intermediate (or precancerous) lesions that have been described in a number of genetic disorders.[98]

Nonhereditary cancers associated with specific deletions in whole chromosomes or chromosomal segments have been identified in meningiomas, carcinomas of the lung, and preleukemias.[180,264,278] In preleukemia, chromosomal changes may precede the development of frank cancer by several years, indicating that the loss of a single gene is insufficient by itself to result in malignancy.

It has been suggested that, since gene deletion cannot cause transformation by itself, one could predict that homologous genes from a nontransformed cell are capable of correcting the alteration in gene activity by genetic complementation.[278] Evidence exists which supports this hypothesis.[242]

The third class of chromosomal abnormality seen in cancers is *duplication of whole chromosomes or chromosomal segments*, i.e., trisomies. These karyotypic abnormalities may coexist with those described above. For example, in chronic myelogenous leukemia, chromosomal duplication commonly occurs during the terminal acute phase of the illness. These duplications involve an extra chromosome 8, Philadelphia chromosome, or duplication of chromosome 17 or 19. Such karyotypic changes are usually a poor prognostic indicator, with death often occurring within 3 months.[263]

Other nonrandom chromosomal duplications have been reported in lymphoproliferative and myeloproliferative disorders, as well as in solid tumors.[211,278] These duplications may precede, or follow, the development of cancer and, thus, need not be directly responsible for the carcinogenic event.

Except in the case of Down's syndrome, trisomies do not appear to be associated with an increased frequency of cancer.[127, 204] The increase in acute leuke-mias seen in Down's patients suggests that an extra chromosome 21 alters the proliferative capacity of a particular cell population, but in these cells, an additional gene is required for neoplastic transformation.[98]

GENE AMPLIFICATION

Many human tumors have increases in the amount of DNA per cell[15] that can simply result from an increase in the number of chromosomes.

Recently, interest in amplified genes has increased by virtue of the identifi-cation of two related, but morphologically distinctive, chromosomal variants thought to represent tandem duplications of whole genes or submicroscopic chromosomal regions. One of these is a homogeneously stained region (HSR), which was first described by Biedler and Spengler.[23] It derives its name from the fact that it is represented by a structurally pale, intermediate staining intensity on a banded chromosome. The second morphologic variant is a double minute (DM) chromosomal fragment which may actually be derived from the HSR.[10, 265] So far, these two chromosomal morphologic variants have only been seen in neoplastic cells. Multiple gene copies have been localized to the HSRs and DMs using *in situ* hybridization techniques. HSRs and DMs have been identified in freshly explanted human tumors and cell lines derived from neuroblastomas.[10, 23, 98, 252, 265]

Of particular interest is the possibility that amplified oncogenes exist in such regions. As the result of chromosome duplication, cells may contain mul-tiple copies of a given gene, including oncogenes. In fact, this has been demon-strated in several human tumors. Human promyelocytic leukemia cell lines have been shown to contain multiple copies of *c-myc*,[55, 57] and a human colon cancer line contains amplified *c-myc*.[3]

MARKER CHROMOSOMES

Marker (abnormal) chromosomes occur commonly in human tumors, either related to the etiology of the neoplastic event or as a secondary phenomenon. The number of marker chromosomes in a given tumor may be as high as several dozen.[210]

The presence or absence of marker chromosomes can sometimes be related to the biology of the tumor. For example, the presence of a marker chromo-some in noninvasive bladder tumors indicates a high probability of recurrence, whereas its absence indicates a high probability of nonrecurrence.[77, 211] The larger the number of marker chromosomes, the more aggressive the tumor is likely to be.[110, 212] Of interest is the fact that, even when the chromosomes from nonneoplastic cells, such as lymphocytes, are examined for chromosomal aber-rations in patients with cancer, one may find increased numbers of gaps, chro-matid breaks, and chromosomal breaks, suggesting that there may be a rela-tionship between somatic chromosome aberrations and cancer risk.[178] However, even if a chromosomal aberration is present, it may underlie the malignant change without being causal since many steps intervene between the initial cellular alteration and unrestrained tumor growth.[271]

Of particular importance is the fact that the presence of karyotypic abnormalities in peripheral lymphocytes or fibroblasts has been used to detect asymptomatic renal cell carcinoma,[51] thus providing one with the possibility of screening patients for occult cancer.

Some chromosomal changes (-5, -7) are thought to reflect possible exposure to toxic agents, such as petroleum products, chemical solvents, and insecticides and pesticides; all have been implicated in the etiology of some cancers.[163]

Because increased gene transcription, with loss of gene activity, can be produced by submicroscopic changes, it is not necessary that every tumor contain visible chromosomal abnormalities. It is possible that this reflects limitations of the previously used banding techniques since Yunis *et al.*[276] have indicated that high resolution chromosomal banding techniques allow one to identify chromosomal rearrangements in every case of acute leukemia. This contrasts with prior observations that karyotypic abnormalities were present in only 50% of acute leukemias.[205]

Since more than one gene is probably involved in the control of cellular differentiation and proliferation, the pattern of gene changes responsible for carcinogenesis in different cancers may differ.

The chromosomal abnormalities described above tend to accumulate in cells as they continue to divide and as individuals age. This suggests that the gene changes produced following transformation contribute to further tumor progression with enhanced ability of the tumor to invade locally and metastasize, eventually killing the patient.

GENETIC INSTABILITY IN TUMOR DEVELOPMENT

Genetic instability is thought to be the basis for Nowell's thesis[181] of "sequential emergence of mutant subpopulations with increasingly malignant properties." The principle is illustrated in those human disorders in which a systemic chromosome instability or aberration seems to predispose the individual patient to subsequent tumor development. There are a number of chromosome breakage syndromes that are associated with a high incidence of tumors and defects in DNA repair or maintenance.[181] Patients with disorders such as ataxia telangiectasia or Fanconi's anemia are abnormally sensitive to chromosonal damage by environmental carcinogens. Patients with Down's syndrome (discussed above) represent an example of genetic instability with a subsequent high risk of tumor development.

One manifestation of genetic instability in neoplasms is the fact that most human tumors are usually aneuploid by karyotypic or DNA analysis. This is usually due to a change in chromosomal number.[271]

The frequency of chromosomal alterations in cancer cell populations is high, and there is great variability in the incidence of chromosomal change and the rate of development of chromosomal aberrations. Some tumors change their karyotype and phenotype fairly rapidly, while others show karyotypic stability over long periods of time.[4, 112]

CLINICAL RELEVANCE OF CHROMOSOMAL ABERRATIONS

Abundant accumulated evidence correlates biologic behavior with karyotypic abnormalities. Aneuploid tumors are often associated with a greater degree of histologic anaplasia, more frequent metastases and a worse prognosis than their diploid counterparts.[89, 183, 270] It has even been shown that in patients with metastatic disease, those whose neoplastic cells are diploid have a better prognosis than those who have metastatic disease in which the neoplastic cells are aneuploid.[270]

Progressive changes in karyotype appear to be the exception in solid tumors.[271] Since some tumors are diploid, without gross chromosomal aberrations, the genetic alteration must occur in individual genes. Even if grossly visible chromosomal changes are evident, the neoplastic event is thought to be a result of a chromosomal aberration affecting a single altered gene.[198] The role of the oncogene, or perhaps the anti-oncogene, clearly indicates the importance of altered function in individual genes and cancer. Chromosomal aberrations in cancer cells might also result from an attack on a localized group of related genes, thereby greatly increasing the probability of neoplastic transformation. Visible chromosomal aberrations may merely serve as signals for the presence of small molecular individual genetic events and could serve as markers for alteration of other gene functions.[271]

DNA REPAIR

Since many substances directly damage cellular DNA, the nucleus is equipped with a series of enzymes that edit DNA bases for their fidelity during DNA replication.[253] We are usually unaware of the function of these enzymes unless they are defective or absent, as in certain diseases such as xeroderma pigmentosum (XP).

Under normal circumstances, when ultraviolet (UV) radiation present in sunlight strikes the DNA of epidermal squamous cells, the interaction causes a distortion in the DNA molecule which creates the formation of thymine dimers. When it comes time for the cellular genetic material to replicate, a specific endonuclease recognizes the abnormal DNA thymine dimers and excises them. The endonuclease breaks the backbone of one DNA strand, and the small region of DNA containing the dimer is removed by an exonuclease. The next step in the repair process is the 5'–3' synthesis of a new strand of DNA, complimentary to the opposite DNA strand. This is achieved by pairing the correct DNA bases, using the opposite DNA strand as a template. The enzyme polynucleotide ligase then joins the ends of the newly formed strand of previously injured DNA, and the repair mechanism is complete.[133]

In XP, the endonuclease that initiates excision of the damaged DNA is missing and failure of the DNA repair mechanisms occurs. Thus, when the DNA is copied, the distorted strand is copied along with the nondistorted strand, eventually leading to the development of numerous skin cancers in the sun-exposed areas of the skin.

DNA repair activity is cell cycle-dependent and may contribute to variation in mutagenesis by environmental agents at certain critical times in the cell cycle. Enzymatic excision of damaged DNA sites is normally low during mitosis and rises in early G_1, remaining fairly constant into the S phase.[54] The potential for incision falls again as the cells approach a rapidly proliferating state. Incision activity (which particularly declines following UV radiation) may leave damaged sites unrepaired.[68]

Viruses, the Nucleus, and Neoplasia

Viruses are attractive investigational oncogenic agents since they are known to produce tumors in experimental situations and they provide a convenient source of foreign genetic material that can account for a permanent genetic difference in the infected cell. The initial interaction of the virus with the cell is probably via specific virus receptors. Once a virus binds to the cell surface, it is capable of inserting its own genetic material into the cytoplasm of the cell. The viral genetic material then translocates to the nucleus to become integrated into the host genome, or it may exist in the nucleus in an unintegrated state.[133]

Cellular transformation is not an inevitable outcome of tumor virus infection. Only certain cell types can be transformed by a particular oncogenic virus (Tables 2.8 and 2.9). If the virus/cell combinations are not correct, then infection may be partially or completely aborted, or the cell may die. Possible interactions as the result of infection by oncogenic viruses are summarized in Table 2.10. Retroviruses are seldom cytolytic, whereas DNA oncogenic viruses commonly are.

One may even identify nuclear viral particles within neoplastic cells (Fig. 2.6). Other nuclear changes include aneuploidy of the infected cell populations, the appearance of nuclear antigens, alterations in DNA binding proteins, and an increase in the polyamine levels. In addition, some viruses such as papilloma virus infections may induce the presence of abnormal mitotic figures.

It is not clear as to how viruses transform cells, but there are several possibilities. The first is a hit-and-run event, in which a viral infection causes a

Table 2.8. Oncogenic RNA Viruses

Virus	Tumor
Mouse mammary tumor virus	Mammary carcinoma
Rous sarcoma virus	Fibrosarcoma (fowl)
Fujinami sarcoma virus	Myxosarcoma (fowl)
Lymphoid leukemia viruses	Lymphoid leukemia
	Erythroblastosis (fowl)
Myeloblastosis viruses	Myeloblastosis (fowl)
Myelocytomatosis viruses	Myelocytomas, renal cell and liver cell carcinoma (fowl)
Erythroblastosis viruses	Erythroblastosis, sarcoma (fowl)
Gross leukemia virus	Lymphoma, leukemia (mice)
Rauscher erythroleukemia virus	Erythroblastosis, leukemia (mice)
Kirsten erythroleukemia virus	Erythroblastosis, leukemia (mice)
Friend erythroleukemia virus	Erythroblastosis, leukemia (mice)
Moloney leukemia virus	T cell leukemia (mice)
Abelson leukemia virus	B cell lymphoma (mice)
Harvey sarcoma virus	Sarcomas (mice and rats)
Kirsten sarcoma virus	Sarcoma (mice and rat)
FBJ sarcoma virus	Osteosarcoma (mice)
Feline leukemia virus	Lymphomas (cats)
Feline sarcoma virus	Fibrosarcoma (cats)
Simian sarcoma virus	Fibrosarcoma (monkeys)
Gibbon ape leukemia virus	Leukemia & lymphoma (monkeys)
Human T cell leukemia/ lymphoma virus	Post-thymic T cell malignancy (human)

by error-prone replication of DNA (either altered nucleotide pools or fidelity-altered polymerases).[253]

Currently, the exact mechanisms of carcinogenic initiation and promotion are not known. However, it appears that, even if the mutagenic effect and activation of oncogenes by chemical carcinogens plays a role in many forms of cancer, this might be important for initiation but insufficient for carcinogenesis.[253]

Two basically different explanations for the mechanisms of neoplastic transformation have been advanced. The first is that the malignant phenotype results from a change in the chemical structure of DNA; the second is that it arises from a nonmutational change in the expression of cellular differentiation. The somatic mutation hypothesis predicts a change in the nuclear DNA sequences or basic structure of DNA, presumably in genes that are crucial to carcinogenesis. Aberrant cellular differentiation predicts that there is no change in the nuclear DNA sequences or structure of DNA but rather, there is a quantitative and qualitative shift in the spectrum of gene expression. The two hypotheses are not mutually exclusive, and it is possible that both mechanisms can give rise to human cancers.[165]

Factors favoring genetic mutations as a cause of cancer include the following: (1) The strongest evidence is that many neoplasms appear to be monoclonally derived, as evidenced by glucose-6-phosphate dehydrogenase studies. (2) There is also a positive correlation between the mutagenic and carcinogenic potential of many environmental chemicals. However, not all mutagens are carcinogens. And, indeed, in an increasingly industrialized society, with exposure to many man-made pollutants, there does not appear to be an increase in the incidence of malignancy.[251] Highly industrialized societies are not particularly cancer prone or cancer ridden.[165] (3) Chemicals that are carcinogenic and can induce malignancy strongly interact with DNA or are metabolized to forms that do.[78, 162, 260] However, these activated carcinogens are usually electrophilic, and they can also react with other cellular macromolecules such as RNA or proteins. Ethionine and hormones are exceptions to the generalization that DNA is the critical target for carcinogenic action. However, it may be that any damage done by these agents creates a base change so small that it is below the level of detection. (4) Human inherited diseases with deficiencies in DNA repair mechanisms, such as XP, have higher levels of malignancy, presumably secondary to damage caused by chemicals, radiation, and other carcinogens.

Features which favor abnormal cellular differentiation include the following: (1) Partial or complete reversion of some malignant tumors to a benign neoplasm (Table 2.11). (2) Neoplastic cells can produce proteins characteristic of early development. Classic examples are the presence of oncofetal antigens such as carcinoembryonic antigen or α-fetoprotein. This is thought to represent reversion of differentiation.

There is abundant evidence that modification of DNA, RNA, and synthetic mutation by carcinogens impairs template activity during transcription or translation (Table 2.12).[261]

Metals are also known to be carcinogenic by one of several mechanisms

TABLE 2.11. TUMORS WITH A TENDENCY TO DIFFERENTIATE[a]

Infantile congeners of Wilms' tumor
Neuroblastoma
Hereditary retinoblastoma
Sacrococcygeal teratomas
Congenital and infantile fibromatosis
Yolk-sac carcinoma in young patients
Hepatoblastoma in infants

[a]Modified from Bolande, R. P., and Vekemans, M. J-J.[30]

TABLE 2.12. CHEMICAL CARCINOGENESIS: MECHANISMS[a]

Random Point Mutations
  Direct: Base substitution, deletion of structural or regulatory genes, frame shift
  Indirect: Induction of error-prone DNA synthesis
Ordered Genes
Rearrangements: transpositions, amplification, deletion, integration of exogenous sequences

[a]Modified from Bolande, R. P., and Vekemans, M. J-J.[30]

TABLE 2.13. GENETIC ABNORMALITIES INDUCED BY METALS

	Ag	As	Be	Cd	Co	Cr	Cu	Hg	Mn	Ni	Ph	Pt	Zn	Sn
Chromosome damage and SCE[a]	X		X	X	X		X	X	X	X		X		
DNA strandbreaks and cross-links	X			X	X	X			X			X		X
DNA polymerase infidelity	X		X	X	X	X	X		X	X		X		
Conversion B-DNA to Z-DNA					X				X	X				

[a]SCE, sister chromatid exchanges

(Table 2.13): (1) The metal cations combine covalently with DNA, causing strand breakage and excisions in specific nucleotide bases leading to frameshift mutations during the repair of DNA damage. (2) Metals may form cross links between DNA and proteins and between the adjacent DNA strands, thereby causing aberrant DNA replication repair. They may also act by causing a transition from B-DNA to Z-DNA, thereby affecting the chromatin structure. DNA is normally formed as a right-handed double helix (B-DNA), but it can adopt a left-handed double helical form (Z-DNA). The Z-DNA configuration is favored by nucleotide sequences with alternating purines and pyrimidines, especially alternating guanine and cytosine molecules. The transition from B-DNA to Z-DNA can affect chromatin structure and result in expression of repressed segments of the genome, such as oncogenes. (3) Metals can also impair the stability of DNA replication by altering the conformation of DNA polymerases at the substrate binding or catalytically active sites, or by modifying template base specificity by disturbing complementary base pairing during DNA replication. (4) Finally, metals may bind histone and nonhistone nuclear proteins, or nucleolar RNA, thereby influencing chromatin structure and gene expression, perhaps by modifying the phosphorylation of regulatory proteins.[245]

HISTONES

Novikoff's hepatocellular carcinoma ascites cells have been found to have a unique nonhistone protein that stimulates nucleolar RNA polymerase activity.[85] In cancer cells, the histones may also possess biochemical modifications. The major modification is the extent to which histones are phosphorylated. This change, in turn, appears to be related to proliferative rates and the cyclic nucleotide concentration.[146]

NUCLEOLAR ANTIGENS

A common nucleolar antigen is found in a broad range of human tumors but not in normal tissue.[35, 42, 47, 48, 61, 70, 269] A nuclear matrix antigen is present in many human malignant cells. These antigens are apparently due to differences in the chromosomal nonhistone protein of normal *vs.* malignant cells.

Antibodies to the antigens can detect immunological changes in chromosomal proteins during chemical carcinogenesis even before the appearance of the malignant phenotype.[47, 70]

Virus-associated antigens may also appear in the nucleus. The best studied include EBV-induced antigens and human papilloma viral (HPV) antigens (also see the Lutzner chapter). These do not signify neoplasia per se, but their presence accompanies malignant transformation. Thus, HPV antigens are seen in nuclei of a variety of human tumors (benign and malignant). In the latter instance, the ability to detect them depends on the degree of maturation of the cells.[82]

PLASMA MEMBRANE ALTERATIONS

The cell membrane is the structure through which cells communicate and interact with one another and with their environment. The plasma membrane of a neoplastic cell has a significantly altered surface when compared to its normal counterpart. The altered surface changes are partially a reflection of changes in the genome. Thus, abnormal gene regulation may account for synthetic and organizational abnormalities of the cell surface molecules that mediate many cellular interactions.[5, 108, 109] Undifferentiated, mitotically active nonmalignant cells share some of these membrane changes with neoplastic cells. The cell surface changes on neoplastic cells help confer an ability to invade, disseminate, implant, survive, and grow at secondary sites (also see chapters by Liotta and Keutner).[84, 174, 199, 257, 262]

Many specific alterations have been described. In general, the surface changes include architectural alterations; surface enzyme, glycolipid, and glycoprotein changes; lost, gained, or changed antigens; altered transport and permeability capabilities; modified adhesiveness and contact inhibition; increased agglutinability by lectins; impaired intracellular communication; and increased secretion and shedding.[28, 31, 46, 67, 81, 84, 113, 128, 131, 133, 174, 175, 187, 188, 199, 262]

Plasma membranes are composed of lipid bilayers, with the membrane proteins present in the lipid bilayer having an ordering effect on membrane lipids. Proteins present at or near the surface of the membrane may penetrate into the lipid layer or bridge the lipid bilayer completely (Fig. 2.7).

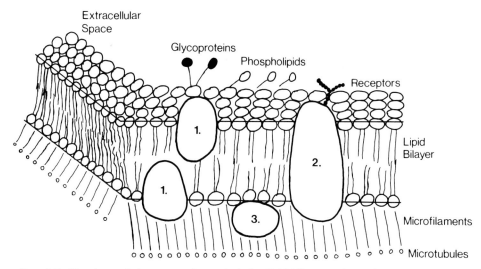

FIG. 2.7. Structure of plasma membrane includes lipid bilayer and membrane proteins. The membrane proteins penetrate into the lipid layer (*1*), bridge the lipid bilayer completely (*2*), or remain near the surface of the membrane (*3*). Surface molecules such as glycoproteins, phospholipids, and receptor molecules are present on the external surface. The inner membrane surface contacts the cytoskeletal system composed of microfilaments and microtubules.

Some architectural changes occur very early in the process of cell transformation and are reversible; these are independent of the increased growth rate.[187]

MICROVILLI

The surface of neoplastic cells becomes quite complicated showing increased ruffling, with increased microprojections, blebs, and microvilli.[31] These surface changes are in a dynamic state of flux, and many of these structures can form and disappear rapidly.[113, 128, 188] Human cancer cells may have numerous microvilli with variable configurations and distributions[166] (Fig. 2.8). Numerous microvilli, however, cannot be considered to be pathognomonic for neoplastic cells.[131, 138] Microvilli increase the surface area of the cancer cells, may increase the exchange of fluids and metabolites across the cell membranes,[67] and may serve as receptors for oncogenic agents.[83]

The acquisition of a microvillus surface can be seen in cervical squamous cells as they are being transformed. A microridge system is normally present on the flat, large, mature benign superficial squamous epithelial cells. With transformation, however, the microridge pattern decreases, and one sees tightly packed microvilli on the surfaces.[83]

REACTION WITH LECTINS

The presence or absence of microvilli in a transformed cell has been related to the increased agglutinability of transformed cells by lectins, for example, by concanavalin A (Con A)[11, 38] (Fig. 2.9). Lectins are multivalent plant molecules that cross-link sugars on adjacent transformed cells. Agglutinability can also

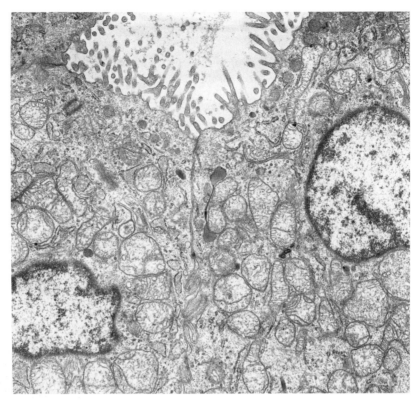

FIG. 2.8. The microvilli present in this serous adenocarcinoma of the ovary are irregularly distributed along the surface. Branched forms are apparent.

be seen in nonmalignant mitotically active cells, again indicating their similarity with malignant cells.

Intracellular cyclic AMP (cAMP) levels have been associated with the presence or absence of microvilli and the degree of agglutinability.[11, 93, 121] As cAMP levels decrease in transformed cells, the number of microvilli and Con A agglutinability increases. Cyclic AMP-treated cells *in vitro* show a decreased number of microvilli and decreased agglutinability.[141] Con A receptor sites in transformed cells form clusters that require receptor migration, allowing polyvalent lectins to agglutinate the cells (Fig. 2.9). This is referred to as "capping." It has been shown that Con A receptor molecules cluster or cap at one pole of transformed cells much more frequently than in untransformed cells[133] (Fig. 2.10). The clumps of transformed cells which are agglutinated by Con A are held together by the interdigitating microvilli.

Endogenous lectins (carbohydrate binding proteins) have been isolated from human tumor cells.[93] These proteins are either calcium dependent or calcium independent. They may be involved in the formation of the cell-cell contacts required for tissue organization and development. Normal cells grown in tissue culture regulate their behavior via their cell contacts. Normally, cell migration stops when one cell membrane contacts another.[31, 133] At the same time, there is a decrease in mitotic rate, and the synthesis of DNA and RNA stops. This is

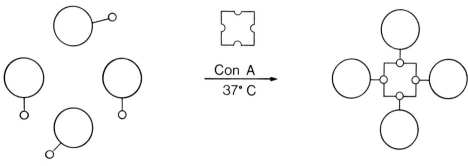

Transformed Cells   Agglutination

FIG. 2.9. Concanavalin A induces aggregation of receptors into clusters. Con A, which is tetravalent, forms cross bridges at contact points between the cells. The agglutination occurs by an increase in the local density of receptors. This receptor movement is mediated through the surface modulation assembly, which includes the receptor, microfilaments, and microtubules.

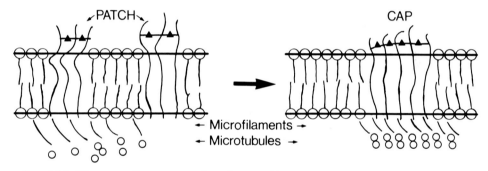

FIG. 2.10. Diagrammatic representation of a cap which forms through the cross-linkage of migrating receptors. This motion is mediated in part by microtubules and microfilaments which lie on the inside of the plasma membrane.

known as contact inhibition. Cancer cells, however, continue to grow and multiply after cell contact has occurred. These cells do not enter the G0 phase, but continue to divide (Fig. 2.11).

The modified pattern of endogenous lectins in human tumor cells may also alter the cells' interaction with normal tissues which, in turn, plays a role in metastasis. The ability to proliferate in an uncontrolled fashion, invade normal tissues, and metastasize to distant sites are characteristics of malignant cells. The surface properties of tumor cells are important in determining this aggressive behavior. Malignant cells can grow autonomously, free of normal growth restraints. Alterations in the surface characteristics change cell-cell interactions and allow cells to escape from their control mechanisms.[175]

FIBRONECTIN

As mentioned, surface enzymes, glycolipids, and glycoproteins are significantly altered in transformed cells. The cell surface glycoprotein, fibronectin (formally called large external transformation substance, LETS), is decreased in transformed cells.[43, 45] Fibronectin is a large protein found in plasma and connective tissue. It has affinity for collagen, heparin, actin, fibrin, and fibri-

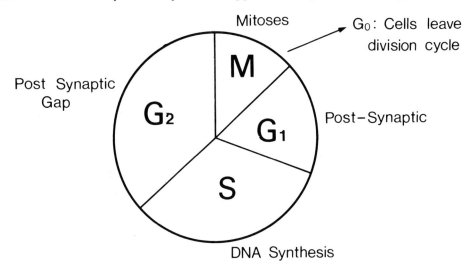

Cancer (Transformed cells) do not enter G_0 state.

Fig. 2.11. Transformation alters the cell so that it no longer undergoes the normal cyclical changes that end in cell division. Transformed cells continue to multiply even when external signals to enter the G_0 phase are present.

nogen and is a nonspecific opsonin in blood.[43,45] Some authors have suggested that fibronectin loss contributes to decreased adhesiveness of malignant cells,[45] thereby allowing for easy separation of individual neoplastic cells from the main tumor mass. The decrease in fibronectin is apparently a late change in the process of cell transformation.[187] Increased plasma levels of fibronectin in cancer patients may cause the increased coagulation disorders observed in cancer patients.[38,73,166]

Portions of the fibronectin molecule have affinity for bacterial species (*Staphylococcus aureus*)[166] and more recently have been shown to bind viral envelope glycoproteins.[124] The interaction between viral glycoproteins and fibronectin may play a role in the opsonization of viruses or in virus-to-cell interactions and may aid the infectability of cells by potentially oncogenic viruses.

In untransformed cells, fibronectin is present over the cell surface. However, in transformed cells, fibronectin is only present in cell contact areas.[43] Decreased fibronectin, and consequent increased tumorigenicity, are present both in fibroblastic and epithelial cells.[44]

Fibronectin plays a role in adhesion in many cell types. The extent of adhesion is related to: (1) the ability of the cell to interact with matrix-bound fibronectin; (2) the synthesis, or lack thereof, of fibronectin; and (3) the lack of deposition of synthesized fibronectin into a soluble matrix around malignant cells. The lack of fibronectin is usually associated with the lack of collagen, laminin, and heparin sulfate.[208] These characteristics appear to be associated with cell migration *in vivo* during embryogenesis; these same characteristics enhance the invasiveness of malignant cells.

Proteolytic Enzymes

The destruction of the extracellular matrix observed during tumor invasion is due to the action of proteolytic enzymes which participate in degradative processes (also see Keutner chapter). The generation of plasmin is an important event in matrix breakdown.[28] Higher levels of degradative enzymes exist in malignant cells when compared with benign lesions and with surrounding normal tissues.[44, 173, 208] Some tumor cells secrete plasminogen activators which convert plasminogen to plasmin.[56, 157, 158] These may not be absolutely necessary for metastatic behavior, but they are important in activating other enzymes.[175] Many other enzymes are degradative such as proteases and glycosidases. The increase in proteases is associated with lost growth regulation and modification of the cell surface. Cell surface enzymatic and adhesive changes can also change tumor implantation properties and the cell's ability to metastasize.

The predominant plasminogen activator is urokinase.[56, 158] A vascular type of activator is also produced,[154] the activity of which is greatly enhanced by fibrin.[37]

Membrane Antigens

Membrane glycolipids are less complex in transformed cells. N-acetylneuraminylgalactosyl ceramide is decreased,[221] and there is a defect in the glucosamine-6-phosphatase molecule, an enzyme which is necessary for the synthesis of long chain proteoglycans. This results in a decreased carbohydrate content of cell surface molecules. Complex sialic acid-containing glycolipids, *i.e.*, gangliosides, disappear after transformation.[14, 32, 72, 103, 104, 156, 272]

High molecular weight glycopeptides are increased in cells transformed by viruses. These large glycopeptides have additional sialic acid residues, a reaction catalyzed by sialic transferase.[72] Surface glycoproteins participate in the adhesion of the tumor cells to a substratum. Since these molecules are poorly glycosylated, they fail to bind to the substrata properly. This failure to connect to the substratum may also involve the connection of the intracellular submembranous system of microfilaments to membrane glycoproteins.[84]

The alteration in glycoproteins and glycolipids affects the metastatic potential of transformed cells as elegantly shown in melanoma cell lines, as well as in other tumors.[14, 32, 103, 104, 272]

Malignant cell transformation is accompanied by the appearance of new cell surface antigens,[80] including: (1) embryonic antigens which are also present on normal embryonic cells; (2) differentiation antigens which are also present on normal syngeneic or allogeneic cells; (3) virus-associated antigens; and (4) tumor-associated antigens which are associated with tumor rejection.

Tumor-associated antigens are markers for the malignant state even if the cell is phenotypically normal. Tumor-associated antigens are usually different from host antigens normally present on the cell surface. The shedding of these antigens may prevent or augment immune responses.[179] These antigens are membrane associated and are different from histocompatibility antigens. They are generally glycoproteins that induce transplantation immunity. Chemical carcinogens can evoke tumor-specific antigens that are specific for an individual tumor, whereas virally-induced neoplasms share viral antigens.[144]

Antigens expressed during fetal life (oncofetal antigens) become apparent during malignant transformation. The best known are α-fetoprotein (AFP)[1] (Fig. 2.12) and carcinoembryonic antigen (CEA) (Fig. 2.13).[99] These antigens are not tumor specific since they are also found in nonneoplastic conditions such as severe hepatitis (AFP) or in heavy smokers (CEA).[133] With the onset of neoplastic transformation, there is an increase or emergence of synthesis of these molecules. They are detected both in the tumor tissue (Fig. 2.12 and 2.13), as well as in the serum.

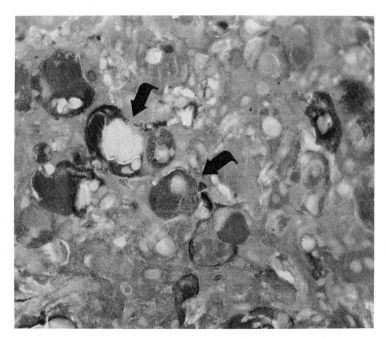

FIG. 2.12. Hepatoma, expressing α-fetoprotein in some of the neoplastic cells (*arrows*).

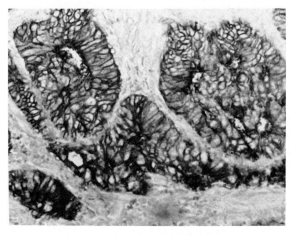

FIG. 2.13. Immunohistochemical localization of carcinoembryonic antigen in a colon carcinoma.

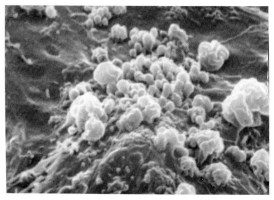

FIG. 2.14. Cell membrane shedding of ovarian carcinoma cell *in vitro*.

Shedding of cell surface material is probably a normal phenomena, but highly malignant cells shed surface material (Fig. 2.14) and antigens more readily than cells of low malignant potential. Blood group substances (antigens) (see chapter by Weinstein *et al.*) can be shed as well as fetal antigens. Occasionally, the shedding of antigens and other glycoproteins into the surrounding media of the tumor can serve as blocking factors that interfere with host immunologic response to neoplastic cells or can elicit weak humoral antibody responses that stimulate tumor growth.

MEMBRANE TRANSPORT AND GROWTH FACTORS

Alterations in membrane permeability allow enhanced transmembrane transport in neoplastic cells. Human tumor cells have an increased capacity for glycolytic consumption of glucose and for diverting biosynthetic precursors into biosynthesis of the pentose phosphate pyrimidines of RNA and DNA. There is also decreased urea metabolism and gluconeogenesis.[259] Neoplastic cells also show increased transport and production of cyclic GMP.

Phorbol esters (tumor promoters) alter permeability, decrease surface charge, and increase potassium uptake by neoplastic cells.[262] Phorbol esters may modify cell surface enzymes such as protein kinase in such a way that they may then act as a specific receptor for the tumor promoters.[24] The substrate for protein kinase is a calcium-dependent lipomodulin which regulates phospholipase A_2, C, and D; the increased phospholipid turnover alters normal cellular feedback systems.

The normal growth of cells is regulated by complex interactions between endogenous substances like polypeptides, steroid hormones, or hormone-like growth factors (Table 2.14),[101, 164] interferons,[149, 193] prostaglandins,[192] and cyclic nucleotides.[90] The coordination of the effects of endogenous growth regulators appears to be moderated via cations, especially calcium, and the calcium-binding protein, calmodulin.[266] Neoplastic cells appear to proliferate independently of the influence of endogenous growth regulators,[71] such as chalones, which inhibit the mitotic activity of cells. The increase in intracellular concentration of cyclic AMP keeps these cells in the G_0 stage of cell division (Fig. 2.11). The primary regulatory defect appears to be late in the G_1 phase of the

TABLE 2.14. HORMONE-LIKE GROWTH FACTORS

Fibroblast growth factor
Epidermal growth factor
Transforming growth factor
Nerve growth factor
Platelet-derived growth factor
Somatomedins
Erythropoietin
Interferons

TABLE 2.15. CALMODULIN EFFECTS

Modifies intracellular levels of cAMP and cGMP
Regulates metabolism of polyamines and prostaglandins
Activates plasma membrane Ca^{2+} pump
Required for DNA synthesis
Stimulates protein kinases
Regulates cyclic nucleotide-dependent kinases
Regulates Ca^{2+}-dependent kinases
Regulates phosphatase activity, including dephosphorylation of histones
Modulates microtubular function

cell cycle prior to DNA synthesis; the period considered to contain Pardu's restriction point. This restriction point is the stage when the daughter cells formed in mitoses must make a commitment to either continue to proliferate or to divide. Normally, the restriction point seems to be under the control of endogenous substances. This contrasts with the neoplastic state, in which the neoplastic cells continue to proliferate in the presence of low calcium, a signal which usually causes cessation of proliferation. This suggests that a mitogenic signal is maintained in the neoplastic cell as it progresses through the G_1-S phase.[116] Calmodulin (CAM) seems to play a major role in the proliferative capability of neoplastic cells. It promotes the progression of the cell through the cell cycle. Increases in CAM levels in cancer cells correlate with increases in tumor growth rate.[159] The effect of CAM in the cells is summarized in Table 2.15.

Transforming growth factors include polypeptides that can confer the transformed phenotype on untransformed cells[241] as measured by the many features ranging from loss of density-dependent inhibition of growth in monolayers to acquisition of anchorage independence.[200] These factors are found in normal embryologic development and, thus, may have a role in normal cellular development. The first of the transforming growth factors to be identified was sarcoma growth factor (SGF).[64,217] SGF caused phenotypic transformation; maintenance of the transformed phenotype was dependent on its continued presence. All of these factors are now known to be a heterogeneous family of polypeptides, present in both neoplastic and nonneoplastic tissues.

RECEPTORS

Expressions of cellular receptors may correlate with the metastatic capability of tumor cells. Studies on the *Fc* receptor for IgG on tumor cells with high and low metastatic capacity indicate that increased numbers of Fc receptors correlate with high metastastic capabilities.[218] Acquisition of these Fc receptors may enable the cells to bind to immune complexes which then mask other tumor antigens and stimulate growth.

We have already stressed that altered cell surface characteristics distinguish neoplastic from nonneoplastic cells. Since the initial interaction of hormones and growth factors is through specific cellular receptors, it is not surprising that qualitative or quantitative changes in hormone responsiveness may coexist with the neoplastic state[49, 209]; multiple new receptors may also be expressed.[160]

The receptors for some of the growth factors, like epidermal growth factor (EGF), platelet-derived growth factor, or insulin are phosphorylated by tyrosine kinases that are activated by oncogenes.[39, 52, 119, 129, 172, 177, 191, 237]

JUNCTIONS

Junctional complexes are defective in cancer cells (Fig. 2.15). In human prostatic cancer cells and cells from benign prostatic hypertrophy, the junctional complexes have been found to be quite different, and defective in the cancer cells as compared to the hyperplastic ones.[235]

Cell junctions are specialized regions that function in intercellular communication, adhesion, and cell recognition. These junctional complexes have three components: (1) a zonula adherens; (2) a desmosome; and (3) a tight junction.[215]

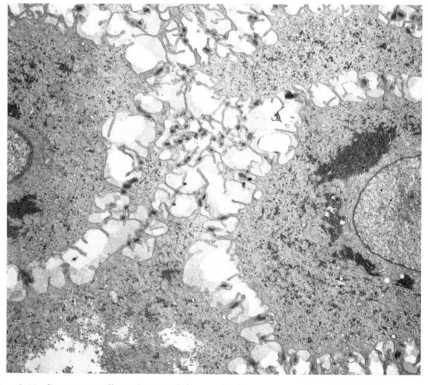

FIG. 2.15. Squamous cell carcinoma of the cervix. Numerous nonkeratinized cells are present, attached through many defective intercellular junctions.

Many cancer cells have decreased numbers of desmosomes,[235] but others have normal numbers.[122, 226] Neoplastic cells can detach and spread despite the presence of a normal complement of desmosomes. Gap junctions, too, are frequently diminished or absent.[147] This results in impaired intercellular communication and impaired metabolic and electrical coupling. The decreased cell-cell coupling observed in some malignant cells may result in a high rate of proliferation.[257] The high proliferative rate could be related to increased negative charge or a lower resting membrane potential[24] of the cells and not necessarily to the level of differentiation.[76] The surface changes of malignant cells may allow these cells to permeate vessels and metastasize.

In summary, the malignant conversion of somatic cells is accompanied by many cell surface changes involving modifications in glycoproteins, glycolipids, surface charge density, surface ion density, enzymes and surface antigens, lectin agglutination, and cell junctions. Contact inhibition, intercellular communication, permeability, membrane transport, and adhesion are also significantly altered.

CYTOSKELETAL CHANGES IN NEOPLASIA

Several decades ago it was appreciated that individual cells had a skeletal framework of their own which included microfilaments (6–8 nm), microtubules (20–25 nm in diameter), and intermediate filaments (10 nm). Certainly, cytoskeletal elements were appreciated in muscle cells with the use of trichrome stains, and tumors derived from muscle cells were also found to contain similar components, albeit arranged in bizarre and unusual configurations.

MICROTUBULES AND MICROFILAMENTS

Microtubules composed of the protein tubulin are usually appreciated in the mitotic spindles (Fig. 2.5) present in the actively proliferating cell populations characteristic of malignant tumors. They are also prominent in ciliated cells and tumors derived from such cells. However, cilia formation is abortive in neoplastic cells (Fig. 2.16),[81, 133] and the arrangement of microtubules within such cilia may be abnormal. Microfilaments on cross-section are small dots with little substructure containing the contractile proteins actin and myosin. In tumors with centriolar abundance, there is an increase in microfilaments.[118] In general, microtubules and microfilaments are present in all eukaryotic cells, even neoplastic ones.

Many neoplastic cells have a full complement of cytoskeletal elements.[176, 184, 254] These elements, however, display rearrangements in normal distribution and organization (Fig. 2.17). Using monospecific antibodies to tubulin, indirect immunofluorescence techniques can help one appreciate significant architectural changes of the microtubules in transformed cells. They are arranged in a network which traverses the cytoplasm from the perinuclear area around and above the nucleus.[184] The marginal cytoplasm contains a meshwork of microfilaments extending into cytoplasmic protrusions. Tissue cultured cells from ascitic fluid of patients with carcinoma of the colon showed unusual rapid expansile-like activity confined to a localized zone around the cell margins. Electron microscopy of these cells revealed the presence of many fine filaments

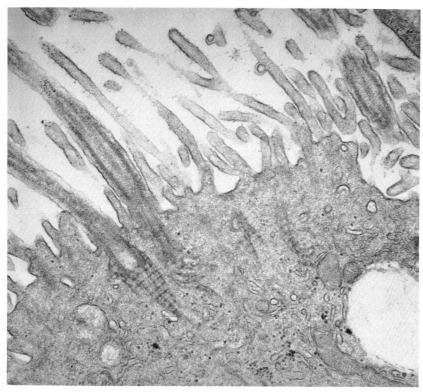

F IG. 2.16. Endometrial carcinoma of the uterus. Notice the abortively formed cilia, as well as ciliary rootlets which do not attach to surface cilia.

throughout the cytoplasm that were concentrated in large bundles beneath the cell membrane. The filaments were actin-like.[88]

During locomotion, leukemia cells assume a characteristic polarized configuration. For instance, blast cells, irrespective of the origin, move in a hand mirror shape. Microfilaments and microtubules have a similar distribution pattern in these polarized cells and in resting cells. However, intermediate filaments occur in two patterns, thin and thick bundles. In polarized cells the intermediate filaments are found in small groups or in single filaments, whereas in resting cells they are present in thick bundles.[22]

Most studies have shown no relationship between microtubule organization and tumorigenic potential. Both tumorigenic and nontumorigenic hybrids may have well organized microtubules. Tumorigenic hybrids, however, have poorly organized microfilaments. Surface fibronectin and microfilaments display close, but not identical, distribution. Surface streaks of fibronectin coincide with the underlying, well-developed microfilament bundles. With time, fibronectin evolves into an autonomous fibrillar network independent of the microfilaments. Disorganization of the microfilament system in tumor cells corresponds to the lack of fibronectin fibrils over the cell surface (Fig. 2.18). Disorganization of the microfilament system significantly influences the cell surface organization.

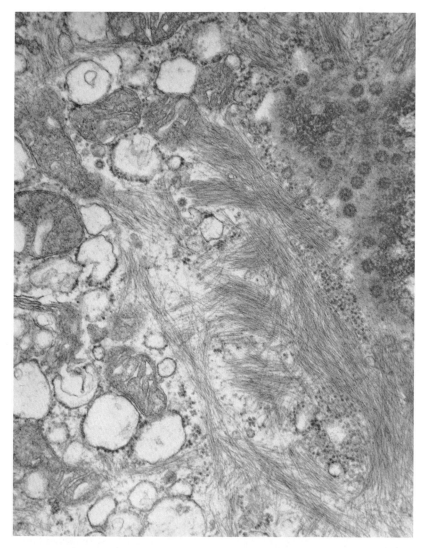

FIG. 2.17. Tangle of microfilaments adjacent to the nucleus in an endometrial carcinoma cell.

Actomyosin plays a major role in the motile forces of neoplastic cells. The role of microtubules, however, is somewhat unclear. Polarization of the microtubules can occur without the help of an ATPase. Polarization of actin-tubulin unit results in unidirectional translocation. Spreading through the surrounding tissues is one of the most prominent features of cancer cells.

The existence of capping implies that the cell possesses structures capable of inducing active movements of receptors. Anchorage modulation triggered by cross-linking of surface glycoprotein receptors is probably mediated by collections of submembraneous structures (*i.e.*, the cytoskeleton). Drugs that disrupt microtubular structure or interfere with their assembly decrease anchorage modulation. Both microtubules and microfilaments are not true cell membrane components, but studies on the control of mobility and distribution of certain cell surface receptors indicate that they are "linked" to surface components.[175, 216, 231]

Microtubule inhibitors decrease the invasiveness of chick embryonic tissue cells *in vitro* and impair direct migration, indicating that this specific migration is dependent on an intact cytoplasmic microtubular system.[155] Alterations of cell behavior resulting in a neoplastic phenotype can be due to the expression of a transforming gene such as the src gene. The cells transformed with this virus component show an alteration in shape, decreased cyclic AMP, and membrane alterations which increases glucose transport. In addition, there is a loss of collagen and cell-specific protein (CSP) secondary to decreased messenger RNA for these proteins. The *src* effect on the cell nucleus alters the synthesis or processing of messenger RNA for CSP and collagen. These two things combined result in decreased adhesion of the cell, increased microvilli production, and increased agglutinability of the cells.

Microfilaments and microtubules interact with viruses at the cell surface membrane, producing a localized alteration for the virus to be extruded and

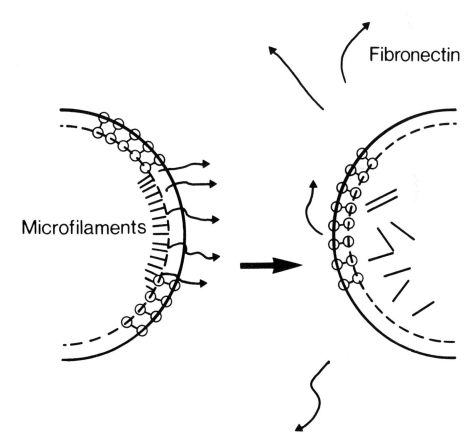

F<small>IG</small>. 2.18. Loss of fibronectin molecules coincides with the disorganization of the microfilament submembrane system.

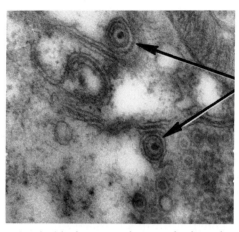

FIG. 2.19. Viruses associated with plasma membrane and submembrane location.

pinched off (Fig. 2.19).[60] The presence of an actin-like protein is associated with purified preparation of murine mammary tumor virus in these surface buds. The actin present in the purified virus preparation is an internal protein of the virion, derived from the host microfilaments.[60]

Cytoplasmic actins maintain cell morphology, motility, and membrane fluidity. Changes in these properties result in disorganized cell arrangement and orientation, uncontrolled cell growth, and an abnormal response to the immediate environment and disrupted cytoskeletal functions.[175] Abnormalities induced by mutation in actin-associated proteins are due to phosphorylation of actin-associated proteins. Increased levels of tyrosine phosphorylase, one of the actin-associated proteins, has been reported.[125,223] An abnormal protein is also present in chemically transformed cells, probably due to a point mutation in the actin gene.[125] Finally, increased levels of endogenous cytochalasin-like inhibitors of F-actin assembly are present in Rous sarcoma virus-transformed cells.[151,159] This alteration can be modulated by viral oncogenes.

Membrane-attached cytoskeletal elements are involved in the phenomena of transmembrane signaling through the plasma membrane. Bidirectional transmembrane flow of information must occur continuously during cell spreading and during coordinated cell locomotion. The actin binding protein vinculin is phosphorylated by the Rous sarcoma virus protein kinase. As previously stated, this alters the integrity of the actin molecules.[25]

Receptors for lectins are under transmembrane control by microtubules and microfilaments.[5] Other agglutinable states, however, appear to be independent of cytoskeletal structure.[223]

It is well established that an extensive cytoplasmic skeletal network ramifies about the cell membrane and the nuclear envelope[18] linking the two structures.[220] Changes in the cell membrane shape may well alter nuclear morphology as well.[220] The linkage of cytoskeletal elements to the cell membrane and the assembling of microtubles may also be impaired.[12,65,74]

Malignant cells from skin cancer, laryngeal carcinoma, and breast cancer contain an increased amount of contractile proteins organized in the form of a microfilamentous apparatus.[150, 161] These contractile proteins are related to locomotion, intracellular transport, and endocytosis. Increased microfilaments (Fig. 2.17) are nonspecific for malignant cells as increased cytoplasmic microfilaments can be seen in nonmalignant states. This includes the increased microfilaments seen in epidermal cells during the healing of an open wound or in hepatocytes during liver regeneration.[92]

Other studies have shown that cells transformed *in vitro* by oncogenic viruses have a decrease in intracytoplasmic microfilaments.[58] There may be no correlation between the amount of actin present and the tendency of tumor to metastasize. The behavioral differences of actin in normal and neoplastic cells may be due to changes in polymerization rather than total quantity.[150]

INTERMEDIATE FILAMENTS

Most recently, attention has been focused on the nature of intermediate filaments. Ultrastructurally, it is difficult to distinguish one type of intermediate filament from another (Fig. 2.20 and 2.21). Five major classes of intermediate filament exist. They include vimentin, desmin, cytokeratins, neurofilament protein, and glial fibrillary acidic protein. Each of the types of

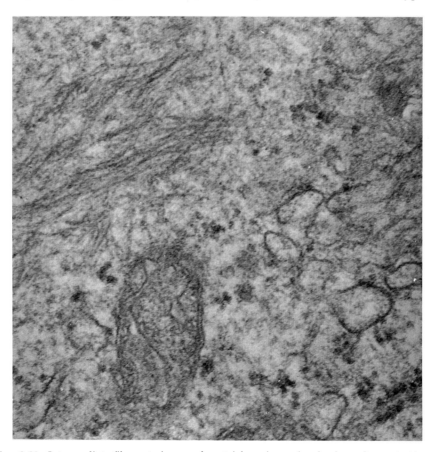

FIG. 2.20. Intermediate filaments in an endometrial carcinoma in a haphazard organization.

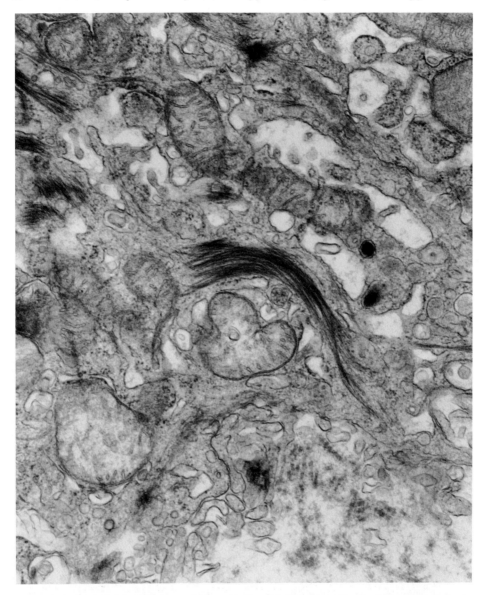

FIG. 2.21. Intermediate filaments which stained positively with antibodies to cytokeratin in the hepatoma. These are forming a compact intracytoplasmic bundle.

intermediate filaments are immunologically specific, as are subclasses of these intermediate filaments.[59, 87, 185, 194, 195]

The most common and most completely studied group is the cytokeratins, of which there are many subclasses.[91, 170, 267] The use of antisera against intermediate filaments is currently quite useful in distinguishing the histogenesis of difficult to diagnose neoplasms since vimentin stains any form of mesenchymal cells; desmin is characteristically present in muscle-derived cells; cytokeratins are present in epithelial cells; neurofilament proteins are present in a neural-derived tissue; and glial fibrillary acidic protein in the glial tissue (Fig. 2.22).

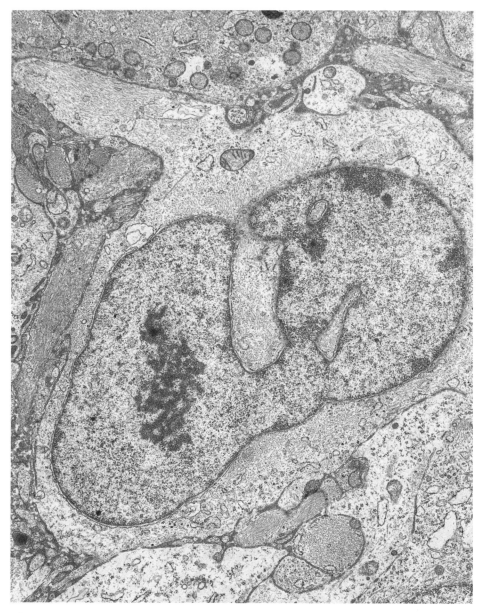

Fig. 2.22. Abundant glial fibrillary acidic protein in this malignant astrocyte from a glioblastoma multiform. Notice cell processes filled with intermediate filaments.

Intermediate filaments are present in normal and neoplastic cells both morphologically and immunologically.

ENDOPLASMIC RETICULUM AND GOLGI APPARATUS

The structure of the endoplasmic reticulum reflects the synthetic capabilities of the neoplastic cell. A differentiated tumor that continues to produce exported cellular products, for example, plasma cell myeloma or a mucinproducing carcinoma, may have a well-developed rough endoplasmic reticulum and may be stimulated to become hyperplastic, with increased production of several metabolic enzymes, particularly of the mixed-function oxidases.

Enzymes associated with the microsomal fraction of cells have an important role in chemical carcinogenesis. For example, hypertrophy of the SER is seen in early stages of experimental nodular hyperplasia of the liver following the administration of carcinogens. In other tumors, a prominent feature of undifferentiated tumor cells may be increased free ribosomes.

Abnormalities of the endoplasmic reticulum in the neoplastic cell have been most extensively studied using models of chemical carcinogenesis. By adding different types of chemical compounds to cells, it is possible to demonstrate that there are significant transcriptional, translational, and regulatory defects in neoplastic cells. Some chemicals interfere directly with the transcription of RNA from the DNA. Viruses may also interfere with the transcriptional ability of cells. Other chemicals may interfere with normal cell translational events in such a way that there is inhibition of protein synthesis, degranulation of the rough endoplasmic reticulum, and disaggregation of polysomes. Viruses may also interfere with translational mechanisms. Finally, oncogenic agents such as viruses or chemicals may result in changes in enzymatic expression or the ability to induce certain enzymes typically used in detoxification processes (cytochrome oxidases). Other chemicals may induce enzymes not normally expressed.

Changes in enzymes, particularly in the area of the Golgi or the Golgi-endoplasmic reticulum lysosomal complexes (GERLS), can result in post-translational modifications of various protein substances (Fig. 2.23) present in the cell, resulting in the expression of altered proteins that may be characteristic of the neoplastic cell but not its normal equivalent. A fairly common example of alteration in post-translational modification is the failure to cleave proteins at the appropriate sites, or complete failure of the cleaving enzymes as seen in the synthesis of unusually large forms of polypeptide hormones (prohormones or preprohormones)[27] or the common "ectopic" production of

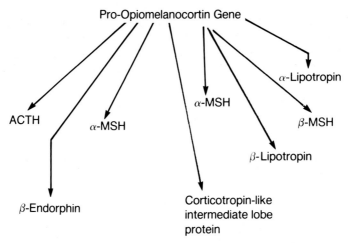

Fig. 2.23. Post-translational modification. Products of the propromelanocortin gene.

TABLE 2.16. TRANSMITTER SUBSTANCE DIVERSITY

Different genes—different peptides
Identical RNA transcripts—alternate splicing
Post-translational modification

hormones by numerous tumors such as medullary carcinomas.[21, 186, 255] In many instances, one can immunocytochemically demonstrate the presence of "ectopic" polypeptide hormones. There are several mechanisms for the generation of hormone diversity (Table 2.16). These hormones are not always associated with the normal physiologic effects of that hormone, presumably because the hormone is larger than usual or it has an unusual conformational structure so that effective binding of the hormone to its receptor on the appropriate target cells may be inhibited.

Other changes in the endoplasmic reticulum may be appreciated ultrastructurally. The changes which are seen reflect the secretory ability of a given neoplasm. For example, in plasmacytomas which are associated with the production of large amounts of immunoglobulins, one often sees an extensively developed network of rough endoplasmic reticulum often with the cisternae containing electron-dense material corresponding to the presence of immunoglobulins. These are the forerunner of Russell bodies. In tumors produced by chemicals that are associated with the induction of the smooth endoplasmic reticulum and the enzymes necessary to convert a noncarcinogenic compound into a carcinogenic one, there is a marked proliferation of the smooth endoplasmic reticulum. Similar proliferations of smooth endoplasmic reticulum are seen in patients with steroid hormone-synthesizing neoplasms.

The induction of rough endoplasmic reticulum or smooth endoplasmic reticulum during the neoplastic transformation and/or proliferation can be appreciated histologically by basophilia in cells in which there is prominent rough endoplasmic reticulum and by cytoplasmic eosinophilia of the cells that contain extensive amounts of smooth endoplasmic reticulum. Ultrastructurally, one can find disorganization of the profiles of endoplasmic reticulum often associated with mitochondria (Fig. 2.24).

Other abnormalities that may be encountered include honeycomb-like structures (Fig. 2.25)[40] or undulating tubules known as ribosomal-lamellar complexes. The latter are seen in cells such as Burkitt's lymphoma or hairy cell leukemia.[203] In addition, one may see accumulations of filaments within endoplasmic reticulum in disorders such as chronic lymphocytic leukemia. The changes are nonspecific and currently are not diagnostically useful in the classification of tumors. Neither are the increased irregular Golgi structures (Fig. 2.26).

Abnormal ER morphologic features may be present in some types of tumors. For example, certain tumors contain whorled arrangements of SER known as "nebenkern." [250]

MITOCHONDRIAL CHANGES

Changes in the respiratory activity of neoplastic cells have been known for a long time, ever since the initial description by Warburg.[258] It is believed that

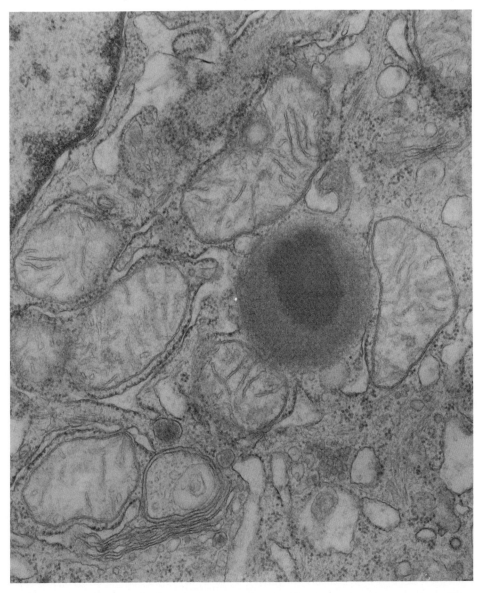

Fɪɢ. 2.24. Transmission electron micrograph of a hepatoma showing the close proximity of the rough endoplasmic reticulum with the mitochondria.

there is an uncoupling of oxidative phosphorylation which partly accounts for the respiratory abnormalities.

Ultrastructurally, one sees various bizarre mitochondrial forms, including mitochondria that appear to be undergoing division, mitochondria that are abnormally large and malformed, and mitochondria with abnormally oriented cristae (Fig. 2.27). They may be longitudinal or assume a zig-zag configuration.

There are a number of tumors that are characteristically associated with a proliferation of mitochondria which is so extensive that it compresses the other

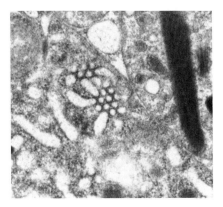

FIG. 2.25. Honeycomb structure in one of the cells of islet cell tumor. The dark bundles represent cytokeratin.

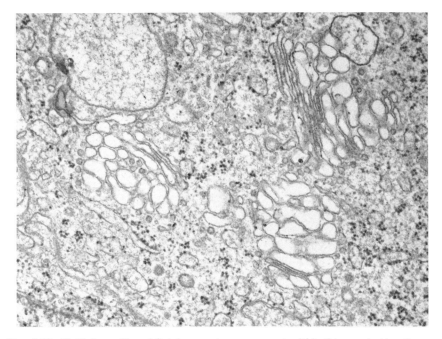

FIG. 2.26. Multiple profiles of Golgi apparatus are present within this neoplastic cell.

cellular organelles, making them almost invisible (Fig. 2.28). These neoplasms are known as oncocytomas and are seen in such places as salivary glands, lungs, or kidneys. Other mitochondrial changes in neoplastic cells are the presence of tubular cristae within the cells of steroid-secreting tumors. This does not represent a phenotypic characteristic of neoplasia but rather reflects the histogenetic cell of origin, since tubular cristae are found in nonneoplastic steroid-synthesizing cells.

Other structural abnormalities include swelling, decreased numbers of cristae, intramitochondrial dense bodies, intercristal fusion, and intramito-

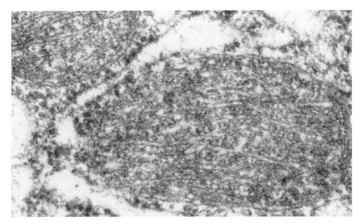

FIG. 2.27. Longitudinally arranged zigzag-shaped cristae are present in the mitochondria of this neoplasm.

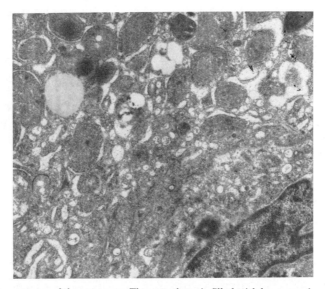

FIG. 2.28. Oncocytoma of the pancreas. The cytoplasm is filled with large numbers of irregularly shaped mitochondria.

chondrial rodlets.[139] Giant mitochondria are noted in some leukemias.[97] Mitochondrial DNA synthesis may also be abnormal.

LYSOSOMES

Because neoplastic cells are often rapidly proliferating and are usually relatively poorly vascularized, despite the synthesis of tumor angiogenesis factor, the central portions become necrotic. Concomitant with tissue or cellular necrosis is an increased number of lysosomes and autophagosomes, as well as myelin figures. The latter represent the cellular digestive products of the phospholipids from various intracytoplasmic organelles, as well as the cell membranes. Some tumors characteristically are associated with vast numbers of cytolysosomes such as tumors that derive from transitional epithelium, as in the urinary bladder or renal pelvis, or Brenner tumors of the ovary. Lysosomal accumulation and crinophagy may occur in a variety of tumors, perhaps secondary to impaired release of secretory granules.[140]

Lysosomes contain a variety of hydrolytic enzymes which may be released as the cells undergo necrosis and may be relatively specific for a particular cell of origin and, therefore, diagnostically useful. Prostatic acid phosphatase is such an example. Muramidase (lysosome) is also useful since it is excreted in the urine in large amounts in patients with monocytic leukemias.

In addition, lysosomes become leaky when cells are infected with viruses leading to increased cellular necrosis, and they may also undergo permeability changes when exposed to chemical agents, particularly hormones.

Lysosomes are important not only for intracellular digestion but also for modification of the extracellular environment, as discussed above. The extracellular secretion of lysosomal enzymes has the ability to modify the cell surface, an event which occurs normally and is not specific for neoplastic cells. However, the lysosomal modifications of the neoplastic cell surface may help to explain why some cells may lose antigenic determinates and escape the ravages of the immune system and immunodestruction. The secretion of lysosomal enzymes is also important in the digestion of the extracellular matrix allowing for increased motility of the already actively ameboid cells in the surrounding tissues (see chapters by Liotta and Keutner). These same enzymes, particularly proteases, may be important in the digestion of collagens, elastin, laminin, and other proteoglycans which allow for the invasion of neoplastic cells into the surrounding supporting tissues.

ACKNOWLEDGMENT

This study was supported in part by the Albuquerque Veterans Administration Hospital.

REFERENCES

1. Abelev, G. I. Alpha-fetoprotein in oncogenesis and its association with malignant tumors. *Adv. Cancer Res. 14:* 295–358, 1971.
2. Advani, H., and Koss, L. G. Diagnostic significance of double sex chromatin bodies in effusions. *Acta Cytol. 22:* 60, 1978.
3. Alitalo, K., Schwab, M., Lin, C. C., and Bishop, J. M. Homogeneous staining chromosomal regions contain amplified copies of an abundantly expressed cellular oncogene (*c-myc*) in malignant neuroendocrine cells from a human colon carcinoma. *Proc. Natl. Acad. Sci. USA 80:*1708–1711, 1983.
4. Arlett, C. F., Lehmann, A. R. Human disorders showing increased sensitivity to the induction of genetic damage. *Annu. Rev. Genet. 12:*95–115, 1978.
5. Asch, B. B., Medina, D., Kretzer, F., Connolly, J. L., Brinkley, B. R. Comparative responses of normal and malignant mouse mammary cells to modulation of surface properties. *Cancer Res. 40:* 2383–2389, 1980.
6. Ashkenzia, Y. E., Goldman, B., and Dotan, A. Rhythmic variation of sex chromatin and glucose-6-phosphate dehydrogenase activity in human oral mucosa during the menstrual cycle. *Acta Cytol. 19:* 62–66, 1975.
7. Atkin, N. B. Triple sex chromatin and other sex chromatin anomalies in tumours of females. *Br. J. Cancer 21:* 40–47, 1967.

8. Atkin, N. B. Sex chromatin positive metastatic melanoma in a male with a favourable prognosis. *Br. J. Cancer 25:* 487–492, 1971.

9. Bachvaroff, R. J., Miller, F., Rapaport, F. T. Alterations in cytoskeletal protein turnover associated with malignant transformation. *Transplant. Proc. 16:* 361–362, 1984.

10. Balaban-Melenbaum, G., and Gilbert, F. Double minute chromosomes and the homogeneously staining regions in chromosomes of a human neuroblastoma cell line. *Science 198:* 739–741, 1977.

11. Bales, B. L., Lesin, E. S., and Oppenheimer, S. B. On cell membrane lipid fluidity and plant lectin agglutinability. A spin label study of mouse ascites tumor cells. *Biochem Biophys Acta 465:* 400, 1977.

12. Ball, E. H., and Singer, S. J. Association of microtubules and intermediate filaments in normal fibroblasts and its disruption upon transformation by a temperature-sensitive mutant of Rous sarcoma virus. *Proc. Natl. Acad. Sci. USA 78:* 6986–6990, 1981.

13. Baradnay, G., Monus, Z., and Kulka. F. Sexchromatin-Untersuchungen in weiblichen Lungenkrebsfällen. *Zentralbl. Allg. Pathol. Pathol. Anat. 111:* 275–276, 1968.

14. Braker, S. A., Stacey, M., Tiper, D. J., and Kirkman, J. H. Some observations on certain mucoproteins containing sialic acid. *Nature, 184:* A68–A69, 1956.

15. Barlogie, B., Johnston, D. A., Smallwood, L., Raber, M. N., Maddox, A. M., Latreille, J., Swartzendruber, D. E., and Drewinko, B. Prognostic implications of ploidy and proliferative activity in human solid tumors. *Cancer Genet. Cytogenet. 6:* 17–28, 1982.

16. Becker, K. L., Martin, B., and Boukhris, R. Effect of exogenous estrogen and progesterone upon sex chromatin frequency. *J. Urol. 109:* 79–81, 1973.

17. Bencosme, S. A., Allen, R. A., and Latta, H. Functioning pancreatic islet cell tumors studied electron microscopically. *Am. J. Pathol. 42:* 1–21, 1963.

18. Bennett, V. The molecular basis for membrane-cytoskeleton association in human erythrocytes. *J. Cell. Biochem. 18:* 49–65, 1982.

19. Berenblum I: The mechanism of carcinogenesis: A study of the significance of co-carcinogenic action and related phenomena. *Cancer Res. 1:* 807–814, 1941.

20. Berger, R., Bernheim, A., Weh, H. J., Flandrin, G., Daniel, M. T., Brout, J. C., Colbert, N. A new translocation in Burkitt's tumor cells. *Hum. Genet. 53:* 111–112, 1979.

21. Bertagna, X. Y., Nicholson, W. E., Sorenson, G. D., Pelhengill, O. S., Mount, C. D., Orth, D. N. Corticotropin, lipotropin, and beta-endorphin production by a human nonpituitary tumor in culture: Evidence for a common precursor. *Proc. Natl. Acad. Sci. USA 75:* 5160–5164, 1978.

22. Bessis, M., Dunn, G. A., Felix, H., Hammerl, G., Isaber, G., Luscher, E. F., Mareel, M., Rungger, T., Brandle, E. *et al.*: Motility, shape, and fibrillar organelles of normal and neoplastic cells. *Eur. J. Cancer 16:* 1–14, 1978.

23. Biedler, J. L., and Spengler, B. A. Metaphase chromosome anomaly: Association with drug resistance and cell-specific products. *Science 191:* 185–187, 1978.

24. Binggel, R., and Weinstein, R. C. Deficits in elevating membrane potential of rat fibrosarcoma cells after cell contact. *Cancer Res. 45:* 235–241, 1985.

25. Birchmeier, W. Cytoskeleton structure and function. *Trends Biochem. Sci. 9:* 192–195, 1984.

26. Bishun, N. P., Smethurst, M., and Williams, D. C. Age, sex chromatin and estrogen receptor status in women with breast cancer. *Cancer Genet. Cytogenet. 4:* 353–355, 1981.

27. Bloom, S. R., and Polak, J. M. (eds.). *Gut Hormones,* ed. 2. New York, Churchill Livingstone, 1981, p. 605.

28. Bogenmann, E., and Jones, P. A. Role of plasminogen in matrix breakdown by neoplastic cells. *J. Natl. Cancer Inst. 71:* 1177–1182, 1983.

29. Bohle, A., Burger, E., Fischbach, H., and Schul, A. Die Bedeutung der Barrshen Körperchen beim Mammakarzinom. *Langenbecks Arch. Klin. Chir. 313:* 393–399, 1965.

30. Bolande, R. P., and Vekemans, M. J-J. Genetic models of carcinogenesis. *Hum. Pathol. 14:* 658–662, 1983.

31. Borek, C., and Fenoglio, C. M. Scanning electron microscopy of surface features of hamster embryo cells transformed *in vitro* by x-irradiation. *Cancer Res. 36:* 1325–1334, 1976.

32. Bryant, M. L., Stoner, G. D., and Metzger, R. D. Protein bound carbohydrate content of normal and tumorous human lung tissue. *Biochim. Biophys. Acta 343:* 226–231, 1974.

33. Busch, H. Molecular lesions in cancer. *Mol. Cell Biochem. 61:* 111–130, 1984.

34. Busch, H., and Smetana, K. *The Nucleolus.* New York, Academic Press, 1970.

35. Bush, H., Gyorkey, F., Busch, R. K., Davis, F. M., Gyorkey, P., and Smetana, K. A nucleolar antigen found in a broad range of human malignant tumor specimens. *Cancer Res. 39:* 3024–3030, 1979.

36. Callahan, R., Drohan, W., Tronick, S., and Schlom, J. Detection and cloning of human DNA sequences related to the mouse mammary genome. *Proc. Natl. Acad. Sci. USA 79:* 5503–5507, 1982.

37. Camiolo, S. M., Markus, G., Evers, J. C., *et al.* Plasminogen activation content of neoplastic and benign human prostate tissues: Fibrin augmentation of an activation activity. *Int. J. Cancer 27:* 191–198, 1981.

38. Caprini, J. A., and Sena, S. F. Altered coagulability in cancer patients. *Cancer 32:* 162–172, 1982.

39. Carpenter, G., King, L. Jr., and Cohen S. Rapid enhancement of protein phosphorylation in A-431 cell membrane preparations by epidermal growth factor. *J. Biol. Chem. 254:* 4884–4891, 1979.

40. Carstens, P. H. B., Alexander, R. W., Ghadially, F. N., Tandler, B., and Toner, P. G. Honeycomb structures in tumor cells. *Ultrastruct. Pathol. 6:* 99–103, 1984.

41. Cavellero, G. Stulla frequenza della cromatina sessuale in un caso di corio-nepithelioma del testicolo. *Pathologica 50:* 215–218, 1958.

42. Chan, P-K., Feyerabend, A., Busch, R. K., and Busch, H. Identification and partial purification of human tumor nucleolar antigen 54/6.3. *Cancer Res. 40:* 3194–3201, 1980.

43. Chen, L. B., Gallimore, P. H., McDougall, J. K., Correlation between tumor induction and the large external transformation sensitive protein on the cell surface. *Proc. Natl. Acad. Sci. USA 73:* 3570–3574, 1976.

44. Chen, L. B., Maitland, N., Gallimore, P. H., and McDougall, J. K. Detection of large external transformation sensitive protein on some epithelial cells. *Exp. Cell Res. 106:* 39–46, 1977.

45. Chen, L. B., Summerhayes, I., Hsieh, P., and Gallimore, P. H. Possible role of fibronectin in malignancy. *J. Supramol. Struct. 12:* 139–150, 1979.

46. Chitra, B. Tumor cell stimulation of collagenase production by fibroblasts. *Biochem. Biophys. Res. Commun. 109:* 1026–1034, 1982.

47. Chiu, J. F., Decha-Umphia, W., Markert, C., and Little, B. W. Immunospecificity of nuclear nonhistone protein-DNA complexes in colon adenocarcinoma. *J. Natl. Cancer Inst. 63:* 313–317, 1979.

48. Chiu, J. F., Hunt, M., and Hnilica, L. S. Tissue-specific DNA-protein complexes during azo dye hepatocarcinogenesis. *Cancer Res. 34:* 913–919, 1975.

49. Cikes, M. Expression of hormone receptors in cancer cells: A hypothesis. *Eur. J. Cancer 14:* 211–215, 1978.

50. Coffin, J. M., Varmus, H. E., Bishop, J. M., Essex, M., Hardy, W. D., Jr., Martin, G. S., Rosenberg, N. E., Scolnick, E. M., Weinberg, R. A., and Vogt, P. K. Proposal for naming host cell derived inserts in retrovirus genomes. *J. Virol. 40:* 953–957, 1981.

51. Cohen, A. J., Li, F. P., Berg, S., *et al.* Hereditary renal cell carcinoma associated with a chromosomal translocation. *N. Engl. J. Med. 301:* 592–595, 1979.

52. Cohen, S., Carpenter, G., King, L., Jr. Epidermal growth factor-receptor-protein kinase interactions. Co-purification of receptor and epidermal growth factor-enhanced phosphorylation activity. *J. Biol. Chem. 25(255):*4834–4842, 1980.

53. Collett, M. S., Erikson, E., Purchio, A. F., Brugge, J. S., and Erikson, R. L. A normal cell protein similar in structure and function to the avian sarcoma virus transforming gene product. *Proc. Natl. Acad. Sci. USA 76:* 3159–3163, 1979.

54. Collins, A. R. S., Downes, C. S., and Johnson, R. T. J. Cell cycle-related variation in UV damage and repair capacity in Chinese hamster. *Cell Physiol. 103:* 179–191, 1980.

55. Collins, S. H., and Groudine, M. Amplification of endogenous *myc*-related DNA sequence in a human myeloid leukemia cell line. *Nature 298:* 679–681, 1982.

56. Corrassant, J. G., Celik, C., Camiolo, S. M., *et al.* Plasminogen activator content of human colon tumors and normal mucosae: Separation of enzymes and partial purification. *J. Natl. Cancer Inst. 65:* 345–351, 1980.

57. Dallas-Favera, R., Bregni, M., Erickson, J., Patterson, D., Gallo, R. C., and Croce, C. M. Human *c-myc* onc gene is located on the region of chromosome 8 that is translocated in Burkitt lymphoma cells. *Proc. Natl. Acad. Sci. USA 79:* 7824–7827, 1982.

58. Damer, D. G., Lue, J., and Neustein, H. B. Comparison of surface material, cytoplasmic filament and intercellular junctions from untransformed and two mouse sarcoma virus-transformed cell lines. *Cancer Res. 34:* 3133–3138, 1974.

59. Damjanov, I. Editorial. Antibodies to intermediate filaments and histogenesis. *Lab. Invest. 47:* 215, 1982.

60. Dansby, C. H., Sheffield, J. B., Tuszynski, G. P., and Warren L. Is there a role for actin in virus budding? *J. Cell Biol. 75:* 593–605, 1977.

61. Davis, F. M., Gyorkey, F., Busch, R. K., and Busch, H. Nucleolar antigen found in several human tumors but not in the nontumor tissues studied. *Proc. Natl. Acad. Sci. USA 76:* 892–896, 1979.

62. Davis, F. M., Tsao, T. Y., Fowler, S. K., and Rao, P. N. Monoclonal antibodies to mitotic cells. *Proc. Natl. Acad. Sci. USA 80:* 2926–2930, 1983.

63. de Klein, A., Van Kessel, A. G., Grosveld, G., Bartram, C. R., Hagemeijer, A., Bootsman, D., Spurr, N. K., Heistekamp, N., Groffen, J., and Stephenson, J. R. A cellular oncogene is translocated to the Philadelphia chromosome in chronic myelogenous leukemia. *Nature 300:* 765–767, 1982.

64. De Larco, J. E., Preston, Y. A., and Todaro, G. J. Properties of a sarcoma growth-factor-like peptide from cells transformed by a temperature-sensitive sarcoma virus. *J. Cell Physiol. 109:* 143–152, 1981.

65. Der, C. J., Ash, J. F., and Starbridge, E. J. Cytoskeletal and transmembrane interactions in the expression of tumorigenicity in human cell hybrids. *J. Cell Sci. 52:* 151–166, 1981.

66. Der, C. J., Krontiris, T. G., and Cooper, G. Transforming genes of human bladder and lung carcinoma cell lines are homologous to the *ras* genes of Harvey and Kirsten sarcoma viruses. *Proc. Natl. Acad. Sci. USA 79:* 3637–3640, 1982.

67. Domejala, W., and Koss, L. G. Configuration of surface of human cancer cells in effusions: A scanning EM study of microvilli. *Virchows Arch. (Zellpathol.) 26:* 27–42, 1977.

68. Downes, C. S., Johnson, R. T., and Collins, A. R. S. Cell cycle-dependent regulation of excision repair of UV damage. *Exp. Cell Res. 142:* 47–56, 1982.

69. Duesberg, P. H. Retroviral transforming genes in normal cells? *Nature 304:* 219–226, 1983.

70. Duhl, D. M., Banar, Z., Briggs, R. C., Page, D. L., and Hnilica, L. S. Tumor-associated chromatin antigens of human colon adenocarcinoma cell lines HT–29 and LoVo. *Cancer Res. 42:* 594–600, 1982.

71. Durkin, J. P., Boynton, A. L., and Whitfield, J. F. The SRC gene product of Rous sarcoma virus rapidly induces DNA synthesis and proliferation of calcium deprived rat cells. *Biochem. Biophys. Res. Commun. 103:* 233–239, 1981.

72. Dvorak, A. M., Robin, R. O., Morgan, E. S., and Dvorak, H. F. Ultrastructure of the cell coat of untransformed and simian-virus 40-transformed fibroblasts. *J. Reticuloendothel. Soc. 25:* 163–177, 1979.

73. Dvorak, H. F., Senger, D. R., and Dvorak, A. M. Fibrin as a component of the tumor stroma: Origins and biological significance. *Cancer Metastasis Rev. 2:* 41–73, 1983.

74. Edelman, G. Surface modulation in cell recognition and cell growth. *Science 16:* 218–226, 1976.

75. Eisenman, R. N., Tachibana, C. Y., Abrams, H. D., and Hann, S. R. *v-myc-* and *c-myc-*encoded proteins are associated with the nuclear matrix. *Mol. Cell Biol. 5:* 114–126, 1985.

76. Elue, R., Brons, J., and Kavitz, K. Surface change modifications associated with proliferation and differentiation in neuroblastoma cultures. *Nature 258:* 616–617, 1975.

77. Falor, W. H., and Ward, R. M. Prognosis in early carcinoma of the bladder based on chromosomal analysis. *J. Urol. 119:* 44–48, 1978.

78. Farber, E. Chemical carcinogenesis. *N. Engl. J. Med. 305:* 1379–1389, 1981.

79. Feldman, R. A., Hanafusa, T., and Hanafusa, H. Characterization of protein kinase activity associated with the transforming gene product of Fujinami sarcoma virus. *Cell 22:* 757–765, 1980.

80. Fenoglio, C. M. Antigens, enzymes and hormones. Their roles as tumor markers in gynecologic neoplasia. *Diagn. Gynecol. Obstet. 2:* 33–42, 1980.

81. Fenoglio, C. M. Ultrastructural features of the common epithelial tumors of the ovary. *Ultrastruct. Pathol. 1:* 419–444, 1980.

82. Fenoglio, C. M., and Ferenczy, A. Etiologic factors in cervical neoplasia. *Semin Oncol. 9:* 349–372, 1982.

83. Fenoglio, C. M., and Lefkowitch, J. H. Herpes simplex virus II and neoplasia of the lower female genital tract. In: *Cancer of the Uterine Cervix*, edited by H. G. Bender and L. Beck, Cancer Campaign of Germany. Stuttgart, West Germany, Gustave Verlag, 1985, pp. 187–198.

84. Fidler, I. J., and Hart, I. R. Recent observations on the pathogenesis of cancer metastasis. In: *Embryonic Development, Part B. Cellular Aspects*, edited by M. Burger. New York, R. Liss, 1982, pp. 601–619.

85. Forger, J. M., Choie, D. D., and Friedberg, E. C. Non-histone chromosomal proteins of chemically transformed neoplastic cells in tissue culture. *Cancer Res. 36:* 258–262, 1976.

86. Franke, W. W., Scheer, U., Krohne, G., and Jarasch, E-D. The nuclear envelope and the architecture of the nuclear periphery. *J. Cell Biol. 91:* 39s–50s, 1981.

87. Franke, W. W., Schmid, E., Osborne, M., and Weber, K. Different intermediate filament proteins distinguished by immunofluorescence microscopy. *Proc. Natl. Acad. Sci. USA 75:* 5032, 1978.

88. Franks, L. M., Riddle, P. N., and Seal, P. Actin-like filaments and cell movements in human ascites tumor cells: An ultrastructural and cinemicrographic study. *Exp. Cell Res. 54:* 157–162, 1969.

89. Frederiksen, P., and Bichel, P. Sequential flow cytometric analysis of the single cell DNA content in recurrent human brain tumours. *Flow Cytometry 4:* 398–402, 1980.

90. Friedman, D. L., *et al.* The role of cyclic nucleotides in the cell cycle. *Adv. Cyclic Nucleotide Res. 7:* 69–114, 1976.

91. Fuchs, E., and Green, H. Multiple keratins of cultured human epidermal cells are translated from different mRNA molecules. *Cell 17:* 573, 1979.

92. Gabbiani, G., Csank-Brasser, J., Schreeberger, J. C., Kapanci, Y., Trenchev, P., and Holborow, E. J. Contractile proteins in human cancer cells. Immunofluorescent and electron microscopic study. *Am. J. Pathol. 83:* 457–468, 1976.

93. Gabius, H. J., Engelhardt, R., Cramer, F., Batge, R., and Wagel, G. A. Pattern of endogenous lectins in a human epithelial tumor. *Cancer Res. 45:* 253–257, 1985.

94. Galloway, D. A., and McDougall, J. K. The oncogenic potential of herpes simplex viruses: Evidence for a 'hit-and-run' mechanism. *Nature 302:* 21–24, 1983.

95. Gav, N. J., and Walker, J. E. Homology between human bladder carcinoma oncogene product and mitochondrial ATP-synthetase. *Nature 301:* 262–264, 1983.

96. Ghadially, F. N., and Parry, E. W. Intranuclear annulate lamellae in Ehrlich ascites tumour cells. *Virchows Arch. Zellpathol. 15:* 131–137, 1974.

97. Ghadially, F. N., and Skinnider, L. F. Giant mitochondria in erythroleukemia. *J. Pathol. 114:* 113–117, 1974.

98. Gilbert, F. Chromosomes, genes and cancer: A classification of chromosome abnormalities in cancer. *J. Natl. Cancer Inst. 71:* 1107–1114, 1983.

99. Gold, P., Freedman, S. O. Demonstration of tumor-specific antigens in human colonic carcinomata by immunologic tolerance and absorption techniques. *J. Exp. Med. 121:* 439–462, 1965.

100. Gonzalez-Crussi, F., Hull, M. T., and Mirkin, D. L. Intranuclear filaments in a soft tissue sarcoma. *Hum. Pathol. 9:* 189–198, 1978.

101. Gospodaarowicz, D. Purification of a fibroblast growth factor from bovine pituitary. *J. Biol. Chem. 250:* 2515–2520, 1975.

102. Goyette, M., Petropoulos, D. J., Shank, P. R., Fausto, N. Expression of a cellular oncogene during liver regeneration. *Science 219:* 510–512, 1983.

103. Grimes, W. J. Sialic acid transferases and sialic acid levels in normal and transformed cells. *Biochemistry 9;* 5083–5091, 1970.

104. Grimes, W. J. Glycosyl transferase and sialic acid levels in normal and transformed cells. *Biochemistry 12:* 990–996, 1973.

105. Groffen, J., Stephenson, J. R., Heisterkamp, N., Bartram, C., de Klein, A., and Grosveld, G.

The human c-abl oncogene in the Philadelphia translocation. *J. Cell Physiol. 3:* 179–191, 1984.

106. Gropp, H., Wulf, U., and Pera, F. Studies on the sex chromatin and the pertinent chromosomal status in breast carcinoma. *Wien Klin. Wochenschr. 76:* 863–869, 1972.

107. Hagy, G., and Broderick, M. Variation of sex chromatin in human oral mucosa during menstrual cycle. *Acta Cytol. 16:* 314–321, 1972.

108. Hakomori, S., and Kannagi, R. Glycosphingolipids as tumor-associated and differentiation markers. *J. Natl. Cancer Inst. 71:* 231–247, 1983.

109. Hakomori, S-I. Blood group glycolipid antigens and their modifications as human cancer antigens. *Am. J. Clin. Pathol. 6:* 635–648, 1984.

110. Han, T., Ozer, H., Sadamoori, N., Emrich, L., Gomez, G. A., Henderson, E. S., Bloom, M. L., and Sandberg, A. A. Prognostic importance of cytogenetic abnormalities in patients with chronic lymphocytic leukemia. *N. Engl. J. Med. 310:* 287–292, 1984.

111. Hanschke, H. J., and Hoffmeister, H. Die zellkernmorphologische Geschlechtsbestimmung beim Bronchialcarzinom der Frau. *Zentralbl. Allg. Pathol. Pathol. Anat. 101:* 99–100, 1960.

112. Harden, D. G. Mechanisms of genetic susceptibility to cancer. In: *Carcinogenesis: Fundamental Mechanisms and Environmental Effects*, edited by B. Pullman, P.O. Tso, and H. Gelboin. New York, Reidel, 1980, pp. 235–244.

113. Hauger, A., and Laerum, O. D. Surface structure of fetal rat brain cells during neoplastic transformation in cell culture. *J. Natl. Cancer Inst. 61:* 1415–1427, 1978.

114. Hayward, W. S., Neel, B. G., and Astrin, S. M. Activation of a cellular *onc* gene by promoter insertion in ALV-induced lymphoid leukosis. *Nature 290:* 475–480, 1981.

115. Heisterkamp, N., Groffen, J., Stephenson, J. R., Spurr, N. K., Goodfellow, P. N., Solomon, E., Carritt, B., and Bodmer, W. F. Chromosomal localization of human cellular homologues of two viral oncogenes. *Nature 299:* 747–749, 1982.

116. Hickie, R. A., Wei, J. W., Blyth, L. M., Wong, D. Y. W., Kaassen, D. J. Cations and calmodulin in normal and neoplastic cell growth regulation. *Can. J. Biochem. Cell Biol. 61:* 934–941, 1983.

117. Hirano, A., and Zimmerman, H. M. Some new cytological observations of the normal rat ependymal cell. *Anat. Rec. 158:* 293-302, 1967.

118. Horvath, E., Kovacs, K., and Ezrin, C. Centrioles and cilia in non-tumourous anterior lobes and adenomas of the human pituitary. *Pathol. Eur. 11:* 81–86, 1976.

119. Hunter, T. Synthetic peptide substrates for a tyrosine protein kinase. *J. Biol. Chem. 257:* 4843–4848, 1982.

120. Hunter, W. G., and Lennox, B. The sex of teratomata. *Lancet 2:* 633–634, 1954.

121. Isselbach, K. I. The intestinal cell surface properties of normal undifferentiated and malignant cells. *Harvey Lect. 69:* 197, 1974.

122. Jesudason, M. L., and Iseri, O. A. Host-tumor cellular junctions and an ultrastructural study of hepatic metastasis of bronchogenic oat cell carcinoma. *Hum. Pathol. 11:* 66, 1980.

123. Johannessen, J. V., Sobrinho-Simoes, M., Finseth, I., Pilström, L. Papillary carcinomas of the thyroid have pore-deficient nuclei. *Int. J. Cancer 30:* 409–411, 1982.

124. Julkuper, I., Vartio, T., Keslzi, C. J. A. Localization of viral envelope glycoprotein sites in fibronectin. *Biochemistry 219:* 425–428, 1984.

125. Kakunaga, T., Leavitt, J., and Hanada, H. A mutation in actin associated with neoplastic transformation. *Fed. Proc. 43:* 2275–2279, 1984.

126. Kallenberger, A., Hagmann, A., Descoenders, C. The interpretation of abnormal sex chromatin incidence of human breast tumors on the basis of DNA measurements. *Eur. J. Cancer 3:* 439–448, 1968.

127. Kaneko, Y., Rowley, J. D., Vatyakojis, D., Chilcote, R., Moohr, J., and Patel, D. Chromosome abnormalities in Down's syndrome patients with acute leukemia. *Blood 58:* 459–470, 1981.

128. Karasaki, S., Simard, A., and DeLamirand, G. Surface morphology and nucleoside phosphatase activity of rat liver epithelial cells during oncogenic transformation *in vitro*. *Cancer Res., 37:* 3516–3525, 1977.

129. Kasuga, M., Zick, Y., Blithe, D. L., Crettaz, M., and Kahn, C. R. Insulin stimulates tyrosine phosphorylation of the insulin receptor in a cell-free system. *Nature 298:* 667–669, 1982.

130. Kempson, R. L., and Bari, N. Uterine sarcomas. Classification, diagnosis and prognosis. *Hum. Pathol. 1:* 331–349, 1970.
131. Kenemans, P., Davina, J. H. M., deHaan, R. W., van den Zander, P., Vooys, G. P., Stalk, J. G., and Stadhouders, A. M. Cell surface morphology in epithelial malignancy and its precursor lesions. *Scanning Electron Microscopy Part 3:* 23–36, 1981.
132. Kimel, V. Clinical-cytological correlations of mammary carcinoma based upon sex-chromatin counts. A preliminary study. *Cancer 10:* 922–927, 1957.
133. King, D. W., Fenoglio, C. M., and Lefkowitch, J. H. *General Pathology: Principles and Dynamics.* Philadelphia, Lea & Febiger, 1983.
134. Kiricuta, I., and Clinici, C. D. Significance of the decrease of sex chromatin incidence in malignant breast tumours. *Morphol. Embryol. 21:* 197–201, 1975.
135. Klein, G. Lymphoma development in mice and humans. *Proc. Natl. Acad. Sci. USA 76:* 2442–2446, 1979.
136. Knudson, A. G., Genetics and the etiology of childhood cancers. *Pediatr. Res. 10:* 513–517, 1976.
137. Knudson, A. G., Jr. Hereditary cancers of men. *Cancer Invest. 1:* 187–193, 1983.
138. Kolata, G. B. Microvilli: A major difference between normal and cancer cells. *Science 88:* 819–820, 1975.
139. Korb, J., and Riman, J. Presence of intramitochondrial bodies in avian leukemia myeloblasts. *Eur. J. Cancer 12:* 959–961, 1976 .
140. Kovacs, K., Horvath, E., Bayler, T. A., Hassaram, S. T., and Ezrin, C. Silent corticotroph cell adenoma with lysosomal accumulation and crinophagy. *Am. J. Med. 64:* 492–499, 1978.
141. Kurth, R., and Bauer, H. Correlation between intracellular cyclic AMP level and membrane antigenicity of normal and malignant cells. *Differentiation 1:* 323–330, 1977.
142. Land, H., Parada, L. F., and Weinberg, R. A. Tumorigenic conversion of primary embryo fibroblasts requires at least two cooperating oncogenes. *Nature 304:* 596–606, 1983.
143. Land, H., Parada, L. F., and Weinberg, R. A. Cellular oncogenes and multistep carcinogenesis. *Science 222:* 771–778, 1983.
144. Law, L. W., Rogers, M. J., and Appella, E. Tumor antigens on neoplasms induced by chemical carcinogens and by DNA- and RNA-containing viruses: Properties of the solubilized antigens. *Adv. Cancer Res. 32:* 201–235, 1980.
145. Leder, P., Battey, J., Lenoir, G., Moulding, C., Murphy, W., Potter, H., Stewart, T., and Taub, R. Translocations among antibody genes in human cancer. *Science 222:* 765–771, 1983.
146. Letnansky, K. The phosphorylation of nuclear proteins in the regenerating and premalignant rat liver and its significance for cell proliferation. *Cell Tissue Kinet. 8:* 423–439, 1975.
147. Loewenstein, W. R. Junctional intracellular communications and the control of growth. *Biochem. Biophys. Acta 560:* 1–65, 1979.
148. Love, R., and Suskind, R. G. Further observations on the ribonucleoproteins of mitotically dividing mammalian cells. *Exp. Cell Res. 22:* 193–207, 1961.
149. Ludwig, C. U., Durie, B. G. M., Salmon, S. E., and Moon, T. C. Tumor growth stimulation *in vitro* by interferons. *Eur. J. Cancer Clin. Oncol. 19:* 1625–1632, 1983.
150. Macartney, J. C., Roxburgh, J., and Currie, R. C. Intracellular filaments in human cancer cell: Histologic study. *J. Pathol. 129:* 13–20, 1979.
151. Magargal, W. W., and Lin, S. Rous sarcoma virus increases endogenous actin-related cytochalasin-like activity in chick embryo fibroblasts. *Fed. Proc. 41:* 1387, 1982.
152. Makowski, D. R., Rothberg, P. G., and Astrin, S. M. The role of promoter insertion in the induction of neoplasia. *Surv. Synth. Pathol. Res. 3:* 342–349, 1984.
153. Manolova, G., and Manolova, Y. Marker bands in one chromosome from Burkitt's lymphoma. *Nature 237:* 33–34, 1972.
154. Marcus, G., Camiolo, S. M., Kohga, S., Madija, J. M., Mittleman, A. Plasminogen activator secretion of human tumors in short term organ culture, including a comparison of primary and metastatic colon tumor. *Cancer Res. 43:* 5517–5525, 1983.
155. Mareel, M. K., and Brabarlle, M. J. Effect of microtubule inhibitors on malignant invasion *in vitro. J. Natl. Cancer Inst. 61:* 787–791, 1978.
156. Mark, J. L. Biochemistry of cancer cells: Focus on cell surface. *Science 165:* 1279–1282, 1974.

157. Markus, G. Plasminogen activators in malignant growth. In: *Progress in Fibrinolysis vol. #6*, edited by J. F. Davidson. Edinburgh, Churchill-Livingstone, 1983, pp. 587–604.
158. Markus, G., Takita, H., Camiolo, S. M. Corrassanti, J. G., Evers, J. C., and Hobika, G. H. Content and characterization of plasminogen activators in human lung tumors. *Cancer Res. 40:* 841–848, 1980.
159. Matsui, T., Yoshinobu, N., Koizumi, T., Nakagawa, T., Kishihara, M., and Fujita, T. Effects of calmodulin antagonists and cytochalasins on proliferation and differentiation of human promyelocytic leukemia cell line HL–60. *Cancer Res. 45:* 311–316, 1985.
160. Matsukura, S., Kakita, T., Sueoka, S., Yoshimi, H., Hirata, Y., Yokota, M., and Fujita, T. Multiple hormone receptors in the adenylate cyclase of human adrenocortical tumors. *Cancer Res. 40:* 3768–3771, 1980.
161. McNutt, N. S. Ultrastructural comparison of the interference between epithelial and stroma in basal cell carcinoma and control human skin. *Lab. Invest. 35:* 132–142, 1976.
162. Miller, E. C., and Miller, J. A. Mechanisms of chemical carcinogenesis. *Cancer 47:* 1055–1064, 1981.
163. Mitelman, F., Nilsson, P. G., Brandt, L., Alimena, G., Gastaldi, R., and Dallapiccola, B. Chromosome pattern, occupation, and clinical features in patients with acute nonlymphocytic leukemia. *Cancer Genet. Cytogenet. 4:* 197–214, 1981.
164. Mobley, W. C., Server, A. C., Ishii, D. N., Riopelle, R. J., and Shooter, E. M. Nerve growth factor. *N. Engl. J. Med. 297:* 1149–1158, 1977.
165. Monnat, R. J., and Loeb, L. A. Mechanism of neoplastic transformation. *Cancer Invest. 1:* 175–183, 1983.
166. Mosher, D. F. Fibronectin. *Prog. Hemostasis Thromb 5:* 111–151, 1980.
167. Muller, R., Harmon, D. J., Tremblay, J. M., Cline, M. J., and Verma, I. M. Differential expression of cellular oncogenes during pre- and postnatal development of the mouse. *Nature 229:* 660–664, 1982.
168. Murray, M. J., Shilo, B., Shih, C., Cowing, D., Hsu, H., and Weinberg, R. Three different human tumor cell lines contain different oncogenes. *Cell 25:* 355–361, 1981.
169. Muschel, R. J., Khoury, G., Lebowitz, P., Koller, R., and Dhar, R. The human c-ras, H oncogene: A mutation in normal and neoplastic tissue from the same patient. *Science 219:* 853–856, 1983.
170. Nagle, R. B., McDaniel, K. M., Clark, W. A., and Payne, C. M. The use of antikeratin antibodies in the diagnosis of human neoplasms. *Am. J. Clin. Pathol. 79:* 458, 1983.
171. Neel, B. G., Jhanwar, S. C., Chaganti, R. S., and Hayward, W. Two human *c-onc* genes are located on the long arm of chromosome 8: *Proc. Natl. Acad. Sci. USA 79:* 7842–7846, 1982.
172. Neil, J. C., Ghysdael, J., Vogt, P. J., and Smart, J. E. Homologous tyrosine phosphorylation sites in transformation-specific gene products of distinct avian sarcoma viruses. *Nature 291:* 675–677, 1981.
173. Nicholson, G. L. Cancer metastasis. Organ colonization and the cell-surface properties of malignant cells. *Biochim. Biophys. Acta 695:* 113–176, 1982.
174. Nicolson, G. L. Cell surface molecules and tumor metastasis. Regulation of metastatic phenotypic diversity. *Exp. Cell Res. 150:* 3–22, 1984.
175. Nicolson, G. L., and Poste, G. The cancer cell: Dynamic aspects and modifications in cell surface organizations. *N. Engl. J. Med. 295:* 197–203, 1976.
176. Nicolson, G. L., *et al.* Transmembrane control of the receptors on normal and tumor cell. Surface changes associated with transformation and malignancy. *Biochim. Biophys. Acta 458:* 1–72, 1976.
177. Nishimura, J., Huang, J. S., and Deuel, T. F. Platelet-derived growth factor stimulates tyrosine-specific protein kinase activity in Swiss mouse 3T3 cell membranes. *Proc. Natl. Acad. Sci. USA 79:* 4303–4307, 1982.
178. Nordenson, I., Beckman, L., Lidin, S., and Stjernberg, N. Chromosomal abberrations and cancer risk. *Hum. Hered. 34:* 76–81, 1984.
179. Nordquest, R. E., Anglon, J. H., and Lerna, M. P. Antigen shedding by human breast-cancer cells *in vitro* and *in vivo. Br. J. Cancer 37:* 776–779, 1978.
180. Nowell, P. C. Cytogenetics of preleukemia. *Cancer Genet. Cytogenet. 5:* 265–278, 1982.
181. Nowell, P. C. Cytogenetics. In: *Cancer: A Comprehensive Treatise*, vol. 1, *Etiology: Chem-*

ical and Physical Carcinogenesis, ed.2, edited by F. F. Becker. New York, Plenum Press, 1982, pp. 3–46.

182. Nowell, P. C., and Hungerford, D. A. A minute chromosome in human granulocytic leukemia. *Science 132:* 1497, 1960.

183. Olszewski, W., Darzynkiewicz, Z., Rosen, P. P., Schwartz, M. K., and Melamed, M. R. Flow cytometry of breast carcinoma. I. Relation of DNA ploidy level to histology and estrogen receptor. *Cancer 48:* 980–984, 1981.

184. Osborn, M., and Weber, K. Display of microtubules in transformed cells. *Cell 12:* 561–571, 1977.

185. Osborn, M., and Weber, K. Biology of disease. Tumor diagnosis by intermediate filament typing: A novel tool for surgical pathology. *Lab. Invest. 48:* 372, 1983.

186. Orth, D. V., Guillemin, R., Ling, N., and Nicholson, W. E. Immunoreactive endorphins, lipotropins, and corticotropins in a human non-pititary tumor: Evidence for a common precursor. *J. Clin. Endocrinol. Metab. 46:* 849–852, 1982.

187. Parey, G., and Hankes, S. P. Detection of an early surface change during oncogenic transformation. *Proc. Natl. Acad. Sci. USA 75:* 3703–3707, 1978.

188. Pasten, I., and Willingham, M. Cellular transformation and the morphologic phenotype of transformed cells. *Nature 274:* 645–650, 1978.

189. Payne, C. M., and Nagle, R. B. An ultrastructural study of intranuclear rodlets in a malignant extracranial neuroepithelial neoplasm. *Ultrastruct. Pathol. 5:* 1–13, 1983.

190. Perucho, M., Goldfarb, M., Shimizu, K., Lama, C., Fogh, J., and Wiggler, M. Human tumor derived cell lines contain common and different transforming genes. *Cell 27:* 467–476, 1981.

191. Pike, L. J., Gallis, B., Casnellie, J. E., Bornstein, P., and Krebs, E. G. Epidermal growth factor stimulates the phosphorylation of synthetic tyrosine-containing peptides by A431 cell membranes. *Proc. Natl. Acad. Sci. USA 79:* 1443–1447, 1982.

192. Powles, T. J., *et al. Prostaglandins and Cancer Proceedings*, First International Conference on Prostaglandins and Cancer, Washington, D.C. New York, A. R. Liss, 1982.

193. Quesada, J. R., and Gutterman, J. U. Interferons and cell growth regulation. *Eur. J. Cancer Clin. Oncol. 20:* 1213–1215, 1984.

194. Ramaekers, F., Puts, J., Kant, A., Moesker, O., Jap, P., and Vooijs, P. Differential diagnosis of human carcinomas, sarcomas and their metastases using antibodies to intermediate-sized filaments. *Eur. J. Cancer Clin. Oncol. 18:* 1251, 1982.

195. Ramaekers, F. C. S., Puts, J. J. G. F., Moesker, O., Kant, A., Huysmans, A., Haag, D., Jap, P. H. K., Herman, C. J., and Vooijs, G. P. Antibodies to intermediate filament proteins in the immunohistochemical identification of human tumours: An overview. *Histochem. J. 15:* 691, 1983.

196. Rao, P. N., and Johnson, R. T. Regulations of the cell cycle in hybrid cells. In: *Control of Proliferation in Animal Cells*, edited by B. Clarkson. Cold Spring Harbor, N.Y., Cold Spring Harbor Laboratory, 1974, pp. 785–800.

197. Reddy, E. P., Reynolds, R. K., Santos, E., Barbacid, M. A point mutation is responsible for the acquisition of transforming properties by the T24 human bladder carcinoma oncogene. *Nature 300:* 149–152, 1982.

198. Redman, M., Jeggo, P., and Wagner, R. Chromosomal rearrangement and carcinogenesis. *Mutat. Res. 98:* 249–264, 1982.

199. Reiber, M., and Reiber, M. S. Effect of malignant transformation and arginine limitation on fibronectin and other cell surface macromolecules of liver epithelial cultures. *Cancer Res. 40:* 2562–2567, 1980.

200. Roberts, A. B., Frolik, C. A., Anzano, M. A., and Sporn, M. B. Transforming growth factors from neoplastic and nonneoplastic tissues. *Fed. Proc. 42:* 2621–2626, 1983.

201. Robertson, D. M., and MacLean, J. D. Nuclear inclusions in malignant gliomas. *Arch. Neurol. 13:* 287–296, 1965.

202. Rosen, P. P., Savino, A., Menedex-Botet, C., Urban, J. A., Mike, V., Schwartz, M. K., and Melamed, M. R. Barr body distribution and estrogen receptor protein in mammary carcinoma. *Ann. Clin. Lab. Sci. 7:* 491–499, 1977.

203. Rosner, M. C., and Golomb, H. M. Ribosome-lamella complex in hairy cell leukemia. Ultrastructure and distribution. *Lab. Invest. 42:* 236–247, 1980.

204. Ross, J. D., Maloney, W. C., and Desforges, J. F. Ineffective regulation of granulopoiesis masquerading as congenital leukemia in a Mongoloid child. *J. Pediatr. 63:* 1–10, 1963.
205. Rowley, J. D. Chromosome abnormalities in cancer. *Cancer Genet. Cytogenet. 2:* 175–198, 1980.
206. Rowley, J. D. Identification of the constant chromosome regions involved in human hematologic disease. *Science 216:* 749–751, 1982.
207. Rowley, J. D. Human oncogene locations and chromosome aberrations. *Nature 301:* 290–291, 1983.
208. Ruoslah, H. E. Fibronectin in cell adhesion and invasion. *Cancer Metastasis Rev. 3:* 43–51, 1984.
209. Saez, J. M., Tell, G. P., and Dazord, A. Human adrenocortical tumors: Alterations in membrane-bound hormone receptors and cAMP protein kinases. In: *Endocrine Control in Neoplasia.* edited by R. K. Sharma and W. E. Criss. New York, Raven Press, 1978, pp. 53–69.
210. Sandberg, A. A. *The Chromosomes In Human Cancer and Leukemia.* New York, Elsevier North-Holland, 1980.
211. Sandberg, A. A. Chromosome studies in bladder cancer. In: *Carcinoma of the Bladder,* edited by J. G. Connolly. New York, Raven Press, 1981, pp. 127–141.
212. Sandberg, A. A. Chromosomal changes in human cancers: Specificity and heterogeneity. In: *Tumor Cell Heterogeneity.* New York, Academic Press, 1982, pp. 367–397.
213. Sandberg, A. A. *Cytogenetics of the Mammalian X Chromosome,* Part B, New York, A. R. Liss, 1983, pp. 459–498.
214. Scarpelli, D. G. Recent developments toward a unifying concept of carcinogenesis. *Ann. Clin. Lab. Sci. 13:* 249–259, 1983.
215. Schneeberger, E. E., and Lynch, R. D. Tight junctions, their structure, composition, and function. *Circ. Res. 55:* 723–734, 1984.
216. Schreiner, G. F., Fujiwana, K., Pollard, T. P., and Unanue, E. R. Redistribution of myosin accompanying capping of surface Ig. *J. Exp. Med. 145:* 1393–1397, 1977.
217. Schumacher, V., Altevogt, P., Fogel, M., Dennis, J., Waller, C. A., Baiz, D., and Schwartz, R. *Invasion Metastasis 2:* 313, 1982.
218. Schumacher, V., and Jacobs, W. Tumor metastases and cell mediated immunity in a model system in DBA/Z mice: VIII. Expression and shedding of Fc gamma receptors in metastatic tumor cell variants. *J. Supramol Struct. 11:* 105–111, 1979.
219. Scolnick, E. M., Papageorge, A. G., and Shih, T. Y. Guanine nucleotide-binding activity as an assay for SRC protein of rat-derived murine sarcoma viruses. *Proc. Natl. Acad. Sci. USA 76:* 5355–5359, 1979.
220. Scott, J. A. The role of cytoskeletal integrity in cellular transformation. *J. Theor. Biol. 106:* 183–188, 1984.
221. Scott, R. E., and Furcht, L. T. Membrane pathology of normal and malignant cells—A review. *Hum. Pathol. 5:* 519–530, 1976.
222. Scully, R. E. Mitosis counting–I. *Hum. Pathol. 7:* 481–482, 1976.
223. Sefton, B. M., and Hunter, T. Vinculin: A cytoskeletal target of the transforming protein of Rous sarcoma virus. *Cell 2:* 165–174, 1981.
224. Sen, A., and Todaro, G. J. A murine sarcoma virus-associated protein kinase: Interaction with actin and microtubular protein. *Cell 17:* 347–356, 1979.
225. Sheldon, S., Speers, W. C., and Lehman, J. M. Nucleolar persistence in embryonal carcinoma cells. *Exp. Cell Res. 132:* 185–192, 1981.
226. Sheriden, J. D., and Johnson, R. G. Cell junctions and neoplasia. In: *Molecular Pathology,* edited by R. A. Good, S. P. Day, and J. J. Yunos. Springfield, Ill. Charles C Thomas, 1975.
227. Sherwin, R. P., Kaufman, C., Dermer, G. R., and Monroe, S. A. Intranuclear rodlets in an intrathyroid tumor associated with hyperparathyroidism. *Cancer 39:* 178–185, 1977.
228. Shih, T. Y., Strokes, P. E., Smythers, G. W., Dhar, R., and Croszlan, S. Characterization of the phosphorylation sites and the surrounding amino acid sequences of the p21 transforming proteins coded for by the Harvey and Kirsten strains of murine sarcoma viruses. *J. Biol. Chem. 257:* 11767–11773, 1982.
229. Shih, T. Y., Weeks, M. O., Gruss, P., Dhar, R., Oroszlan, S., and Scolnick, E. M. Identification of a precursor in the biosynthesis of the p21 transforming protein of Harvey murine sarcoma virus. *J. Virol. 42:* 253–261, 1982.

230. Shih, T. Y., Weeks, M. O., Young, H. A., and Scolnick, E. M. Identification of a sarcoma virus-coded phosphoprotein in nonproducer cells transformed by Kirsten or Harvey murine sarcoma virus. *Virology 96:* 64–79, 1979.

231. Shohan, J., and Sachs, L. Differential cyclic changes in the surface membrane of normal and malignant transformed cells. *Exp. Cell Res. 85:* 8–14, 1974.

232. Shriver, K., and Rohrschneider, L. Organization of pp60 SRC and selected cytoskeletal proteins within adhesion plaques and junctions of Rous sarcoma virus-transformed rat cells. *J. Cell Biol. 89:* 525–535, 1981.

233. Siegesmund, K. A., Dutta, C. R., and Fox, C. A. The ultrastructure of the intranuclear rodlet in certain nerve cells. *J. Anat. 98:* 93–97, 1964.

234. Silverberg, S. G. Reproducibility of the mitosis count in the histologic diagnosis of smooth muscle tumors of the uterus. *Hum. Pathol. 7:* 451–454, 1976.

235. Sinha, A. A., Bentley, M. D., and Blackard, C. E. Freeze fracture observations on the membranes and junctions of human prostatic carcinoma and benign prostatic hypertrophy. *Cancer 40:* 1182–1188, 1977.

236. Siracky, J. Sex chromatin in gynecologic cancer: Incidence and limitations of its clinical interpretation. *Acta Cytol. 16:* 105–110, 1972.

237. Smart, J. E., Oppermann, H., Czernilofsky, A. P., Purchio, A. F., Erikson, R. L., and Bishop, J. M. Characterization of sites for tyrosine phosphorylation in the transforming protein of Rous sarcoma virus (pp60v-src) and its normal cellular homologue (pp60c-src). *Proc. Natl. Acad. Sci. USA 78:* 6013–6017, 1981.

238. Smetana, K., Daskal, Y., Gyorkey, F., Gyorkey, P., Lehane, D. E., Rudolph, A. H., and Busch, H. Nuclear and nucleolar ultrastructure of Sezary cells. *Cancer Res. 37:* 2036–2042, 1977.

239. Smethurst, M., Bishun, N. P., Fernandez, P., Allen, J., Burn, J. I., Alaghband-Zadh, J., and Williams, D. C. Steroid hormone receptors and sex chromatin frequency in breast cancer. *J. Endocr. Invest. 4:* 455–457, 1981.

240. Sobrinho-Simoes, M. A., and Goncalves, V. Nuclear bodies in papillary carcinomas of the human thyroid gland. *Arch. Pathol. 98:* 94–99, 1974.

241. Sporn, M., *et al.* Retinoids and suppression of the effects of polypeptide transforming factors—A new molecular approach to chemoprevention of cancer. In: *Molecular Actions and Targets for Cancer Chemotherapeutic Agents*, edited by A. C. Sartorelli, J. S. Lazo, and J. R. Bertino. New York, Academic Press, 1981, pp. 541–554.

242. Stanbridge, E. J., Der, C. J., and Doerson, C. H., *et al.* Human cell hybrids: Analysis of transformation and tumorigenicity. *Science 215:* 252–259, 1982.

243. Sumi, S. M., and Reifel, E. Unusual nuclear inclusions in astrocytoma. *Arch. Pathol. 92:* 14–19, 1971.

244. Summers, W. P., Grogan, E. A., Shedd, D., Robert, M., Liu, C. R., and Miller, G. Stable expression in mouse cells of nuclear neoantigen after transfer of a 3.4-megadalton cloned fragment of Epstein-Barr virus DNA. *Proc. Natl. Acad. Sci. USA 79:* 5688–5692, 1982.

245. Sunderman, F. W. Recent advances in metal carcinogenesis. *Ann. Clin. Lab. Sci. 14:* 93–122, 1984.

246. Tabin, C. J., Bradley, S. M., Bargmann, C. I., Weinberg, R. A., Papageorge, A. G., Scolnick, E. M., Dhar, R., Lowry, D. R., and Chang, E. H. The mechanism of activation of a human oncogene. *Nature 300:* 143–149, 1982.

247. Tani, E., Ametani, T., Ishijima, Y., Higashi, N., and Fujihara, E. Intranuclear para-crystalline fibrillar arrays in human glioma cells. *Cancer Res. 30:* 1210–1217, 1971.

248. Temin, H. M. Do we understand the genetic mechanisms of oncogenesis? *J. Cell Physiol. 3:* 1–11, 1984.

249. Therman, E., Sarto, G. E., and Buchler, D. A. The structure and origin of giant nuclei in human cancer cells. *Cancer Genet. Cytogenet. 9:* 9–18, 1983.

250. Tomiyasu, U., Hirano, A., and Zimmerman, H. M. Fine structure of human pituitary adenoma. *Arch. Pathol. 95:* 287–292, 1973.

251. Totter, J. R. Spontaneous cancer and its possible relationship to oxygen metabolism. *Proc. Natl. Acad. Sci. USA 77:* 1763–1767, 1980.

252. Trent, J. M. Cytogenetic analysis of human tumor cells cloned in agar. In: *Cloning of Human Stem Cells*, edited by S. E. Salmon. New York, A. R. Liss, 1980, pp. 165–177.

253. Trosko, J. E., and Chang, C-C. Error-prone DNA repair and replication in relation to malignant transformation. *Transplant. Proc. 16:* 363–365, 1984.
254. Tucker, R. W., Sanford, K. K., and Frankel, F. R. Tubulin and actin in paired non-neoplastic and spontaneously transformed cell lines *in vitro. Cell 13:* 629–642, 1978.
255. Uribe, M., Fenoglio-Preiser, C. M., Grimes, M., and Feind, C. Medullary carcinoma of the thyroid gland: clinical, pathological and immunohistochemical features with review of the literature. *Am. J. Surg. Pathol.,* 9: 577–594, 1985.
256. Vogel, F., and Motulsky, A. G. *Human Genetics: Problems and Approaches.* Berlin, Springer-Verlag, 1979.
257. Wallach, D. F. H. Generalized membrane defects in cancer. *N. Engl. J. Med. 280:* 761–767, 1969.
258. Warburg, O. On the origin of cancer cells. *Science 123:* 309–314, 1956.
259. Weber, G. Enzymology of cancer cells. *N. Engl. J. Med. 296:* 541–550, 1979.
260. Weinstein, I. B. Current concepts and controversies in chemical carcinogenesis. *J. Supermol. Struct. Cell Biochem. 17:* 99–120, 1981.
261. Weinstein, I. B. The scientific basis for carcinogen detection and primary cancer prevention. *Cancer 47:* 113–1141, 1981.
262. Wenner, C. E., Tomei, L. D., and Leister, K. J. Tumor promoters: An overview of membrane-associated alterations and intracellular events. *Transplant. Proc. 16:* 381–385, 1984.
263. Whang-Peng, J., Cannelos, G. P., Carbone, P. P., and Tjis, H. H. Clinical implications of cytogenetic variants in chronic myelogenous leukemia. *Blood 32:* 755–766, 1968.
264. Whang-Peng, J., Kao-Shan, C. S., Lee, F. C., Bunn, P. A., Carney, D. N., Gazdar, A. F., and Minna, J. D. Specific chromosome defect associated with human small cell lung cancer: Deletion 3p (14–23). *Science 215:* 181–182, 1982.
265. Whang-Peng, J., Kao-Shan, C. S., Lee, E. C., Bunn, P. A., Carney, D. N., Gazdar, A. F., Portlock, C., Minna, J. D. Deletion 3p (14–23): Double minute chromosomes, and homogeneously staining regions in human small-cell lung cancer. In: *Gene Amplification,* edited by R. T. Schimke. Cold Spring Harbor, New York, Cold Spring Harbor Laboratory, pp. 107–113, 1982.
266. Whitefield, J. F., MacManus, J. P., Boynton, A. L., Durkin, J., and Jone, A. Functional regulation at the cellular and molecular levels. In: *Proceedings of Conference,* Ithaca, N.Y., edited by R. A. Coiradinold. New York, Elsiever-North Holland, 1982, pp. 61–87.
267. Winter, H., Schweizer, J., and Goerttler, K. Keratin polypeptide composition as a biochemical tool for the discrimination of benign and malignant epithelial lesions in man. *Arch. Dermatol. Res. 275:* 27, 1983.
268. Winters, W. D., and Sykes, J. A. Intranuclear crystalline zebra structures induced in human tumour cells by adenovirus type 5. *J. Gen. Virol. 40:* 675–679, 1978.
269. Wojkowiak, Z., Duhl, D. M., Briggs, R. C., Hnilica, L. S., Stein, J. L., and Stein, G. S. A nuclear matrix antigen in HeLa and other human malignant cells. *Cancer Res. 42:* 4546–4552, 1982.
270. Wolley, R. C., Schreiber, K., and Koss, L. G. DNA distribution in human colon carcinomas and its relationship to clinical behavior. *J. Natl. Cancer Inst. 69:* 15–22, 1982.
271. Wolman, S. R. Cytogenetics and cancer. *Arch. Pathol. Lab. Med. 108:* 15–19, 1984.
272. Yogeeswam, G., Stein, B. S., and Sebastian, H. Altered cell surface organization of gangliosides and sialylglycoproteins of mouse metastatic melanoma variant lines selected *in vivo* for enhanced lung implantation. *Cancer Res. 38:* 1336–1344, 1978.
273. Young, H. A., Shih, T. Y., Scholnick, E. M., Rashfeed, S., and Gardner, M. B. Different rat-derived transforming retroviruses code for an immunologically related intracellular phosphoprotein. *Proc. Natl. Acad. Sci. USA 76:* 3523–3527, 1979.
274. Yunis, J. J. Specific fine chromosomal defects in cancer. *Hum. Pathol. 12:* 503–515, 1981.
275. Yunis, J. J. The chromosomal basis of human neoplasia. *Science 221:* 227–236, 1983.
276. Yunis, J. J., Bloomfield, C. D., and Ensrud, K. All patients with acute non-lymphocytic leukemia may have a chromosomal defect. *N. Engl. J. Med. 1305:* 135–139, 1981.
277. Yunis, J. J., and Soreng, A. L. Constitutive fragile sites and cancer. *Science 226:* 1199–1204, 1984.
278. Zang, K. D., and Singer, H. Chromosomal constitution of meningiomas. *Nature 216:* 84–85, 1967.

Chapter 3

Oncogenes and Cancer

THOMAS B. TOMASI

INTRODUCTION

The story of oncogenes (derived from the Greek word onkos, meaning mass or tumor) begins with the discovery of retroviruses. Retroviruses have genomes of single-stranded RNA and replicate via a double-stranded DNA intermediate which is inserted into the host cell genome. Expression of the retroviral genome in its simplest form involves RNA → DNA → RNA protein. However, the process is extremely complicated, and there are significant gaps in our knowledge of some of the steps involved. The typical replication-competent retrovirus (Fig. 3.1) contains three sets of genes: *gag*, *pol*, and *env* bounded on either side by repeated sequences called long terminal repeats (LTRs) which are not translated into proteins but contain important control elements as will be discussed below. The *gag* genes are translated into four or five proteins which are components of the core of the virion; *pol* encodes the enzyme reverse transcriptase; and the *env* gene products (usually two) are proteins (often glycoproteins) of the envelope of the particle. The reverse transcriptase is responsible for converting RNA into a complementary DNA. When in the early 1970s reverse transcriptase was first discovered independently by Howard Temin and David Baltimore, the central "dogma" was DNA makes RNA makes protein. Thus the name reverse transcriptase was used to signify that DNA could be made " backwards" from RNA.

The first retrovirus to be thoroughly explored was the Rous sarcoma virus (RSV). Peyton Rous reported in 1911[102] that a filterable agent produced sarcomas in chickens, an observation for which Dr. Rous was awarded a Nobel Prize in 1966. The gene responsible for the transforming and tumorigenic properties of RSV was identified in the early 1970s[127] and was called the *src* (for sarcoma) gene. It was structurally different from any of the other genes of RSV (*gag*, *pol*, *env*), and its presence in the viral genome was required for the production of tumors. This was first shown by mutant viruses with specific deletion of the *src* gene, which was correlated with a loss of transforming potential.[7] Subsequently the construction of clones of deletion mutants of

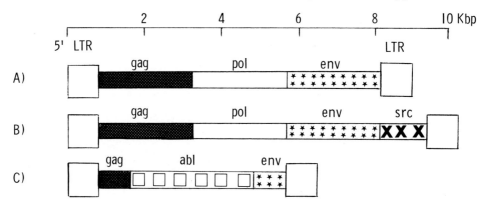

FIG. 3.1.   Retrovirus genome. (*A*) Replication competent, nondefective helper virus. Does not contain oncogene sequences. (*B*) Replication competent, nondefective Rous sarcoma virus. Acute transforming virus containing *onc* gene (*src*) but retaining normal viral genes needed for replication. (*C*) Replication defective Abelson murine leukemia virus. Contains *onc* gene (*abl*) which replaces part or all of the normal viral genes. Genome of defective virus usually shorter than helper virus.

other viruses also showed that the ability to produce tumors was correlated with the presence or absence of an oncogene or "*onc*" gene.[1] The fact that a single gene, was responsible for the transforming potential of a virus was a significant advance in our understanding of cancer. It was on this background that Huebner and Todaro[56] proposed the oncogene hypothesis of cancer. They theorized that normal cells harbored genes homologous to the viral transforming genes which could be activated by carcinogenic agents. The seminal idea of this hypothesis was that cellular genes could, when appropriately activated, lead to cancer. Temin's protovirus hypothesis[126] was similar to the oncogene hypothesis but made the critical distinction that qualitative changes occurred in normal genes (*c-oncs*, or proto-oncogenes) to render them transforming. Thus, the basic difference between the two theories still serves as a point of controversy: Are quantitative changes in normal gene products sufficient for transformation under natural conditions or are mutations or alterations in the structure of gene products required? This point will be discussed below in more detail.

The oncogene hypothesis was remarkably predictive of the subsequent unexpected discovery[120] that the *src* gene was present in normal uninfected chicken cells. It was shown experimentally (by hybridization studies with *src*-specific c-DNA probes) that normal avian DNA, and subsequently also a variety of other vertebrates, contained sequences related to the transforming genes of RSV. This was the first experimental evidence that normal cells contain genes which are closely related to those responsible for virally produced tumors in animals.

TYPES OF TRANSFORMING RETROVIRUSES

Three classes of oncogenic retroviruses have been described which differ in the mechanism(s) by which they induce transformation (outlined in Table 3.1).

Acute transforming viruses of animals which produce tumors in 2–3 weeks

TABLE 3.1. THREE MECHANISMS BY WHICH RETROVIRUSES TRANSFORM CELLS

1. Acute transforming virus, *e.g.*, Rous sarcoma virus contains an oncogene, *v-onc*
2. Slow transforming virus, *e.g.*, avian leukosis virus, promoter (LTR) insertion, activation of *c-onc*
3. Human T cell leukemia virus, *e.g.*, HTLV I, II, BLV, *trans* acting factor increases transcription from viral promoter and certain cellular genes (*e.g.*, IL-2 receptor)

are not transmitted in the germ line or by infection, and are almost always replication-defective. The hallmark of this group is the presence of a structurally distinct *onc* gene which is not essential to viral survival but is critical to transformation. Indeed, most commonly, *onc* genes replace one or more viral genes required for replication and thus, in order to reproduce, acute transforming viruses require the presence of a nondefective "helper" virus. Helper viruses provide the missing viral genes deleted by the integration of the *onc* gene. Acute transforming viruses infect many cells, and the resulting tumors are thus polyclonal in nature. They can produce tumors in cultured cells and a variety of tumor types have been identified in animals, including sarcomas, lymphomas, leukemias, and carcinomas. About 20 different *v-oncs* have been described in acute retroviruses. Some *v-oncs* are associated predominantly with one type of cancer (for example, *v-abl* with lymphoid tumors) while others such as MC 29 (containing *v-myc*) are associated with multiple tumors including sarcomas, myeloid tumors, and carcinomas.

A key question is how *v-oncs* are acquired by acute retroviruses. Did they arise from cellular oncogenes (*c-onc*) or vice versa? Abundant evidence reviewed by Bishop[7] suggests that *v-oncs* were derived from *c-oncs*. Although the details are not entirely clear, a current model is that retroviral DNA integrates near one of the 20 or so *c-oncs* (see Ref. 103 for chromosomal locations of *c-onc*). A deletion and rearrangement occurs which fuses the *c-onc* gene with viral DNA. A primary RNA transcript is made which is then spliced to remove the introns present in the *c-onc*. This "chimeric" RNA containing viral and cellular sequences in continuity is then packaged into a virion by the information contained in another intact "helper" provirus. Since each virus particle contains two RNA molecules, some of the particles will therefore contain one hybrid RNA and an infused RNA. Nonhomologous recombination occurs between the two strands and creates a transforming genome. Two types of viral genomes are formed as shown in Fig. 3.1. In the RSV genome the *src* gene is present 3' to the *env* gene and, therefore, it does not delete critical viral genes necessary for replication. Thus, certain of the RSV strains are replicative competent viruses. However, with almost all other acute transforming viruses, the fusing of the *c-onc* gene with the viral genome deletes segments that are required for replication. In many cases the *v-onc* gene product is composed of *gag* and/or *env* sequences in addition to the *v-onc*. For example, the *v-abl* product of certain murine B cell lymphomas is a protein of molecular weight 160,000 designated p160 *gag-abl* because it consists of amino acid sequences derived from both the *gag* and *abl* portions of the retroviral RNA genome. There is some evidence that the *gag* sequences are not merely accidents of recombination but play an important role in transformation[88].

Using mutant plasmids to transfect fibroblasts and lymphoid cells, it was shown that *gag*-deficient genomes were unable to transform lymphocytes, a major target of Abelson induced leukemia. It is interesting that *gag* sequences can sometimes be detected on the surfaces of cells,[17] while the *v-abl* sequences are located inside the plasma membrane. The p160 *gag-abl,* like many other transforming proteins, has covalently bound lipid and some evidence[54] suggests that it may be attached to the *gag* sequences. In RSV and perhaps other *v-oncs* which are not fusion products with *gag* or *env,* the lipid which may be necessary for membrane association and tumorigenicity,[42, 65] is directly bound to the N-terminal sequences.

Since viral oncogenes are derived from cellular DNA sequences by transduction involving two nonhomologous recombinations, the question arises as to whether *v-onc* and *c-onc* are identical. Structural data shows very significant homologies between many *v-oncs* and *c-oncs;* however in all cases examined to date, the genes are not identical. Besides the fusion products mentioned above, there may be deletions and mutations. For example, the coding regions of *c-src* and *v-src* show scattered mutations over 1–2% of the sequences and the C-terminal 14 amino acid of pp60^{c-src} are replaced by different 12 amino acids in pp60^{v-src}. Thus it appears that there are significant qualitative (structural) differences between viral and cellular oncogenes, and it has been suggested that these, rather than quantitative changes, may be the reason that viral *onc* genes readily transform cells while cellular proteins do so only under special circumstances (see discussion below).

As discussed above, the viral genome includes control regions contained in the LTRs. They appear to be necessary for the formation of circular DNA, which may be a step (as yet unproven) in integration similar to the circular DNA viruses in lambda phage, which are essential for integration and replication. LTRs contain important regulatory elements, including promoters and enhancers[70] and the signals for transcriptional termination. It has recently been reported,[15] using recombinant genomes of the human T cell leukemia virus (HTLV), that target cell specificity of the T cell virus is determined by the LTRs. Examples of the tissue expression of genes are those of the lymphadenopathy-associated viruses (LAV) associated with acquired immune deficiency syndrome (AIDS) and infecting T cells and the restricted transcription of immunoglobulin genes to B cells.[90] Several regulatory molecules, such as hormones and metals, modulate gene expression by activating (or repressing) regulatory elements in LTRs. For example, the increased expression of murine mammary tumor virus (MMTV) induced by glucocorticoids is mediated by an interaction with transcriptional enhancers in the LTR[85] and metal ions, such as cadmium and zinc, regulate the activity of the metallothionine gene, probably by interacting with similar types of control regions in the eukaryotic genome.[128] The protein product of the gene regulated by metals (metallothionine) chelates and detoxifies these metals, and thus this activation is biologically useful.

The second class of oncogenic retroviruses is the slow transforming viruses. The best-studied example is the avian leukosis virus (ALV) which results in tumors in chickens 4–12 months after injection. Unlike acute transforming virus, ALV is not capable of transforming cells in culture and does not contain genes homologous to normal cellular sequences, and the resultant tumors are clonal in origin. Hayward *et al.*[51] have shown that ALV integrates adjacent to a normal cellular gene (the *c-myc* gene) in bursal lymphocytes. Various lengths of ALV-DNA integrate, but the LTR is always included, and the level of expression of RNA transcripts of *c-myc* increases to 100–300 copies/cell. Since viral promoter sequences are present in the LTR, the mechanism of ALV tumorigenesis has been termed promoter insertion. Activation of *c-myc* by proximal action of ALV promoters was the first example of tumors resulting from activation of a normal gene and is thought (but not proven) to be a major mechanism in carcinogenesis by slow-acting viruses.

Integration of retroviruses is thought to be a random event; hence, in any population of lymphocytes the statistical likelihood that the proviral LTR will integrate adjacent to, for example, *c-myc* sequences is small. This would presumably explain (a) the long latent period associated with slow viruses, (b) why the oncogenic potential of ALV seems to reside within an area which does not encode a viral protein, (c) why the only viral sequences consistently detected in the B cell tumors produced by ALV are the terminal nucleotides of the LTR covalently linked to the *c-myc* gene, and (d) the clonal nature of ALV-induced tumors. The presence of integrated proviral DNA sequences at "preferred" sites is not necessarily the result of a preference for site-specific integration sequences, but rather the selective growth advantage given a single cell and its clonal progeny when a provirus happens to integrate adjacent to the appropriate cellular (*c-myc*) sequence.

The concept of insertional mutagenesis as a mechanism of *in vivo* carcinogenesis is supported by *in vitro* experiments in which mouse *c-mos*[8] and normal human *c-Ha-ras*[13] were shown to transform NIH 3T3 cells, but only if linked to upstream retroviral LTRs. The transformants also form tumors in nude mice,[13] and transformed cells express high levels of the normal gene product.

The third class of oncogenic retroviruses are represented by the recently described T cell leukemia viruses. The genome of the T-cell leukemia viruses (HTLV I and II) contains a unique sequence located between the 3' end of the *env* gene and the 3' LTR (see Fig. 3.2).[50] The 1500-nucleotide sequence contains two regions: a 500 base-pair, nonconserved region and a 1000-nucleotide sequence which is conserved (76% identical) between HTLV I and HTLV II. Unlike with an oncogene, no relation to a normal cellular sequence and the conserved region could be identified. This region could code for a protein of molecular weight of about 40,000, and a protein possibly originating from this sequence has been identified in HTLV-infected cells. In addition, transacting factors induced by HTLV infection have been reported to substantially augment expression of viral genes and promote viral replication.[116] The conserved sequence found in the 3' region has not been found in other retroviruses, with the possible exception of bovine leukemia virus (BLV), and it is interesting that BLV has been shown to have other characteristics similar to HTLV.[41] A speculative scenario is that the conserved sequence encodes a 40,000-dalton transacting factor which activates transcription by interacting with the HTLV

STRUCTURE OF HTLV

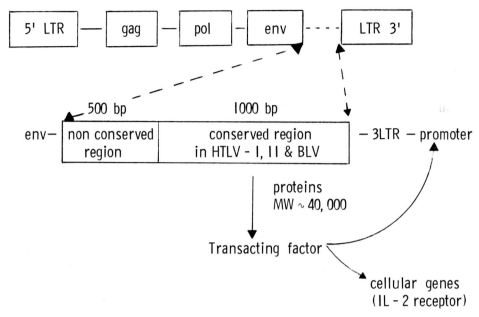

FIG. 3.2.   Structure of HTLV.

LTR. This enhances expression of viral genes and possibly other cellular genes (such as IL-2 or IL-2 receptors) which may be involved in transformation. Transacting factor(s) would explain the absence of specific integration sites in HTLV, which are required for insertional mutagenesis mechanisms. It should be noted that transacting factors, although not found in other retroviruses, have been identified as transcriptional regulatory factors in adenoviruses[9] and SV40.[43,60] Thus, the structure of HTLV (and possibly BLV) suggests a new subgroup of viruses distinct from acute and slow-transforming viruses. Whether HTLV III, which has been associated with the lymphadenopathy-associated virus (LAV) and the acquired immune deficiency syndromes (AIDS), has a similar structure has not been established. However, this virus is distinctly different from HTLV I and II in that it promotes T cell death rather than proliferation, produces a major core protein (p25) which is cross-reactive with a protein product of the virus of equine infectious anemia (and is not related to the p24 of HTLV I and II), and induces the production by human T helper (T4) cells of a potent immunosuppressive factor.[67] LAV and presumably HTLV III can also be propagated in Epstein-Barr virus (EBV)-infected B cells and therefore suggests that B cells may serve as an important reservoir for the blood-borne virus. This could be related to the high incidence of B cell lymphomas in AIDS patients.[112]

ONCOGENE EXPRESSION IN HUMAN TUMORS

The finding of cellular sequences homologous to known viral transforming genes suggests that a variety of other tumors induced by chemicals, x-ray, and

UV light, or of apparent spontaneous origin, might involve activation and/or alteration in *c-onc* genes. Two general approaches have been used to look for an association of oncogenes with human tumors. One involves surveys of large groups of tumors using DNA probes derived from *v-onc* genes. The techniques most frequently utilized are dot-blot or northern blot hybridization of RNA extracted from the tumors. In some instances, Southern blot analysis of tumor DNA has also been carried out to determine if the activated *onc* genes are amplified. A second technique explores the ability of tumor DNA to transform certain "normal" cell lines, both by the usual criteria for transformation *in vitro* as well as by the production of tumors in nude mice. In many studies, cell lines derived from human tumors have been used as possible sources for transforming DNA. However, several reports[38, 124] show significant differences in early *vs.* late passage cell lines in the structure of oncogenes, including point mutations and translocations, and in the ability to transform and produce tumors in nude mice. This has prompted the use of fresh tissue directly from tumors in more recent transfection experiments.

Extensive studies by Slamon *et al.*[115] included the examination of 20 different types of fresh human tumor from 54 patients. The technique employed RNA extracted from tumors blotted onto nitrocellulose paper and hybridized to 15 different ^{32}P-labeled *v-onc* probes. Whenever possible, normal tissue was obtained from the same patient. In most cases, the elevations noted in *onc* gene expression were of the order of 2- to 10-fold, as compared to those of the corresponding normal tissue. Of the 54 cases studied almost all of the tumors showed elevated expression of one or more (usually at least two *c-onc* genes). Only 2 of the 54 tumors listed were negative for any of the 15 *v-onc* gene probes used. Three patterns were observed: (*a*) four oncogenes were expressed in increased levels, as compared to normal tissues in nearly all tumors (*c-myc, c-fos, H-ras,* and *K-ras*); (*b*) five oncogenes were infrequently expressed (*c-abl, c-fes, c-fms, c-myb,* and *c-src*). Some of these *c-oncs* showed selective expression in certain tumors. For example, *c-myb, c-abl, c-fes,* and *c-src* in hematopoietic tumors, others such as *c-fms* were present in 18 of 54 tumors with no obvious specific tumor associations; (*c*) six oncogenes showed no increase in expression in any of the tumors tested in this particular series (*c-erbA, c-erbB, c-mos, c-sis, c-rel,* and *c-yes*). However, studies from other groups have shown that some of these latter genes appear to be activated in certain tumors. It should also be mentioned that although studies of fresh tissues are important for the reasons stated above, tumors and normal tissues may contain markedly different cell types. For example, 1 g of normal colon tissue may contain markedly different numbers of epithelial cells than 1 g of malignant colon tissue. Also malignant tissues may be infiltrated with a variety of inflammatory cells which may vary in their *onc* gene content. Techniques, such as *in situ* hybridization to tissue sections, may be important in detecting transcripts in particular locations and in specific cell types. Only with hematopoietic clonal malignancies are there homogeneous populations of cells, and even in this instance, the appropriate control (the same cell type at the same stage of differentiation) may be difficult to obtain. Rosson and Tereba[100] examined 30 cases of childhood hematopoietic malignancies by dot-blot hybridization of tumor RNA. Expression of *c-myc, c-rel,* and *c-ras* RNA occurred in almost all tumors, regardless of type, and although there was some variation, overall they were not significantly elevated, compared to normal cells. These results suggest that comparable *onc* gene expression in leukemic and normal cells occurs with several oncogenes. Thus, if these particular genes are involved in these leukemias they are operating in conjunction with other factors. Some differential expression (*myb, erb, src*) was also noted, but normal control cells at the same stage of differentiation are needed in order to evaluate the significance of these changes in relation to the malignant phenotype. In contrast to this study, it was shown that 10 of 67 patients with leukemia showed elevations (10–30×) of *myc* RNA, as compared to those of normal peripheral blood leukocytes (PBL).[101] Elevations most commonly occurred in acute leukemia where DNA rearrangements, including the *c-myc* gene, were noted. Whether the expression of other oncogenes is increased in those cases with normal levels of *c-myc* expression is unknown. Moreover, more than one oncogene may be elevated in a given tumor,[100,115] and there may be changes in oncogene expression following treatment when a patient undergoes remission.

Another member of the *myc* gene family, the *N-myc* gene, has recently been implicated in tumors of neural tissues, including neuroblastomas and retinoblastomas. Brodeur *et al.*[10] found that 40% of 63 fresh neuroblastoma tissues expressed increased *N-myc* and that the gene was significantly (40-fold) amplified. Importantly, amplification was one of the best indicators of prognosis with lower levels of amplification signifying a better prognosis. Increased levels of *N-myc* RNA were found in all of 10 primary retinoblastomas. The occurrence of activated *N-myc* in all tumors, even those at a very early stage of their development, suggests that *N-myc* could be involved in the etiology of the disease. On the other hand, in the neuroblastomas, less than half had elevated *N-myc* in mRNAs, suggesting that it may be a secondary (albeit possibly an important) event. Both diseases are associated with chromosomal abnormalities: Neuroblastomas with abnormalities on chromosome 1, while in retinoblastomas deletions occur on chromosome 13. In retinoblastoma (and perhaps other childhood tumors) there is thought to be a loss of suppressor genes.[78] It is postulated that suppressor genes reside on each homologue of chromosome 13 and function in some as yet unknown way to inhibit an "expressor gene" (perhaps an oncogene), the activation of which promotes the development of tumors. Thus, a balance between the expressor and suppressor genes may determine tumorigenicity, as suggested in certain animal systems.[137] Several other childhood diseases (Wilms' tumor and familial renal cell carcinoma) may well fit this model. It is also feasible that suppressor elements operate in the adult.[63,118]

DNA-mediated gene transfer is a powerful approach in the analysis of transforming genes in human tumors. Certain immortalized cell lines, such as the NIH 3T3 cell, are able to incorporate and express genes of donor genomic DNA when presented to the recipient cell as a coprecipitate with calcium phosphate.[135] Weinberg *et al.*[129] first demonstrated a transforming gene in methylcholanthrene-treated cells when their DNA was transfected into NIH 3T3 cells. Subsequently a variety of studies,[21,64,89,129] using transfection of genomic DNA into recipient NIH 3T3 cells, have identified transforming elements in various rodents and human tumor cell lines and in some fresh solid tumors. As discussed below, using recombinant DNA technology, the DNA responsible for transformation has been isolated from the tumors, molecularly cloned and sequenced. It should be emphasized again that the use of fresh tumor DNA[89] derived from solid tumors is particularly relevant in view of the changes in gene organization that occur during culture. Although the set of oncogenes identified by transfection techniques overlaps that discovered by the studies of retroviruses discussed above, there is a striking predominance of three genes (all belonging to the *ras* gene family) which are detected by transfection assays. Pulciani *et al.*[89] and Santos *et al.*[107] examined 96 human tumor and tumor cell lines for their ability to transform (many of these were fresh solid tumors), and several transforming genes were identified. In this series, only one tumor (the EJ/T24 bladder carcinoma) carried an *H-ras* transforming gene, whereas in eight different carcinomas and sarcomas a *K-ras* gene was detected by transfection. In earlier studies the isolation of the active transforming gene from the human bladder EJ/24 carcinoma revealed its close homology with the Harvey sarcoma virus, an acute transforming virus of rats containing the *v-H-ras* oncogene. Like other *v-oncs*, this gene had a normal cellular counterpart, *c-H-ras*. The normal gene was, however, nontransforming in the 3T3 transfection assay. Isolation by molecular cloning from the bladder tumor cell lines and a comparison of the DNA sequence of the tumor *ras* gene with a normal cellular gene led to the striking finding of a single nucleotide substitution.[95,123] A point mutation occurred in codon 12 and altered the 12th amino acid of the p21 *ras* gene protein, replacing a glycine with a valine. It was speculated that the loss of glycine at residue 12 could lead to a significant conformational change in the protein. A precedent exists for other single amino acid changes having profound effects on protein function, the best known example being sickle cell hemoglobin. In regard to the functional properties of mutated *H-ras* and *K-ras* genes, a recent study[39] indicated no difference in subcellular localization, affinity of GTP binding, or post-translational acylation. It is possible that the mutational activation of p21 is a consequence of alterations in its interactions with other cellular proteins, rather than a change in the intrinsic biochemical activities of the protein. However, further work on the biochemical properties of the mutant *vs.* normal *ras* gene protein are necessary before any firm conclusions are drawn.

On the basis of computer models of the p21 protein, changes in the 12th amino acid might be expected to result in very significant structural alterations in the molecule.[95] One of the implications of these findings is that changes at position 12 may represent a precise target for mutagenesis, resulting in carcinogenesis. This thesis has been examined in the following manner: as pointed out above, transformation by *H-ras* is relatively rare, at least as determined by transfection assays. The 12th codon of *c-ras* is GGC, and this is preceded by the dinucleotide CC. The sequence CCGG is a restriction site for cleavage by two restriction endonuclease enzymes. Mutant *ras* gene DNA would therefore have a different restriction pattern than normal DNA on Southern blot analysis using a *c-ras* probe which spans the region of interest. Using this technique, Feinberg *et al.*[38] examined 29 human cancers (20 primary tumors and 9 cell lines). The tumors included 10 bladder Ca, 9 colon Ca, and 10 lung Ca. None of the tumors showed evidence of mutation at codon 12, although a mutation at the third base of the 12th codon would not have been detected by this technique.

It is of interest that premalignant but benign papillomas induced by chemical carcinogens (DMBA initiator followed by TPA promoter) showed activated *c-H-ras* genes by transfection and elevated levels of *ras* transcript, as compared to normal epidermis. Elevated *H-ras* levels were not found in hyperplastic epidermis. The proportion of papillomas having transforming activity (>25%) was much larger than the number of benign tumors progressing to frank malignancy (5–7%). This suggests that *H-ras* activation is a relatively early event and that progression to malignancy requires additional events. Whether the *H-ras* gene was mutated in the benign papilloma was not determined. However, it should be noted that other data suggest that under conditions of strong promotion (using viral LTRs linked to *c-H-ras*) normal ras DNA transforms NIH 3T3 cells. Thus it has not been excluded that mutation, possibly at position 12 or 61 (see below), may be a later event closer to the malignant phenotype.

A similar analysis of *Ki-ras* gene has been undertaken.[107] The 12th codon is GGT and is not part of a known restriction endonuclease cleavage site. However, replacing the first G with a C creates GAGCTC, which is recognized by the enzyme Sac I. Replacing the second G with a C results in a GCTGC and creates a Fnu4HI site. Thus new restriction sites are produced near the 12th codon and Southern blot analysis, with an appropriate DNA probe, (such as a *v-ras* probe which includes the first exon) can be used to detect these two mutations. There are six possible mutations at codon 12; however, none of the other four mutations of the 12th triplet would generate restriction polymorphism. Using this method, mutations were found in *K-ras* in two tumor cell lines (a bladder and a lung carcinoma), both resulting in arginine replacing glycine at position 12 of the p21 gene product. Eight primary lung carcinomas were also examined. One showed a similar mutation in fresh tumor tissue but not in normal bronchial tissue or PBL from the same patient, i.e., a tumor-specific mutation. The DNA from this tumor, but not from normal tissue of the same patient, transformed 3T3 cells in the transfection assay.

Another method of detecting mutant genes is to determine whether their gene product is structually altered either by sequence analysis (which is often difficult because of the amount of pure protein needed) or by physical properties such as electrophoretic mobility. Two lung and two colon carcinoma cell lines containing activated *K-ras* genes (by transfection) expressed abnormal p21 proteins detected by their altered electrophoretic mobility.[27] In these experiments p21 *K-ras* proteins, labeled in culture with 35^S methionine, were precipitated with a monoclonal anti-p21 antibody and analyzed by sodium dodecyl sulfate (SDS)-polyacrylamide gel electrophoresis. Three of the proteins were similar in electrophoretic mobility but distinct from normal p21 *K-ras*. The fourth protein had a unique electrophoretic mobility. All four proteins were identified in transfected NIH 3T3 cells, and the transformed cell expressed the altered p21 species. The nature of the mutation in these tumors was not elucidated by restriction enzyme or sequence analysis.

A third member of the *ras* family *(N-ras)* was first identified in a neuroblastoma cell line.[114] The *H-ras*, *K-ras*, and *N-ras* genes have an overall similar structure, share regions of homology, and produce a similar p21 GTP binding protein as their gene product. Nevertheless, the three genes show significant sequence differences from one another and from their viral *ras* gene counterparts, which are of rat origin.

Studies of the *N-ras* gene derived from the neuroblastoma cell line revealed only one nucleotide difference from the normal *ras* gene. The 61st amino acid encodes a glutamine in the normal *N-ras (c-N-ras)* which is replaced by a lysine in the transforming *N-ras* protein.[125] No differences were found in the products of normal and transforming genes at position 12. It is of interest that Yuasa *et al.*[138] have reported a transforming *H-ras* protein with a substitution of leucine for glutamine at position 61. It may, therefore, be pertinent that the only point mutations so far described are at positions 12 or 61 in the *ras* family. Threonine at position 59 is the site of autophosphorylation by GTP so that position 61 is close to the GTP binding site. On the other hand, various substitutions of glycine number 12 (with valine, aspartic acid, arginine, serine, or cystine in different tumors) have been reported to activate transformation, and there is some theoretical evidence[133] that glycine 12 may be involved in the GTP site.

The number of mutations (productive of amino acid changes) that may be generated in the *ras* gene family is 42 (6 at codon 12 and 8 at codon 61). However, few *ras* genes have been shown to have mutations at the two vulnerable points: codons 12 and 61. Only four of these mutations give rise to restriction enzyme polymorphism. Thus, extensive sequence studies are necessary to determine the presence or absence of mutant *ras* genes. However, *ras* genes activated and detected by transfection assays have been found in only about 25% of the tumors examined (expecially colon, lung, urinary bladder, and gall bladder), although increased levels of *ras* gene transcripts are common in many tumors, as described above.[115]

The relatively low incidence of transformation by transfection analysis in the *ras* family is unlike that found in ALV-induced B cells in chickens, where approximately 90% of the tumors have a transforming gene *(Blym-1)* detected by transfection. Using the chicken *Blym-1* gene as a hybridization probe, homologous genes have been identified in six Burkitt's lymphomas, suggesting that the transforming element in human B cells may also be related to the *Blym* genes. A human *Blym-1* transforming gene has also been isolated from a Burkitt's lymphoma, and the gene sequence predicts a protein of 58 amino acids, which is 33% identical with that of the chicken *Blym-1* gene. The human gene also shows homology with the amino terminal portion of the transferrin protein. Although the *Blym-1* gene is transforming and has homologies to a normal cellular gene or family of genes, it differs from other *onc* genes (even those such as *erb B* and *sis*, which both encode proteins related to growth processes) in that a viral homologue *(v-onc)* has not been identified. The only other human *onc* gene (other than the *ras* family and *Blym-1*) that has been reported to transform NIH 3T3 cells is a DNA clone of *c-sis* obtained from the Hut 102 cell line. Hut 102 is a cell line derived from a cutaneous T cell lymphoma infected with HTLV and is unusual in that it expresses high levels of *c-sis* transcripts. *Sis* gene activation has previously been reported in five of six sarcoma cell lines, three of five glioblastoma lines[36] but not in hematopoietic cells. As pointed out below, this might be expected since the *c-sis* product, the platelet-derived growth factor (PDGF) acts predominantly on mesenchymal cells (such as fibroblasts), which have receptors for the platelet-derived growth factor. The predominance of certain *onc* genes, especially those of the *ras* family, detected by the transfection assays now in use could be a result of the techniques employed, and further exploration using different transfection methods is needed.

THE MULTISTEP NATURE OF CARCINOGENESIS

At least two distinct steps, initiation and promotion, are known to be involved in the multistep process of carcinogenesis.[86] The ability of a single event in the transfection studies discussed above (presumably the introduction of an oncogene) to result in transformation seems contrary to established principles of tumor biology. It is known that transformation of normal cells is a result of at least two processes: immortalization (or establishment), which results in the ability of the cells to grow essentially indefinitely in culture (EBV, adenovirus Ela, and polyoma virus large T antigen may perform this function), and a second event which leads to *in vitro* transformation and *in vivo* tumorigenesis (adenovirus Elb and polyoma middle T antigen may provide this signal). Since NIH 3T3 cells are already immortalized, they would thus be susceptible to single hit factors which would not ordinarily transform completely normal cells. The fact that NIH 3T3 cells are useful in oncogene studies may well be because they have already traveled some distance along the pathway to malignancy. In contrast, studies by Land *et al*.[66] have shown the requirement for at least two cooperating factors in the transformation of normal (rat embryo) fibroblasts. Thus, the *EJ-3 ras* bladder oncogene has a limited capacity to induce proliferation in normal rat fibroblasts and these cells do not become tumorigenic in syngeneic hosts. Since the *myc* gene is commonly found in association with other *onc* genes in human tumors (including several EJ tumor cell lines) the two genes (*myc* and *H-ras*) were introduced together into normal fibroblasts; the combination led to transformation and the production of tumors in nude mice. Extension of this concept of cooperation between two oncogenes, one leading to immortalization (or establishment), the other to transformation, have led to the recognition of complementation groups. These groups are based on their ability to cooperate with either EJ *ras* or *myc* in the transformation of normal fibroblasts. For example, cotransfection with DNA containing *myc* and polyoma virus middle T leads to transformation. Also a truncated form of polyoma large T DNA behaves like *myc* in its ability to cooperate with EJ *ras* DNA in producing transformation in normal cells. A cooperation between adenovirus Ela and *ras* in inducing transformation has also been reported.[105] Based on these data, the complementation groups outlined in Table 3.2 were constructed with the full realization that the multistep process of carcinogenesis may well involve additional steps and factors that the simplistic two oncogene hypothesis implies. Although the number of discrete steps in carcinogenesis is unknown (estimates from 2 to 7 have been made), it

TABLE 3.2. COMPLEMENTATION IN TUMORIGENESIS

Immortalization (Establishment)[a]	Transformation
myc	mutant *ras* genes
polyoma large T	polyoma middle T
E1a	E1b

[a]The class of genes involved in immortalization encodes products that are nuclear binding factors while those implicated in transformation are localized in the plasma membrane.

seems likely that a limited number of steps are necessary. If each in itself is a rare genetic event (particularly considering the occurrence of back mutations), then the long latency period required for most cancers is understandable. The exceptions, as discussed above, are the inherited tumors resulting from germ line mutations, such as in retinoblastoma, where one of the two or more switches needed to detonate the malignant process have been closed at conception.

THE ONCOGENE-ENCODED PROTEINS

Of the estimated 30,000 or so genes in a human cell which code for specific proteins, probably less than 100 are normal cellular proto-oncogenes. Evidence for this comes from the observation that the same oncogenes are being found repeatedly in human tumors, suggesting that the number is relatively small. Proto-oncogenes could become oncogenic by mutation, elevated expression (dosage), or inappropriate activation at the wrong time in the life cycle of the cell. The proteins encoded by oncogenes (about 15–20 have been identified) which ordain the transformation of a normal cell into a tumor cell have little in the way of common structural features which suggest a common mechanism of tumor induction. The first oncogene protein described was derived from *v-src* and was identified in 1978 by Brugge and Erickson.[11] Both the viral and cellular proteins have a molecular weight of 60,000 (p60^{src}) and in their phosphorylated form are designated pp60^{src}. pp60^{src} has been found to be a protein kinase which transfers phosphate groups from ATP to other proteins.[18,69] About 90% of normal cell protein-bound phosphate is serine, 10% threonine, and less than 1% tyrosine. Only 1 in 2000 protein phosphates in a normal cell are linked to tyrosine. Kinase activity of *src* is thus unusual in that it phosphorylates tyrosine[58] and is thus termed a tyrosine kinase (TK). TK activity was subsequently found in seven other oncogene products. The small amount of TK activity found in normal cells is probably mainly derived from the *c-src* protein. Amino acid sequence analysis calculated from the nucleotide sequences of the genes revealed that the domain responsible for TK activity lies in the C-terminal 220 amino acids of pp60^{src}. Homologous domains are present in the other *onc* gene products having TK activity usually, although not always, in the C-terminus of the protein. All of the tyrosine kinase proteins have a plasma membrane (and/or cytoskeleton) location: this has not been definitely established for the *fps* gene product. In addition, five other *onc* gene products (*erb B, fms, raf, mil, mos*) lacking TK activity contain areas homologous with those *onc* genes possessing TK domains. These gene products may therefore have some similar function or may subsequently be shown to have TK activity by other methods. It is important to note that phosphorylation-dephosphorylation are common regulatory control mechanisms for cellular metabolic pathways, and it is not surprising, therefore, that *onc* genes could regulate cell function by phosphorylation. The relative predominance of tyrosine phosphorylation, as opposed to threonine or serine, is unexplained. The question as to whether the quantitative increase in phosphorylation of certain normal cellular proteins is sufficient to transform or whether there are unique protein phosphorylations characteristic of the malignant state is at present unsolved. It would be particularly important to compare the phosphorylation targets of transformed cells with those of normal cells and also with normal cells activated by certain mitogenic or growth-promoting factors involved in normal development. Although these questions cannot be answered as yet, some information on the target proteins of TK oncogenes is available. Because of the changes in morphology that occur in transformed cells, one of the first sites examined was cytoskeletal structure. Of 10 cytoskeletal proteins examined, only vinculin contained phosphotyrosine, and the number of phosphorylated tyrosines was increased 20-fold in RSV-infected cells.[57] Vinculin is normally localized to the plasma membrane and to adhesion plaques. Bundles of actin filaments criss-cross the cell and terminate in these plaques. Thus vinculin may serve to connect the cell membrane with the internal cytoskeletal structural elements. pp60^{src} has also been localized in adhesion plaques and in areas of cell-cell contact by immunofluorescence.[99] Phosphorylation of vinculin, and possibly other plaque proteins, could alter actin and stress fibers, resulting in the disorganization of cell morphology which is characteristic of transformation. These changes are also correlated with a striking loss of fibronectin surrounding the cell as well as with a decrease in cell adhesions. Thus far three TK oncogene products have been identified in similar locations. However, it is premature to draw conclusions relating the ability to transform, TK activity, and location within the cell. For example, RSV mutants lacking pp60^{src} in adhesion plaques have been described[98] which are anchorage-independent and induce tumors in animals. Also the *fps* and *fes* gene products have TK activity and are not found in adhesion plaques. An important factor which has not been fully explored is the relationship of transformation caused by these viruses (as well as *src* mutants) to the surrounding matrix cell surface fibronectin, which may play a key role in growth and invasive properties of the cell.

A new oncogene target reported by Sugimato *et al.*[122] for the *src* kinase and Macara *et al.*[71] for the *ros* kinase in phosphatidylinositol. As shown in Figure 3.3, this system serves as a "second messenger" for transducing signals resulting from the binding of certain hormones and growth factors (see discussion below).

Of the protein targets for phosphorylation discussed above, only vinculin is phosphorylated in normal cells. This suggests the possibility that RSV, and perhaps other acute transforming oncogenes, may result in the phosphorylation of new and inappropriate cellular targets. This may be due either to quantitative differences (much more pp60^{src} in RSV-infected cells) or to structural differences between the *v-onc* and *c-onc* proteins. As pointed out earlier, all known *v-onc* genes differ in structure from their cellular homologues; therefore, target specificity (and oncogenicity) may be based on these structural differences. Experiments constructing appropriate vectors with *c-oncs*,

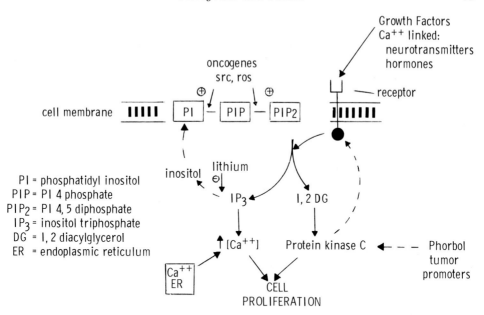

FIG. 3.3.   Oncogenes, inositol lipids, and growth factors: new 2nd messenger system.

under the influence of strong promoters, may answer the question of whether qualitative or quantitative exchanges explain the transformation phenomenon.

GROWTH FACTORS AND ONCOGENES

Under normal circumstances growth is controlled and, as with many other biological systems (e.g., bleeding-clotting), there must exist complex feedback mechanisms which control normal cell proliferation. Tumor cells fail to respond to normal regulatory signals and incessantly proliferate. Some growth factors such as epidermal growth factor (EGF), insulin and insulin-like growth factors (IGF-I) or somatomedin C and IGF-II have a fairly broad target cell range while others, like platelet-derived growth factor (PDGF), affect a restricted number of cell types (largely cells of mesenchymal origin such as fibroblasts and neuroglial cells). Still others, such as interleukin 2 (T cell growth factor) apparently exert a highly cell-specific effect. The growth factors that have been most extensively studied and appear to be related to oncogene activity are PDGF and EGF. Normal cells become arrested in G_0/G_1 phase of the cell cycle in the absence of exogenous growth factors while transformed cells may traverse the cell cycle in the absence of exogenous growth factors. Such autonomous growth may result from the constitutive expression and autocrine stimulation by growth factors involved in the normal proliferative pathway.[52] As shown in Figure 3.4, the elements involved in normal mitogenesis include several growth factors, the cell receptor for the growth factors, and a mechanism for transducing membrane events to signals that regulate genes in the nucleus. Abnormalities at one or more points along this pathway may lead to uncontrolled proliferation. Oncogenes of normal cells may function in one or more of the various steps along this route. For example, the predicted amino

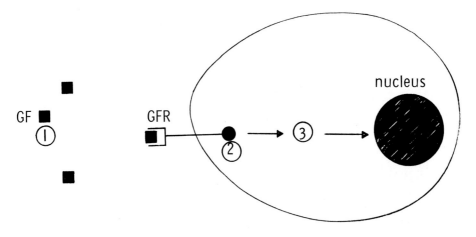

Fig. 3.4.   Possible interrelation of growth factor-mediated mitogenesis and malignant transformation.

acid sequence of *c-sis* protein is identical with one of the chains of PDGF, and since there is significant homology between the chains, it is possible that these two genes arose by duplication from a common ancestral precursor with subsequent evolutionary divergence.[59] PDGF is a major polypeptide growth factor in serum derived from the alpha granules of platelets during blood clotting and is intimately involved in wound healing and connective tissue repair. PDGF, when bound to specific cell receptors, stimulates TK activity with phosphorylation of intracellular proteins, modulation of EGF binding, accumulation of intracellular cyclic AMP, and morphological changes in the cytoskeleton and cell membrane. It induces the expression of *c-myc* RNA and a 29KD nuclear protein in fibroblasts. The protein produced by the oncogene of the simian sarcoma virus (SSV), which was derived from a fibrosarcoma of a pet woolly monkey, is encoded by the *v-sis* gene, and the p28^{sis} gene product is closely homologous, although not identical to, the PDGF B chain. Whether the few substitutions found are due to differences between the monkey and human *c-sis* genes, or reflect mutations in *v-sis* not occurring in the monkey *c-sis*, would be important to establish. In any case, lysates of fibroblasts transformed by SSV contain PDGF-like proteins whose mitogenic activity is completely blocked by antisera to PDGF.[28] Other transformed cell lines, including

SV-40 transformed BHK cells,[31] and a human osteosarcoma cell line (U-20S) have been found to release a growth factor similar to PDGF.[53] In addition, factors present in conditioned media from human clonal glial cells[80] and a rhabdomyosarcoma cell line[5] have immunological reactivity with anti-PDGF antibodies. Importantly *sis*-related RNA transcripts have been found in five human sarcoma and three glioblastoma cell lines but not in cell lines from other tumors.[36] The finding of *sis* transcripts and products restricted to cells of mesenchymal origin (which are responsive to PDGF) is of importance in regard to the hypothesis of autocrine stimulation. The PDGF receptor is an integral membrane protein, and like the EGF receptor, the binding domain is on the exterior of the cell, while the domain possessing TK activity is on the interior (cytoplasmic) surface.

If p28[sis] acts as a PDGF agonist (stimulating PDGF receptors from within or externally after secretion), then it might be expected that the application of large amounts of PDGF to normal cells could lead to a transformed phenotype. Indeed there are some phenotypic changes in fibroblasts and glial cells treated *in vitro* with PDGF that resemble those found in transformed cells.[52] PDGF also stimulates the synthesis of certain proteins thought to be characteristic of transformed cells.[108] A recent study of Assaian *et al.*[3] reports that human platelet extracts induce anchorage-independent growth which results from a concerted action of three peptide growth factors—PDGF, TGF-β, and a newly described analogue of EGF. PDGF alone does not transform normal rat kidney cells. TGF-β increases the number of EGF receptors as well as altering their downregulation while the EGF analogue (a TGF-α-like molecule) binds to EGF receptors and exerts an EGF effect. These data are consistent with the reports of Wharton *et al.*[132] that PDGF controls proliferation by modulating the response to other growth factors. Thus the interaction of three platelet peptides in the presence of plasma can transform fibroblasts. Whether these cells are capable of producing tumors has not yet been reported.

When EGF binds to its receptor, at least two discrete events occur: internalization of the complex in vesicles and stimulation of TK activity. The relationship between these two events is unclear. As with the PDGF receptor, the TK domain of the EGF receptor is located on the inner (cytoplasmic) aspect of the cell membrane. Stimulation by EGF is associated with a marked increase (about 10-fold) in the phosphotyrosine content of cellular proteins. Phosphorylation of p42 has also been identified in PDGF-treated as well as virally transformed cells. The addition of EGF leads to a 2- to 3-fold increase in phosphorylation of the EGF receptor (autophosphorylation) and of an 81K protein, which is not phosphorylated by RSV.[22] A protein kinase cascade with one kinase activating another in sequence is an interesting possibility.

About 12 to 24 hours after EGF binds to the cell surface, DNA synthesis begins. It has been assumed, that these cellular events are triggered by intercellular messengers, perhaps phosphorylated proteins, or even cellular *onc* genes such as *c-myc*. A recent study also suggests that the EGF receptor has a direct effect on DNA.[76] If the receptor does have two effector activities, presumably the TK activity would be an early event at the cell membrane, activated by binding of ligand (EGF), while the interaction with DNA would be a late mitogenic effect. The separation into distinct early phosphorylation and endocytosis and late DNA, RNA, and protein synthesis events is consistent with the selective induction of the early phase of the mitogenic response by cross-linking EGF receptors with antibodies.[110]

Several potentially important relationships between growth factors and *onc* genes exist: (1) The common property of tyrosine kinase activity of several of the growth factor receptors and a group of oncogenes, summarized in Figure 3.5. (2) Certain common target proteins (*e.g.*, p42) for phosphorylation by both growth factors and *v-onc* genes. (3) The apparent identity of *c-sis* with the gene that encodes normal PDGF, and the similarity of the transforming product of the simian sarcoma virus p28^{sis} to PDGF.[32, 97] (4) The close similarity of the EGF receptor with the *erb-B* gene product.[33] *erb-B* encodes a truncated form of the EGF receptor which retains the transmembrane and cytoplasmic TK domain but lacks the external EGF binding site. It has been postulated that the truncated receptor is continually active, which in turn leads to uncontrolled proliferation and tumorigenesis. (5) Several transforming peptides [initially called sarcoma growth factors, now termed transforming growth factors (TGFs)] are found in the conditioned medium from a variety of transformed rodent and human cell lines. TGF-α, which is distinct from but shows homologies with EGF and binds to the EGF receptor, is mitogenic, while TGF-β does not bind to the EGF receptor but has transforming activity which is enhanced 100-fold by EGF.[2] The transforming activity present in crude conditioned media from cultures of a variety of animal and human tumors is thus a result of the combined action of TGF-α and TGF-β (or EGF and TGF-β). Several human tumor cells have been reported to produce TGFs[72,96] which are capable of

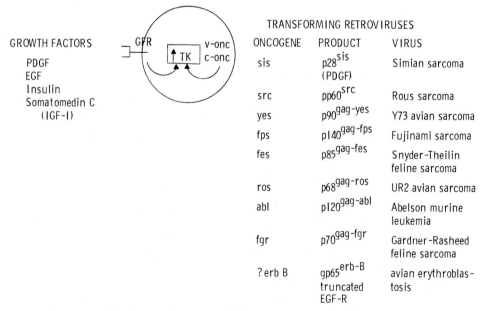

Fig. 3.5.   Tyrosine kinase activity of growth factor receptors and oncogenes.

phosphorylating tyrosine on EGF receptors. The tumor-enhancing effect of EGF noted in several different systems[40,49] could be due to potentiation of small amounts of TGFs. It has also been noted that EGF synergizes with PDGF and insulin or somatomedin C in stimulating a proliferative response. It has, in fact, been suggested that a primary action of PDGF is to increase the sensitivity of fibroblasts to EGF.[132] Fetal bovine serum contains platelet-derived TGF-like compounds in small amounts[16] which may be responsible for the capacity of high concentrations of fetal serum to induce colonies in soft agar of nontransformed mouse and rat cells. (6) EGF enhances guanine nucleotide binding and increases phosphorylation of the *ras* gene product p21 by GTP. Gilman[44] has recently discussed a speculative, but intriguing relationship between the *ras* gene products and G proteins. G proteins are guanine-binding proteins which are embedded in the plasma membrane and which appear to communicate signals (either stimulatory or inhibitory) from the cell surface receptor binding of hormones, neurotransmitters, and other ligands to the adenyl cyclase system. The *ras* protein not only binds GTP and is a membrane protein but shows a provocative albeit restricted homology with one member of the G family (transducin). Thus the *ras* gene protein could, as postulated for the G protein, be a component of a transmembrane signal transmitting system. Thus, abnormal activity resulting from mutations or marked elevations of the *ras* gene product may lead to deregulation, perhaps substituting a continuous signal for a normally transient one. Interesting is the fact that *ras* transformed cells have reduced numbers of EGF receptors, presumably due to receptor occupancy by TGF-α.[61] (7) The activation of *c-myc* by PDGF[62] as discussed below. (8) The stimulation of the inositol phospholipid system by EGF, PDGF, and by the products of the *v-src* and *v-ros* transforming genes.[74,122] (9) Other homologies between growth factors and *onc* gene products that have been reported but are more tenuous, although intriguing, include the following: (a) *Blym-1* gene product with transferrin[30]; (b) Polyoma middle T antigen with gastrin, a hormone which stimulates secretion and cell proliferation[4]; (c) *c-myc* and *v-myc* genes with the interleukin-2 genes[81]; (d) HTLV and interleukin-2.[55] This homology is between the DNA of the viral LTRs and three regions in the 5′ sequence flanking the IL 2 gene. The fourth homology region is between the viral LTR and a sequence within the second intron.

THE FUNCTION OF ONCOGENES IN NORMAL CELLULAR PROCESSES

As discussed above, elevated cellular or proto-oncogene expression has been detected in many human malignancies, and alteration or activation of a cellular *onc* gene is thought to predispose or directly lead to the transformed state. Quantitative alterations due to increased transcription may arise from gene amplification,[24,111] chromosomal rearrangements or the insertion of promoter-enhancer elements of transcription in the vicinity of a proto-oncogene.[51,94] Alternately, qualitative alterations in genes may occur as a result of chromosomal rearrangements involving the proto-oncogene[23,26,48,84] or mutations and other structural changes within the proto-oncogene itself.[79,95] Analysis of proto-oncogenes in many different tumor cell lines has revealed that expression of certain of these genes tends to occur sporadically in multiple tumors. More-over, with certain exceptions this expression is not limited to any one type of tumor. When the DNA from particular tumors which display high levels of expression of certain proto-oncogenes is used to transform NIH 3T3 cells in gene transfer experiments, a DNA fragment other than the expressed proto-oncogene can be responsible for the transformation.[29,82] These observations raise critical issues regarding the role that proto-oncogenes play in tumori-genesis. Is a "high" level of proto-oncogene expression directly related to the transformed state necessary but not sufficient for transformation or, alter-nately, does this level simply reflect what would be "normal" for a cell frozen at a particular stage of differentiation? Clearly, conclusions regarding the role that proto-oncogenes play in malignant cells cannot be formulated until their role is elucidated in normal cells.

The fact that proto-oncogene transcription occurs in normal cells[6,117] and that these genes are highly conserved throughout evolution suggests a role for these genes in differentiation, growth, and development. It was initially theor-ized that expression of each proto-oncogene might be tissue-specific, but Gonda *et al.*[46] discovered that transcription of *c-myc*, *c-erb*, and *c-src* was detectable at various levels in nearly all cells and tissues tested. Similar re-sults have been obtained in analyzing the expression of *c-Ha-ras*, *c-Ki-ras*, and *c-yes*.[77,113] Other proto-oncogenes display more tissue-specific expression. For instance, *c-myb* expression is restricted to tissues of hematopoietic origin.[46,130,131] The observation that the *c-fps* protein (NCP 98) is present in bone marrow and spleen has led Hanafusa *et al.*[75] to suggest that this protein is specifically involved in hematopoietic differentiation. While the *c-abl* proto-oncogene is expressed in multiple tissues, the only cells with detectable *c-abl* products (NCP 159) are thymocytes and other lymphoid cells.[77] Recently, Muller *et al.*[77] have determined that levels of *c-fos* transcripts (homologous to the transforming gene of FBJ murine osteosarcoma virus) are 100-fold greater in fetal membranes than in any other tested tissue and only cells of mesen-chymal origin (skin, bone, and muscle) exhibited significant expression of *c-fos* in the postnatal mouse.[77] Thus, while certain types of proto-oncogenes may be constitutively expressed, others may be more selectively expressed, and their protein products may be key determinants of growth and differentiation in specific tissues.

Analyses of normal tissues and tumor cell lines imply that certain proto-oncogenes are in fact differentially expressed in certain developmental stages. The first demonstration was in HL 60 cells, an established promyelocytic leukemia cell line. This cell line expresses high levels of *c-myc*, *c-myb* and *c-abl*.[130,13] When these cells are chemically induced to differentiate with reti-noic acid or DMSO, expression of *c-myc* and *c-myb* dramatically decreased while *c-abl* remained unchanged.[130] A murine myeloid leukemia line, WEHI 3B (D+ subline) can be induced with granulocyte-colony-stimulating factor plus low concentrations of actinomycin D to differentiate into mature monocytes.[45] Induction is associated with a substantial decrease in *c-myb* and *c-myc* (10-fold) while *c-fos* transcripts increase 11-fold. The transition of undifferentiated cells to promonocytes resulted in slight or negligible decreases in *onc* gene levels, so that only when the most mature changes occurred (after 4–5 days in culture) did *c-myc* and *c-myb* substantially decrease. This maturation was associated with morphological characteristics typical of monocytes, esterase positivity, and a loss of growth in clonogenic soft-agar assays. Other early myeloid cell lines contain comparable levels of *c-myc* and *c-myb* RNA while mature normal macrophages have high levels of *c-fos* RNA. This suggested that the results with WEHI 3B may reflect changes in *onc* genes which occur during normal myeloid differentiation. However, in this study the changes in the expression of these *onc* genes (*c-myc* and *c-myb*, which show significant relatedness)[92] were late, and considerable differentiation occurred even in the presence of high levels of *c-myc* and *c-myb* RNA. In this regard AMV (avian myeloblastosis virus, which carries the *v-myb* gene) can transform progenitor macrophages only after they have evolved into mature adherent macrophage cells.[35] It seems likely, therefore, that the changes in *c-myc* and *c-myb* expression may be a result of the differentiation and perhaps the proliferative stage rather than the cause of the differentiation. Similarly, we have found[136] that the transition from the immature, nonadherent to the adherent, mature macrophage is accompanied by a significant fall in *c-src* RNA levels. This may be important since pp60[c-src] is found in adhesive plaques and changes could alter adhesion and morphological properties of these cells.

Two other recent examples of differential proto-oncogene expression have also been described in normal cells. First, hepatocytes regulate the expression of *c-H-ras* RNA by increasing transcription within 12–24 hours after injury (by chemicals or stimulation of liver regeneration after partial hepatectomy), and subsequently (72 hours later) expression rapidly decreases.[47] Secondly, Muller *et al.*[77] determined that *c-abl* expression in murine embryo tissues rises steadily up to day 10 and decreases dramatically after day 11. Simultaneous determinations of *c-H-ras* have revealed unaltered expression, implying that the differential expression of *c-abl* is important in embryogenesis.

A clear example of the relation of *c-onc* genes in normal metabolic pathways comes from studies of *c-myc* expression. As pointed out, altered *c-myc* expression is observed in tumors of diverse origin but is also found in normal tissues. In the *onc* gene, cooperative interactions discussed by Land *et al.*,[66] *c-myc* appeared to be required for transformation of normal fibroblasts by contributing an establishment or immortalization function but was not in itself sufficient for transformation. Thus, *c-myc* may be related to the ability of cells to enter the initial phase of the proliferative response, referred to by Pledger *et al.*[87] as competence. Quiescent cells briefly exposed to PDGF become "competent" to replicate their DNA but do not "progress" through G_0/G_1 into the S phase unless plasma containing somatomedin C (IGF-1) and EGF is added.[121] In fact more recent studies[68] suggest that while PDGF renders cells competent and initiates G_1, that EGF and IGF-1 (the latter can be replaced by high levels of insulin) are the major hormones controlling progression through mid- and late G_1, respectively. Thus, if oncogenes are involved in normal proliferation one might expect to find evidence of expression of oncogenes during different phases of the cell cycle. Evidence from two laboratories[12,62] suggests that this may be the case, since *c-myc* can be detected early (during the competent phase) and *c-K-ras* in the mid-late progressive events.

When BALB/c 3T3 cells are exposed to PDGF (together with platelet-poor plasma, EGF, and insulin), there is a rapid (within 3 hours) 40-fold increase in *c-myc* RNA. EGF and insulin alone, which are late acting, have no effect. A similar (10- to 20-fold) increase in *c-myc* RNA within 1–2 hours is seen after lipopolysaccharide (LPS) or conA stimulation of whole spleen cells. This precedes by 6–12 hours any changes in DNA or RNA synthesis. Maximum *c-myc* expression occurs in 2–9 hours and returns to baseline by 60 hours, at which time tritiated thymidine incorporation is maximal. Thus *c-myc* is an early G_1 transcript. The addition of protein inhibitors, such as cyclohexamide, enhances *c-myc* expression 3- to 5-fold, suggesting that *c-myc* is "superinducible," possibly due to the removal of a normal repressor protein that acts as a feedback inhibitor or possibly by means of changes in the half-life of message. Therefore, *c-myc* appears to be normally regulated by those mitogens that induce competence in quiescent cells and to be involved in the first of the two phases required for transition from G_0 to the S phase. Presumably, *c-myc* products, at least in the amounts observed in cells stimulated by mitogens, are not sufficient for continued proliferation, and the addition of second-step factors is required. In ALV (avian leukosis virus)-induced B cell tumors, plasmacytomas, Burkitt's lymphomas, as well as other tumors having elevated *c-myc*, one limiting factor (the early phase of transit through G_0/G_1) is removed which may give the cells a proliferative advantage. The persistent elevation of *c-myc* products may also prevent cycling cells from becoming quiescent, *i.e.*, from entering G_0. Thus, an inappropriate temporal expression of *c-myc* may be as important as the absolute levels of the *c-onc* genes. Moreover, as indicated above, elevations of *c-myc* expression are not always found in Burkitt's or ALV-induced tumors, and *in vitro* studies suggest that other genes, in addition to *c-myc*, are necessary for transformation. Campisi *et al.*[12] have shown that the A31 embryonic fibroblast line is immortal (but not tumorigenic), and when in G_0 (caused by deprivation of serum) *c-myc* expression is low. When serum is added, *c-myc* RNA is increased 20-fold in early G_1 while *c-K-ras* expression does not begin until mid to late G_1. In BPA31 and DA31 cell lines which are tumorigenic variants of A31 (chemically transformed *in vitro* by benzopyrene or dimethylbenzoanthrene, respectively), *c-myc* expression is constitutive and equivalent to that of normal proliferating cells; both quiescent and growing cells have essentially similar *c-myc* levels. Thus, *c-myc* has lost its cell cycle-dependent regulation in the tumorigenic varieties of the A31 cells. This could result from a loss of transacting repressor in the chemically transformed cells. However, *c-K-ras* remains cell cycle-dependent in tumorigenic cells. Since *c-K-ras* appears in mid G_1, it may be controlled by EGF, which acts at this point, in the cell cycle. Some workers[106] have linked defective terminal differentiation to tumorigenesis, and the finding with the A31 is consistent with this hypothesis.

MECHANISMS OF EXPRESSION OF ONCOGENES

The following is a brief summary of several mechanisms (most have been discussed in detail above) which may lead to altered oncogene expression (see Table 3.3).

TABLE 3.3. MECHANISMS OF ONCOGENE ACTIVATION

Insertional mutagenesis
Translocations
Amplification
Mutations

GENE AMPLIFICATION

This can sometimes be determined microscopically as homogeneously staining regions (HSRs) on chromosomes and by the presence of double minutes. HSRs are regions lacking the normal banding patterns which consist of large tandem arrays of the genes. Double minutes are small pieces of chromosomes containing several copies of the amplified gene, are extra chromosomal, and appear to be self replicating. Since they lack centromeres, they segregate erratically. Gene amplification can occur, however, without morphologically observable evidence. It is best detected by quantitation of copy number by Southern blots of DNA derived from cell lines or fresh tissue or by dot-blot or solution hybridization. Since amplification is known to occur during normal development, the finding of an amplified gene does not necessarily signify malignancy; it could be that the malignant cell is frozen at a particular point in differentiation at which amplification normally occurs. Amplified *myc* genes have been found in a human myeloid cell line, HL-60, as well as in stored uncultured tumor cells from the same patient.[19,24] It is unknown whether normal cells from this patient have an amplified *c-myc* gene. Other fresh myeloid leukemias and the K562 myeloid cell line do not have amplified *c-myc*, but c-myc has been reported to be amplified in small cell carcinomas of the lung (8 of 18) and in a neuroendocrine tumor; *N-myc* is also amplified in some neuroblastomas.[73,109] However, overall amplification is found in a relatively small percentage of tumors. Also a 6- to 10-fold amplification of some genes (*e.g.,c-H-ras*) have been found in certain strains of normal mice and hamsters.[14]

INSERTIONAL MUTAGENESIS

This has been discussed above for tumors induced by slow viruses and includes the promoter insertion model as well as the effect of the enhancer-like elements contained in LTRs.

CHROMOSOMAL TRANSLOCATION

Changes in the position of *c-onc's* by movement of chromosomal segments may presumably activate *onc* genes or inactivate repressor genes by exposing or removing them from regulatory influences, for example, strong promoter or enhancer elements. Translocation may move only a part of a *c-onc* gene (*c-myc* in mouse plasmacytomas), thus removing upstream regulatory elements normally attached to the gene.[119] In addition, movement of the whole *c-onc* gene to a new site may set the stage for mutations in critical control regions. For example, Rabbitts *et al.*[91] have shown multiple mutations in exon 1 (a noncoding but possible regulatory region) of the *c-myc* gene in a Burkitt's lymphoma: these mutations presumably occurred during or after the translocation and could (by affecting interactions with transacting regulatory factors) alter the expression of the coding regions (exons 2 and 3). Regulatory factors are proposed to normally interact with exon 1 or perhaps the conserved region 5' to exon 1.

In many cases it is difficult to determine whether translocations are a primary event leading to malignancy or a result of the malignant process. However, the consistency with which some translocations are seen in specific tumors indicates a definite association. Changes in gene expression resulting from a specific translocation could endow a cell of a specific lineage and at a particular stage in differentiation with a selective proliferative advantage, while subsequent events would initiate the development of malignancy. The literature on translocations and cancer is extensive, and for an excellent review, I suggest the following: Refs. 104 and 109, and Chapter 4 by J. J. Yunis.

MUTATIONS

These include a variety of mutations in oncogenes, the most notable of which are those at codons 8 and 61 of the *ras* gene discussed above in detail. Much remains to be clarified in this area, and many, if not most, so-called *c-onc* genes found in transformed cell lines and in fresh tumor tissue may carry subtle but important mutations in either coding or noncoding regulatory regions. Moreover, a subtle change in structure may affect critical functions such as the attachment of lipid, which determines membrane insertion, the binding or activity of regulatory substances such as GTP, or the interaction with other cellular proteins involved in growth control. Both hypomethylation of genes and alteration ("loosening") of chromatin structure and changes in histone and nonhistone proteins have been implicated as regulatory mechanisms in gene control (for review, see Ref. 25). Hypomethylation of the *c-H-ras* gene was detected in six of eight carcinomas (five colons and one lung) when tumor tissue was compared to adjacent normal tissue.[37] Interestingly, *c-K-ras*, which is more commonly implicated in carcinomas by transfection studies, was fully methylated. Also, other genes are hypomethylated, such as gammaglobulin and growth hormone, which would not be expected to be expressed in a colon carcinoma so that the significance of observed methylation patterns in tumors is not as yet clear. There is, however, no doubt that methylation is related to gene expression.[93] Importantly, methylated genes will not be expressed in DNA transfection or following microinjection.[20,134] Thus, it may be that transforming genes will only be detected by the commonly employed transfection assays, unless the genes have lost methyl groups. Although both the degree of methylation and the structure of the chromatin surrounding the *onc* gene may be immediate events determining *onc* gene activation, the critical question is what determines these changes and how close are they to the primary transforming event.

SUMMARY

There is substantial evidence that the carcinogenic potential of acute transforming viruses resides in viral oncogenes (*v-onc*), although other parts of the viral genome (*gag-env*) may be critical to the tumorigenic potential of certain viruses. *v-oncs* have been acquired from *c-oncs*, but they are not isogenic with them, and deletions and mutations have occurred which may be important in determining oncogenesis. How slow viruses produce cancer is less clear, but promoter insertion seems to be established in most cases of B cell tumors produced by avian leukosis virus (ALV) and regulatory elements (probably enhancers) in LTRs appear to be necessary in other cases. In fact, the common insertional element of slow viruses which appears to be involved in muta-genesis is its LTR.

In human tumors, the question as to whether purely quantitative changes in the level of expression of normal *c-oncs* are sufficient for tumorigenesis has not been definitely answered. Some *in vitro* evidence involving linkage of *c-oncs* to strong promoters, such as those in LTRs or SV-40, have suggested that quanti-tative changes are sufficient. However, not only were these experiments car-ried out using NIH 3T3 cells, which are already immortalized (although not transformed), but linkage of these same promoters to other *c-oncs* does not cause transformation. The results of the simultaneous injection of two onco-genes suggest that indeed carcinogenesis is a multistep phenomenon (a fact known for many years from earlier initiator-promoter studies) and that there may be a need for a cooperating set of oncogenes and/or other unknown fac-tors, *i.e.*, an interaction between oncogenes such as *c-myc* that results in immortalization and another *c-onc*, such as *ras*, that initiates the transformed state.

The finding of elevated transcripts of *c-oncs* in a large variety of tumors (although a few tumor-specific relationships have been found in hematopoietic malignancies) may be indicative of nonspecificity. Moreover, not all tumors of the same type have increased expression of *c-oncs*. Recent studies have shown that *c-oncs* are expressed normally during the cell cycle; *c-myc* and *c-fos* early in G_0/G_1 in the induction of "competence" and *c-ras* in mid to late G_1 during "progression." This leads to the question of whether the changes in tumors are primary or represent the normal processes involved in continuous growth and proliferation. Most tumors, except for the clonal hematopoietic malignancies, contain a variety of cells (including infiltrating normal cells) which are at different stages of differentiation. Even with clonal hematopoietic tumors, appropriate controls (cells at the same stage of differentiation) are seldom available. This is critical in evaluating whether an elevated *c-onc* gene tran-script or its product is a result of the particular normal differentiation stage at which the cell has become frozen by the malignant process or is characteristic of the malignancy state. However, in many cases where *c-onc* genes are exam-ined in transformed cells, they are found to be altered either in their coding or noncoding regions, for example, *c-myc* in Burkitt's cell lymphoma. In addition, genes other than the one which is increased may be critical in transformation; the Blym-1 gene appears to be the transforming element in ALV-induced B cell lymphomas which characteristically have *c-myc* elevations.

The finding of mutations in the transforming *c-ras* genes localized to specific areas (codon 8 or 61 resulting in 42 possible mutations that could conceivably be related to transformation) is intriguing and obviously has some relationship to malignancy. However, the relation is not a direct one since many, if not most, tumors of the same histological type do not have such mutations. Moreover, except in NIH 3T3 cells, transformation of normal cells involves other factors, such as a second oncogene, as discussed above. Nevertheless, structural alterations in *c-oncs* are likely candidates as participants in tumorigenic events.

Four basic mechanisms have been described in which oncogenes may be "activated": insertional mutagenesis by viral LTRs; translocations of *onc*-genes to other regions where control is altered (similar in effect to insertional mutagenesis); mutations, such as with the *ras* oncogenes; and direct infection with intact viruses, such as the T cell leukemia virus (HTLV), which does not contain an oncogene but does produce a virally encoded product which may act as a *trans*-acting regulatory element. This could in fact be a transforming factor which "turns on" both viral expression and perhaps other normal cellular genes (such as the IL-2 receptor) which regulate cell growth.

The remarkable relationship between oncogenes and normal genes involved in growth and differentiation has given us an early glimpse into the mechanisms by which normal cells control growth and into the potential location of defects that may occur in malignancy. It seems likely that many, if not most, oncogenes may function by simulating normal growth factors, probably either by the continuous and inappropriate production of structurally normal growth factors or functionally active factors that do not correspond to normal control signals. The failure of these growth factors to be normally regulated may be in the gene itself (due to structural defects in regulatory sequences) or in mutations that provide abnormal products with altered distributions, functions, and/or abilities to be downregulated.

Finally, an exciting area just beginning to be explored is the function of those conserved *c-oncs* in normal cellular differentiation. The studies relating *c-onc* expression to the normal cell cycle, discussed above, and the changes in relative expression of several *c-oncs* during differentiation has opened a new field in the study of normal growth and development.

ACKNOWLEDGMENT

This work was supported in part by NIH Grants HD 17013 and CA 22105.

REFERENCES

1. Aaronson, S. A., Reddy, E. P., Robbins, K., Devare, S. G., Swan, D. C., Pierce, J. H., and Tronick, S. R. Retroviruses, onc genes, and human cancer. In: *Human Carcinogenesis*, New York, Academic Press, 1983, p. 609.
2. Anzano, M. A., Roberts, A. B., Smith, J. M., Sporn, M. B., and DeLarco, J. E. Sarcoma growth factor from conditioned medium of virally transformed cells is composed of both type α and type β transforming growth factors. *Proc. Natl. Acad. Sci. 80:* 6264, 1983.
3. Assaian, R. K., Grotendorst, G. R., Miller, D. M., and Sporn, M. B. Cellular transformation by coordinated action of three peptide growth factors from human platelets. *Nature 309:* 804, 1984.
4. Baldwin, G. S., Gastrin and the transforming protein of polyoma virus have evolved from a common ancester. *FEBS Lett. 137:* 1, 1982.
5. Betsholtz, C., Heldin, C. H., Nister, M., Ek, B., Wasteson, A., and Westermark, B. Synthesis of a PDGF-like growth factor in human glioma and sarcoma cells suggests the expression of the cellular homologue of the transforming protein of simian sarcoma virus. *Biochem. Biophys. Res. Commun. 117:* 176, 1983.

6. Bishop, J. M. Cellular oncogenes and retroviruses. *Annu. Rev. Biochem. 52:* 301, 1983.
7. Bishop, J. M. A. Retroviruses. *Annu. Rev. Biochem. 47:* 35, 1978.
8. Blair, D. G., Oskarsson, M: Activation of the transforming potential of a normal cell sequence: a molecular model for oncogenesis. *Science 212:* 941, 1981.
9. Brady, J., Bolen, J. B., Radonovich, M. M., Salzman, N., and Khoury, G. Stimulation of simian virus 40 late gene expression by simian virus 40 tumor antigen. *Proc. Natl. Acad. Sci. (USA) 81:* 2040, 1984.
10. Brodeur, G. M., Saeger, R. C., Schwab, M., Varmus, H. E., and Bishop, J. M. Amplification of N-myc in untreated human neuroblastomas corelates with advanced disease stage. *Science 224:* 1121, 1984.
11. Brugge, J. S., and Erikson, R. L. Identification of a transformation-specific antigen induced by an avian sarcoma virus. *Nature 269:* 346, 1977.
12. Campisi, J., Gray, H. E., Pardee, A. B., Dean, M., and Sonenshein, G. E. Cell-cycle control of c-myc but not c-ras expression is lost following chemical transformation. *Cell 36:* 241, 1984.
13. Chang, E. H., Furth, M. E., and Scolnick, E. M. Tumorigenic transformation of mammalian cells induced by a normal human gene homologous to the oncogene of Harvey murine sarcoma virus. *Nature 297:* 479, 1982.
14. Chattopadhyay, S. K., Chang, E. H., Lander, M. R., Ellis, R. W., Scolnick, E. M., and Lowy, D. R. Amplification and rearrangement of onc genes in mammalian species. *Nature 296:* 361, 1982.
15. Chen, I. S. Y., McLaughlin, J., and Golde, D. W. Long terminal repeats of human T-cell leukemia virus II genome determine target cell specificity. *Nature 309:* 276, 1984.
16. Childs, C. B., Proper, J. A., Tucker, R. F., and Moses, H. L. Serum contains a platelet-derived transforming growth factor. *Proc. Natl. Acad. Sci. USA 79:* 5312, 1982.
17. Coffin, J. M., Varmus, H. E., Bishop, J. M., Essex, M., Hardy, W. D., Jr., Martin, G. S., Rosenberg, N. E., Scolnick, E. M., Weinberg, R. A., and Vogt, P. K. Proposal for naming lost cell-derived inserts in retrovirus genomes. *J. Virol. 40:* 953, 1981.
18. Collett, M. S., and Erikson, R. L. Protein kinase activity associated with the avian sarcoma virus src gene product. *Proc. Natl. Acad. Sci. USA 75:* 2021, 1978.
19. Collins, S., and Groudine, M. Amplification of endogenous myc-related DNA sequences in a human myeloid leukaemia cell line. *Nature 298:* 679, 1982.
20. Compere, S. J., and Palmiter, R. D. DNA methylation controls the inducibility of the mouse metallothionine-1 gene in lymphoid cells. *Cell 25:* 233, 1981.
21. Cooper, G. M. Cellular transforming genes. *Science 218:* 801, 1982.
22. Cooper, J. A., and Hunter, T. Similarities and differences between the effects of epidermal growth factor and Rous sarcoma virus. *J. Cell Biol. 91:* 878, 1981.
23. Dalla-Favera, R., Martinotti, S., Gallo, R. C., Erickson, J., and Croce, C. Translocation and rearrangements of the c-myc oncogene locus in human undifferentiated B-cell lymphomas. *Science 219:* 963, 1983.
24. Dalla-Favera, R., Wong-Staal, F., and Gallo, R. C. Onc-gene amplification in promyelocytic leukaemia cell line HL-60 and primary leukaemic cells of the same patient. *Nature 299:* 61, 1982.
25. Darnell, J. E. Variety in the level of gene control in eukaryotic cells. *Nature 297:* 365, 1982.
26. deKlein, A., vanKessel, A. G., Grosveld, G., Bartram, C. R., Hagemeijer, A., Bootsma, D., Spurr, N. K., Heisterkamp, N., Groffen, J., and Stephenson, J. R. A cellular oncogene is translocated to the Philadelphia chromosome in chronic myelocytic leukaemia. *Nature 300:* 765, 1982.
27. Der, C. J. and Cooper, G. M. Altered gene products are associated with activation of cellular ras^k genes in human lung and colon carcinomas. *Cell 32:* 201, 1983.
28. Deuel, T. F., Huang, J. S., Huang, S. S., Stroobant, P., and Waterfield, M. Expression of a platelet-derived growth factor-like protein in simian sarcoma virus transformed cells. *Science 221:* 1348, 1983.
29. Diamond, A., Cooper, G. M., Ritz, J., and Lane, M. A. Identification and molecular cloning of the human Blym transforming gene activated in Burkitt's lymphoma. *Nature 305:* 112, 1983.
30. Diamond, A., Devine, J. M., and Cooper, G. M. Nucleotide sequence of a human Blym transforming gene activated in a Burkitt's lymphoma. *Science 225:* 516, 1984.
31. Dicker, P., Pohjanpelto, P., Pettican, P., and Rozengurt, E. Similarities between fibroblast-derived growth factor and platelet-derived growth factor. *Exp. Cell Res. 135:* 221, 1981.

32. Doolittle, R. F., Hunkapiller, M. W., Hood, L. E., Devare, S. G., Robbins, K. C., Aaronson, S. A., and Antoniades, H. N. Simian sarcoma virus onc gene, v-sis, is derived from the gene (or genes) encoding a platelet-derived growth factor. *Science 221:* 275, 1983.

33. Downward, J., Yarden, Y., Mayes, E., Scrace, G., Totty, N., Stockwell, P., Ullrich, A., Schlessinger, J., and Waterfield, M. D. Close similarity of epidermal growth factor receptor and v-erb-B oncogene protein sequences. *Nature 307:* 521, 1984.

34. Duesberg, P. H. Retroviral transforming genes in normal cells? *Nature 304:* 219, 1983.

35. Durban, E. M., and Boettiger, D. Replicating, differentiated macrophages can serve as in vitro targets for transformation by avian myeloblastosis virus. *J. Virol. 37:* 488, 1981.

36. Eva, A., Robbins, K. C., Andersen, P. R., Srinivasan, A., Tronick, S. R., Reddy, E. P., Ellmore, N. W., Galen, A. T., Lauterberger, J. A., Papas, T. S., Westin, E. H., Wong-Staal, F., Gallo, R. C., and Aaronson, S. A. Cellular genes analogous to retroviral onc genes are transcribed in human tumour cells. *Nature 295:* 116, 1982.

37. Feinberg, A. P., and Vogelstein, B. Hypomethylation of ras oncogenes in primary human cancers. *Biochem. Biophys. Res. Commun. 111:* 47, 1983.

38. Feinberg, A. P., Vogelstein, B., Droller, M. J., Baylin, S. B., and Nelkin, B. D. Mutation affecting the 12 amino acid of the c-Ha-ras oncogene product occurs infrequently in human cancer. *Science 220:* 1175, 1983.

39. Finkel, T., Der, C. J., and Cooper, G. M. Activation of ras genes in human tumors does not affect localization, modification, or nucleotide binding properties of p21. *Cell 37:* 151, 1984.

40. Fisher, P. B., Bozzone, J. H., and Weinstein, I. B. Tumor promoters and epidermal growth factor stimulate anchorage-independent growth of adenovirus-transformed rat embryo cells. *Cell 18:* 695, 1979.

41. Gallo, R. C., and Wong-Staal, F. Retroviruses as etiologic agents of some animal and human leukemias and lymphomas and as tools for elucidating the molecular mechanism of leukemogenesis. *Blood 60:* 545, 1982.

42. Garber, E. A., Krueger, J. G., Hanafusa, H., and Goldberg, A. R. Only membrane-associated RSV src proteins have amino-terminally bound lipid. *Nature 302:* 161, 1983.

43. Gaynor, R. B., Hillman, D., and Berk, A. J. Adenovirus early region 1A protein activates transcription of a nonviral gene introduced into mammalian cells by infection or transfection. *Proc. Natl. Acad. Sci. USA 81.* 1193, 1984.

44. Gilman, A. G. G proteins and dual control of adenylate cyclase. *Cell 36:* 577, 1984.

45. Gonda, T. G., and Metcalf, D. Expression of myb, myc, and fos proto-oncogenes during the differentiation of a murine myeloid leukaemia. *Nature 310:* 249, 1984.

46. Gonda, T. J., Sheiness, D. K., and Bishop, J. M. Transcripts from the cellular homologs of retroviral oncogenes: Distribution among chicken tissues. *Mol. Cell. Biol. 2:* 617, 1982.

47. Goyette, M., Petropoulos, C. J., Shank, P. R., and Fausto, N. Expression of a cellular oncogene during liver regeneration. *Science 219:* 510, 1983.

48. Groffen, J., Heisterkamp, N., Stephenson, J. R., vanKessel, A. G., deKlein, A., Grosveld, G., and Bootsma, D. c-sis is translocated from chromosome 22 to chromosome 9 in chronic myelocytic leukemia. *J. Exp. Med. 158:* 9, 1983.

49. Harrison, J., and Auersperg, H. Epidermal growth factor enhances viral transformation of granulosa cells. *Science 213:* 218, 1981.

50. Haseltine, W. A., Sodroski, J., Patarca, R., Briggs, D., Perkins, D., and Wong-Staal, F. Structure of 3' terminal region of type II human T lymphotropic virus: Evidence for new coding region. *Science 225:* 419, 1984.

51. Hayward, W. S., Neel, B. G., and Astrin, S. M. Activation of a cellular onc gene by promoter insertion in ALV-induced lymphoid leukosis. *Nature 290:* 475, 1981.

52. Heldin, C. H., and Westermark, B. Growth factors: Mechanism of action and relation to oncogenes. *Cell 37.* 9, 1984.

53. Heldin, C. H., Westermark, B., and Wasteson, A. Chemical and biological properties of a growth factor from human cultured osteosarcoma cells: Resemblance with platelet-derived growth factor. *J. Cell. Physiol. 105:* 235, 1980.

54. Henderson, L. E., Krutzsch, H. C. and Oroszlan, S. Myristyl amino-terminal acylation of murine retrovirus proteins: An unusual post-translational protein modification. *Proc. Natl. Acad. Sci. USA 80:* 339, 1983.

55. Holbrook, N. J., Lieber, M., and Crabtree, G. R. DNA sequence of the 5' flanking region of

the human interleukin 2 gene: Homologies with adult T-cell leukemia virus. *Nucleic Acids Res. 12:* 5005, 1984.

56. Huebner, R. J., and Todaro, G. J. Oncogenes of RNA tumor viruses as determinants of cancer. *Proc. Natl. Acad. Sci. USA 64:* 1087, 1969.

57. Hunter, T. The proteins of oncogenes. *Sci. Am. 251:* 70, 1984.

58. Hunter T., and Sefton, B. M. Transforming gene product of Rous sarcoma virus phosphorylates tyrosine. *Proc. Natl. Acad. Sci. USA 77:* 1311, 1980.

59. Johnson, A., Heldin, C. H., Wasteson, A., Westermark, B., Beuel, T. F., Huang, J. S., Seeburg, P. H., Gray, A., Ullrich, A., Scrace, G., Stroobant, P., and Waterfield, M. D. The c-sis gene encodes a precursor of the B chain of platelet-derived growth factor. *EMBO J. 3:* 921, 1984.

60. Jones, N., and Shenk, T. An adenovirus type S early gene function regulates expression of other early viral genes. *Proc. Natl. Acad. Sci. USA 76:* 3665, 1979.

61. Kamata, T., and Feramisco, J. R. Epidermal growth factor stimulates guanine nucleotide binding activity and phosphorylation of ras oncogene proteins. *Nature 310:* 147, 1984.

62. Kelly, K., Cochran, B. H., Stiles, C. D., and Leder, P. Cell-specific regulation of the c-myc gene by lymphocyte mitogens and platelet-derived growth factor. *Cell: 35:* 603, 1983.

63. Klinger, H. P., and Shows, T. B. Suppression of tumorigenicity in somatic cell hybrids. II. Human chromosomes implicated as suppressors of tumorigenicity in hybrids with Chinese hamster ovary cells. *J. Natl. Cancer Inst. 71:* 559, 1983.

64. Krontiris, T. G., and Cooper, G. M. Transforming activity of human tumor DNAs. *Proc. Natl. Acad. Sci. USA 78:* 1181, 1981.

65. Krueger, J. G., Garber, E. A., Goldberg, A. R., and Hanafusa, H. Changes in amino-terminal sequences of pp60src lead to decreased membrane association and decreased in vivo tumorigenicity. *Cell 28:* 889, 1982.

66. Land, H., Parada, L. F., and Weinberg, R. A. Oncogenes. *Nature 304:* 596, 1983.

67. Laurence, J., and Mayer, L. Immunoregulatory lymphokines of T hybridoma from AIDS patients: Constitutive and inducible suppressor factors. *Science 225:* 66, 1984.

68. Leof, E. B., Wharton, W., VanWyk, J. J., and Pledger, W. J. Epidermal growth factor (EGF) and somadomedin C regulate G1 progression in competent BALB/c-3T3 cells. *Exp. Cell Res. 141:* 107, 1982.

69. Levinson, A. D., Opperman, H., and Levintow, L. Evidence that the transforming gene of avian sarcoma virus encodes a protein kinase associated with a phosphoprotein. *Cell 15:* 561, 1978.

70. Levinson, B., Khoury, G., VandeWoude, G., and Gruss, P. Activation of SV40 genome by 72-base pair tandem repeats of Moloney sarcoma virus. *Nature 295:* 568, 1982.

71. Macara, I. G., Marinetti, G. V., and Balduzzi, P. C. Transforming protein of avian sarcoma virus UR2 is associated with phosphatidylinositol kinase activity: Possible role in tumorigenesis. *Proc. Natl. Acad. Sci. USA 81:* 2728, 1984.

72. Marquardt, H., and Todaro, G. J. Human transforming growth factor. *J. Biol. Chem. 257:* 5220, 1982.

73. Marx, J. Oncogenes amplified in cancer cells. *Science 223:* 40, 1984.

74. Marx, J. L. A new view of receptor action. *Science 224:* 271, 1984.

75. Mathey-Prevot, B., Hanafusa, H., and Kawai, S. A cellular protein is immunologically crossreactive with and functionally homologous to the Fujinami sarcoma virus transforming protein. *Cell 28:* 897, 1982.

76. Mroczkowski, B., Mosig, G., and Cohen, S. ATP-stimulated interaction between epidermal growth factor receptor and supercoiled DNA. *Nature 309:* 270, 1984.

77. Muller, R., Slamon, D. J., Tremblay, J. M., Cline, M. J., and Verma, I. M. Differential expression of cellular oncogenes during pre- and postnatal development of the mouse. *Nature 299:* 640, 1982.

78. Murphree, A. L., and Benedict, W. F. Retinoblastoma: Clues to human oncogenesis. *Science 223:* 1028, 1984.

79. Muschel, R. J., Khoury, G., Lebowitz, P., Koller, R., and Dhar, R. The human c-Ras$^{H}_{1}$ oncogene: A mutation in normal and neoplastic tissue from the same patient. *Science 219:* 853, 1983.

80. Nister, M., Heldin, C. H., Wasteson, A., and Westermark, B. A glioma-derived analog to

platelet-derived growth factor: Demonstration of receptor competing activity and immunological cross-reactivity. *Proc. Natl. Acad. Sci. USA 81:* 926, 1984.

81. Ohno, S., and Yazaki, A. Simple construction of human c-myc gene implicated in B cell neoplasms and its relation with avian v-myc and human lymphokines. *Scanit. J. Immunol. 18:* 373, 1983.

82. Ozanne, B., Wheeler, T., Zack, J., Smith, G., and Dale, B. Transforming gene of a human leukaemia cell is unrelated to the expressed tumour virus related gene of the cell. *Nature 299:* 744, 1982.

83. Parker, R. C., Varmus, H. E., and Bishop, J. M. Expression of v-src and chicken c-src in rat cells demonstrates qualitative differences between pp60^{v-src} and pp60^{c-src}. *Cell 37:* 131, 1984.

84. Payne, G. S., Bishop, J. M., and Varmus, H. E. Multiple rearrangements of viral DNA and an activated host oncogene in bursal lymphomas. *Nature 295:* 209, 1982.

85. Pfahl, M., McGinnis, D., Hendricks, M., Groner, B., and Hynes, N. E. Correlation of glucocorticoid receptor binding sites on MMTV proviral DNA with hormone inducible transcription. *Science 222:* 1341, 1983.

86. Pierce, G. B., Shikes, R., and Fink, L. M. *Cancer: A Problem in Developmental Biology.* Englewood Clifts, NJ, Prentice Hall, 1978.

87. Pledger, W. J., Stiles, C. D., Antoniades, H. N., and Scher, C. D. Induction of DNA synthesis in BALB/c 3T3 cells by serum components: Reevaluation of the commitment process. *Proc. Natl. Acad. Sci. USA 74:* 4481, 1977.

88. Prywes, R., Foulkes, J. G., Rosenberg, N., and Baltimore, D. Sequences of the A-MuLV protein needed for fibroblast and lymphoid cell transformation. *Cell 34:* 569, 1983.

89. Pulciani, S., Santos, E., Lauver, A. V., Long, L. K., Aaronson, S. A. and Barbacid, M. Oncogenes in solid human tumors. *Nature 300:* 539, 1982.

90. Queen, C., and Baltimore, D. Immunoglobulin gene transcription is activated by downstream sequence elements. *Cell 33:* 741, 1983.

91. Rabbitts, T. H. Forster, A., Hamlyn, P., and Baer, R. Effect of somatic mutation within translocated c-myc genes in Burkitt's lymphoma. *Nature 309:* 592, 1984.

92. Ralston, R., and Bishop, J. M. The protein products of the myc and myb oncogenes and adenovirus E1a are structurally related. *Nature 306:* 803, 1983.

93. Razin, A., and Riggs, A. DNA methylation in gene function. *Science 210:* 604, 1980.

94. Rechavi, G., Givol, D., and Canaani, E. Activation of a cellular oncogene by DNA rearrangement: Possible involvement of an IS-like element. *Nature 300:* 607, 1982.

95. Reddy, E. K., Reynolds, R. K., Santos, E., and Barbacid, M. A point mutation is responsible for the acquisition of transforming properties by the T24 human bladder carcinoma oncogene. *Nature 300:* 149, 1982.

96. Reynolds, F. H., Todaro, G. J., Fryling, C., and Stephenson, J. R. Human transforming growth factors induce tryosine phosphorylation of EGF receptors. *Nature 292:* 259, 1981.

97. Robbins, K. C., Antoniades, H. N., Devare, S. G., Hunkapiller, M. W., and Aaronson, S. A. Structural and immunological similarities between simian sarcoma virus gene product(s) and human platelet-derived growth factor. *Nature 305:* 605, 1983.

98. Rohrschneider, L. R. and Rosok, M. J. Transformation parameters and pp60^{src} localization in cells infected with partial transformation mutants of Rous sarcoma virus. *Mol. Cell. Biol. 3:* 731, 1983.

99. Rohrschneider, L. R., Rosok, M. J., and Gentry, L. E. Molecular interaction of the src gene product with cellular adhesion plaques. *Prog. Nucleic Acid Res. Mol. Biol. 29:* 233, 1983.

100. Rosson, D., and Tereba, A. Transcription of hematopoietic-associated oncogenes in childhood leukemia. *Cancer Res. 43:* 3912, 1983.

101. Rothberg, P. G., Erisman, M. D., and Diehl, R. E. Elevated expression of the c-myc in human acute leukemia and Burkitt's lymphoma. Manuscript in preparation, 1985.

102. Rous, P. A sarcoma of the fowl transmissible by an agent separable from the tumor cells. *J. Exp. Med. 13:* 397, 1911.

103. Rowley, J. D. Identification of the constant chromosome regions induced in human hematologic malignant disease. *Science 216:* 749, 1982.

104. Rowley, J. D. Biological implications of consistent chromosomal rearrangements in leukemias and lymphomas. *Cancer Res. 44:* 3159, 1984.

105. Ruley, H. E. Adenovirus early region 1A enables viral and cellular transforming genes to transform primary cells. *Nature 304:* 602, 1983.

106. Sachs, L. Constitutive uncoupling of pathways of gene expression that control growth and differentiation in myeloid leukemia: A model for the origin and progression of malignancy. *Proc. Natl. Acad. Sci. USA 77:* 6152, 1980.

107. Santos, E., Martin-Zanca, D., Reddy, E. P., Pierotti, M. A., DellaPorta, G., and Barbacid, M. Malignant activation of a K-ras oncogene in lung carcinoma but not in normal tissue of the same patient. *Science 223:* 661, 1984.

108. Scher, C. D., Dick, R. L., Whipple, A. P., and Locatell, K. L. Identification of a BALB/c-3T3 cell protein modulated by platelet-derived growth factor. *Mol. Cell. Biol. 3:* 70, 1983.

109. Schimke, R. Gene amplification in cultured animal cells. *Cell 37:* 705, 1984.

110. Schreiber, A. B., Libermann, T. A., Lax, I., Yarden, Y., and Schlessinger, J. Biological role of epidermal growth factor-receptor clustering. *J. Biol. Chem. 258:* 846, 1983.

111. Schwab, M., Alitalo, K., Varmus, H. E., and Bishop, J. M. A cellular oncogene (c-Ki-ras) is amplified, overexpressed, and located within karyotypic abnormalities in mouse adrenocortical tumour cells. *Nature 303:* 497, 1983.

112. Seligmann, M., Chess, L. Faley, J. L., Fanci, A. S., Lachmann, P. J., L'Age-Stehr, J., Ngu, J., Pincheng, A. J., Rosen, F. S., Spiro, T. J., and Wybran, J. AIDS-immunologic reevaluation. *N. Engl. J. Med. 311:* 1286, 1984.

113. Shibuya, M., Hanafusa, H., and Balduzzi, P. C. Cellular sequences related to three new onc genes of avian sarcoma virus (fps, yes, and ros) and their expression in normal and transformed cells. *J. Virol. 42:* 143, 1982.

114. Shimizu, K., Goldfarb, M., Perucho, M., and Wigler, M. Isolation and preliminary characterization of the transforming gene of a human neuroblastoma cell line. *Proc. Natl. Acad. Sci. USA 80:* 383, 1983.

115. Slamon, D. J., deKernion, J. B., Verma, I. M., and Cline, M. J. Expression of cellular oncogenes in human malignancies. *Science 224:* 256, 1984.

116. Sodroski, J., Patarca, R., Perkis, D., Briggs, D., Lee, T-H., Essex, M., Coligan, J., Wong-Staal, F., Gallo, R. C., and Haseltine, W. A. Sequence of the envelope glycoprotein gene of Type II human T lymphotropic virus. *Science 225:* 421, 1984.

117. Spector, D. H., Smith, K., Padgett, T., McCombe, P., Roulland-Dussoix, D., Moscovici, C., Varmus, H. E., and Bishop, J. M. Uninfected avian cells contain RNA related to the transforming gene of avian sarcoma viruses. *Cell 13:* 371, 1978.

118. Stanbridge, E. J., Der, C. J., Doersen, C. J., Nishimi, R. Y., Peehl, D. M., Weissman, B. E., and Wilkinson, J. E. Human cell hybrids: Analysis of transformation and tumorigenicity. *Science 215:* 252, 1982.

119. Stanton, L. W., Watt, R., and Marcu, K. B. Translocation, breakage and truncated transcripts of c-myc oncogene in murine plasmacytomas. *Nature 303:* 401, 1983.

120. Stehelin, D., Varmus, H. E., and Bishop, J. M. DNA related to the transforming gene(s) of avian sarcoma viruses is present in normal avian DNA. *Nature 260:* 170, 1976.

121. Stiles, C.D., Capone, G. T., Scher, C. D., Antoniades, H. N., VanWyk, J. J., and Pledger, W. J. Dual control of cell growth by somatomedins and platelet-derived growth factor. *Proc. Natl. Acad. Sci. USA 76:* 1279, 1979.

122. Sugimato, Y., Whitman, M., Cantley, L. C., and Erikson, R. L. Evidence that the Rous sarcoma virus transforming gene product phosphorylates phosphatidylinositol and diacylglycerol. *Proc. Natl. Acad. Sci. USA 81:* 2117, 1984.

123. Tabin, C. J., Bradley, S. M., Bargmann, C. I., Weinberg, R. A., Papageorge, A. G., Scolnick, E. M., Dhar, R., Lowy, D. R., and Chang, E. H. Mechanism of activation of a human oncogene. *Nature 300:* 143, 1982.

124. Tainsky, M. A., Cooper, C. S., Giovanella, B. C., and VandeWoude, G. F. An activated ras[N] gene: Detected in late but not early passage human PA1 teratocarcinoma cells. *Science 225:* 643, 1984.

125. Taparowsky, E., Shimizu, K., Goldfarb, M., and Wigler, M. Structure and activation of the human N-ras gene. *Cell 34:* 581, 1983.

126. Temin, H. M. The protoviruses hypothesis: Speculations on the significance of RNA-directed DNA synthesis for normal development and for carcinogenesis. *J. Natl. Cancer Inst. 46:*

III, 1971.

127. Vogt, P. K. Spontaneous segregation of nontransforming viruses from cloned sarcoma viruses. *Virology 46:* 939, 1971.

128. Walters, R. A., Enger, D. M., Hildebrand, C. E., and Griffith, J. K. Genes coding for metal-induced synthesis of RNA sequences are differentially amplified and regulated in mammalian cells. *J. Supramol. Struct. (Suppl.)5:* 439, 1981.

129. Weinberg, R. A molecular basis of cancer. Sci. *Am. 249:* 126, 1983.

130. Westin, E. H., Gallo, R. C., Arya, S. K., Eva, A., Souza, L. M., Baluda, M. A., Aaronson, S. A., and Wong-Staal, F. Differential expression of the amv gene in human hematopoietic cells. *Proc. Natl. Acad. Sci. USA 79:* 2194, 1982.

131. Westin, E. H., Wong-Staal, F., Gelmann, E. P., Dalla-Favera, R., Papas, T. S., Lautenberger, J. A., Eva, A., Reddy, E. P., Tronick, S. R., Aaronson, S. A., and Gallo, R. C. Expression of cellular homologues of retroviral onc genes in human hematopoietic cells. *Proc. Natl. Acad. Sci. USA 79:* 2490, 1982.

132. Wharton, W., Leof, E., Olashaw, N., O'Keefe, E. J., and Pledger, W. J. Mitogenic response to epidermal growth factor (EGF) modulated by platelet-derived growth factor in cultured fibroblasts. *Exp. Cell. Res. 147:* 443, 1983.

133. Wierenga, R. K., and Hol, W. G. J. Predicted nucleotide-binding properties of the p21 protein and its associated cancer variant. *Nature 302:* 842, 1983.

134. Wigler, M., Levy D., and Perucho, M. The somatic replication of DNA methylation. *Cell 24:* 33, 1983.

Chapter 4

Chromosome and Oncogene Rearrangements in Leukemia and Lymphoma

JORGE J. YUNIS

Using high-resolution chromosome analysis,[18] we have found that the malignant cells of most tumors in 372 consecutive cancer patients have a specific chromosomal defect.[19,22-25] These abnormalities are more often represented by a translocation or loss of a chromosome band. Less commonly, a trisomy or inversion is found. In the lymphohematopoietic malignancies, such defects are so important in the disease process that they have made it posible to subdivide acute nonlymphocytic leukemia (ANLL) into distinct categories with prognosis varying from poor to long survival, regardless of the standard French-American-British Cooperative Group (FAB) classification.[23]

For example, using high-resolution examination of chromosomes from bone marrow specimens of 105 consecutive adult patients with *de novo* ANLL, we found that 93% of the patients showed a chromosomal defect. Seventeen separate categories were identified, and 12 of them represented a specific recurrent defect.[23] Three categories emerged as having independent prognostic significance: (1) patients with an inversion 16, diagnosed as either M2, M4, or M5b by the morphological FAB classification, who showed a uniform and sustained complete remission with a median survival of 25 months; (2) patients with complex chromosomal abnormalities diagnosed variously as M1, M2, M4, M5a, and M6 who carried a very poor prognosis with a median survival of 2.5 months; and (3) patients with a trisomy 8 as a single defect who showed an intermediate prognosis with a median survival of 10 months. With the recent availability of different types of treatment for *de novo* ANLL, high-resolution chromosomal analysis can become an essential tool in selecting specific types of therapy for groups of ANLL patients with differing prognoses.[23]

High-resolution chromosomes in non-Hodgkin's lymphomas (NHLs) may also yield useful information. In a study of lymphomatous tissue from 128 patients, 95% showed a chromosomal abnormality, and 64% of them had a specific defect that identifies distinct NHL subgroups. In most instances of lymphomas of the B-cell type, one of eight specific defects was found.[24,25] They included (1) a t(8;14) in most if not all patients with Burkitt's and small, noncleaved non-Burkitt's lymphoma and in a subgroup of immunoblastic lymphoma[24]; (2) a t(14;18) in 80% of the patients with follicular, small, cleaved, mixed small and large cell, and large cell lymphomas[24,25]; and (3) a t(11;14), del 11q, or trisomy 12 in the majority of patients with small lymphocytic cell lymphoma.[11,25] Furthermore, when follicular, small, cleaved cell and small lymphocytic cell lymphomas were accompanied by additional chromosomal defects, the clinical course of the affected patients appeared to be worse.[6,25]

Diffuse large cell lymphoma is believed to represent an amalgam of disorders with varying prognoses.[11,25] Although half of the patients have a deletion 6q, there are patients with a t(8;14), a t(11;14), or a t(14;18). It is conceivable that, as in acute leukemias, these patients would respond differently to treatment, depending on the type of primary chromosomal defect found.

Little was known about the possible molecular mechanisms involved in the chromosomal rearrangements until 1982, when a rearranged and activated cellular oncogene *myc* (*c-myc*) was discovered in Burkitt's lymphoma.[10] In this disease of B-lymphoid cells, a reciprocal chromosomal translocation t(8;14) with breakpoints at bands 8q24.1 and 14q32.3 is often found. In such instances, the oncogene *c-myc* moves from its normal location at band 8q24.1 and becomes activated when rearranged with the constant genes of the immunoglobulin heavy chain (IgH) at band 14q32.3. Less often *c-myc* rearranges with the kappa or lambda immunoglobulin light chain genes of a chromosome 2 or 22 [t(2;8) (p11;q24.1) and t(8;22) (q24.1;q11.2)], respectively.[10,18]

Evidence is accumulating to suggest that one of the two breakpoints in a translocation is the site of a proto-oncogene that becomes abnormally active when rearranged with a second site carrying a very active gene in a specific cell type, here termed a cell-differentiation gene, (see also the chapter by Tomasi). Such a rearrangement can be visualized as a crucial event that sets a stem cell toward a malignant path.[21] In this regard, a recent study has shown that a transcribed DNA sequence, termed *bcl*-1, is normally located at band 11q13.3 but rearranges with the IgH locus of chromosome 14 in the t(11;14) (q13.3;q32.3) found in small lymphocytic cell lymphoma.[16] In the t(14;18) (q32.3;q21.3) of follicular lymphomas, a putative oncogene from 18q21.3 (*bcl*-2) was also found rearranged with chromosome 14.[15] Interestingly, in these two B-cell lymphomas *bcl*-1 and *bcl*-2 generally become rearranged upstream of the J region of the IgH locus of chromosome 14, while *c-myc* in Burkitt's lymphoma generally rearranges upstream of a constant gene. Since *bcl*-1 and *bcl*-2 can become activated by an enhancer element found between the J and the switch region of the IgH genes, and *c-myc* appears to be activated by transacting factors,[4] it can be postulated that enhancers or enhancer-like elements not only help to activate a rearranged oncogene but may help determine the stage of cell differentiation that occurs in a given malignancy. This concept can now be tested in other non-Hodgkin's lymphomas since 65% of them involve a rearrangement with band 14q32.3,[18] and it opens the way for further cloning of chromosomal breakpoints of previously unknown proto-oncogenes.

In leukemias, structural chromosomal defects may also be linked to proto-oncogenes mapped to specific chromosome bands or subbands. One example is the t(9;22) (q34.1;q11.21) in chronic myelogenous leukemia, where the cellular proto-oncogene abl from band 9q34 translocates to a chromosome 22. An abnormal transcript of *abl* has been found in this disorder.[1] Also, the proto-oncogenes *erb A* (17q21.3;22),[7] *mos* (8q22.1),[12] and *H ras* 1 (11p14.1-14.2),[8] have been localized at or near the described breakpoints in acute promyelocytic leukemia with t(15;17)(q22; q11.2-q22), acute myelogenous leukemia with t(8;21) (q22.1q22.3), and T-cell acute lymphocytic leukemia with t(11;14) (p13-14.2;q11-13), respectively. All in all, 8 of 17 proto-oncogenes have been found to map at or close to known cancer chromosome breakpoints.[18,26] However, a proto-oncogene rearrangement or activation has not been demonstrated, except for *myc* and *abl*. In myelogenous leukemias, as in lymphomas and lymphoid leukemias, one of the two breakpoints of a translocation, inversion or deletion, may highlight a region where an active gene of cells of differentiated activity is localized,[21] although this also remains to be determined.

Despite these findings and observations, it is likely that a primary genomic rearrangement by itself would not generally lead to an immediate expression of malignancy. Other regulatory steps of cell proliferation and differentiation may need to be affected to commit a stem cell toward one or another type of malignancy.[2,10] One example in this regard is the finding of a t(14;14) (q11;q32.3) in T-cell chronic lymphocytic leukemia,[17] a chromosomal abnormality also seen with relative frequency in the normal lymphocytes of patients with ataxia telangiectasia, some of whom develop a T-cell lymphoma or leukemia from the t(14;14) cell clone several months or years later.[9]

A second and more general example pertains to the fact that in the well-studied leukemias and lymphomas the primary chromosomal abnormality is often shared among related disorders.[18] For instance, the t(8;14) (q24.1;q32.3) observed in Burkitt's lymphoma is also found in small cell non-Burkitt's lymphoma, a subgroup of immunoblastic lymphomas and B-cell acute lymphocytic leukemia.[13,24] What may in part explain why cells with a shared chromosomal defect differentiate into one or another type of related tumor is the finding of different activated transforming genes in human pre-B, B (Burkitt's lymphoma), and mature B (myeloma) cell malignancies. This suggests that such genes could be involved in differentiation-specific control of cell proliferation.[2] One such gene is *Blym-1*, which encodes a small protein of 65 amino acids and shows significant homology to the amino-terminal region of the transferrin family of proteins. Recently this gene was found to be activated in Burkitt's lymphoma.[3]

In addition to proto-oncogenes, 16 heritable chromosomal fragile sites (*h-fra*) have been identified.[14] *H-fra* are usually expressed heterozygously as a gap, break, or displacement of a chromosome segment at a specific site, and they are found with a frequency of less than 0.2% each in the general population. Except for *h-fra* 10q25.2, 16q22.1, and 17p12, the expression of these sites is related to inhibition of thymidylate synthetase, resulting in thymidine deprivation. They are expressed by culturing cells in media lacking folic acid and thymidine or by exposing them to a thymidylate synthetase inhibitor such as fluorodeoxyuridine.[14] *H-fra* 7p11.2, 11q13.3, 11q23.3, 12q13.1, and 16q22.1 have been found to coincide with a breakpoint of three specific translocations, one inversion and one deletion in leukemias and non-Hodgkin's lymphomas.[18,20,21,26] Further, an *h-fra* 11q13.3 (where *bcl*-1 is located) was found in the normal blood cells of three of three patients with small lymphocytic lymphoma and t(11;14) (q13.3;q32.3); an *h-fra* 12q13.1 was found in the normal blood cells of one patient with T-cell diffuse mixed cell lymphoma and t(12;14) (q13.1;q32.3) and an *h-fra* 16q22 was found in the normal cells of four of five patients with acute myelomonocytic leukemia and inv(16)(p.13.1;q22.1)(p13.11;q22.2).[19,24]

This suggests that some individuals may be genetically predisposed to develop a given type of malignancy.[20] An even more intriguing observation is the recent discovery of a family of 51 constitutive fragile sites (*c-fra*) located at very precise points in fine bands of the human and primate genome.[26] The expression to 2.2 mM caffeine (a DNA repair inhibitor that serves as a mutagen enhancer) during the last 6 hours of culture.[5,20] They are expressed homozygously in most or all individuals, and some individuals have a higher expression of certain sites. In addition, 20 *c-fra* map at or close to one of the two breakpoints found in 24 of the 31 specific structural chromosome defects known in cancer, including solid tumors.[26]

In a preliminary study of *c-fra* expression in patients with leukemia or lymphoma and with specific chromosomal abnormalities in their malignant cells, we have observed: (1) an elevated expression (14 and 14.5%, respectively) of *c-fra* 7q31.2 in the normal blood cells of two of two patients with ANLL and deletion 7q31.2q36.3; (2) an elevated *c-fra* 8q21.1 of 10.5% in the normal blood cells of a patient with ANLL and t(8;21) (q22.1;q22.3); (3) an elevated *c-fra* 16q22.1 expression of 21% in the normal blood cells of a patient with ANLL and inv(16)(p13.11;q22.1); and (4) an elevated *c-fra* 18q21.3 expression of 13% in the normal blood cells of one of two patients with follicular small cleaved cell lymphoma and a t(14;18) (q32.3;q21.3).[26] If these results are confirmed, they would suggest that under some conditions there is a higher expression than normal (3–10%) of a specific *c-fra* that may help predispose them to certain malignancies.

It is remarkable that when the 17 proto-oncogenes, 16 heritable fragile sites, and 51 constitutive fragile sites mapped to specific bands or small chromosomal regions are considered together,[26] they coincide with at least one of the two breakpoints involved in all of the 22 specific structural chromosome defects identified thus far in leukemias and non-Hodgkin's lymphomas.[20,26] Only a few of these apparent correlations are being successfully elucidated at the molecular level, but there is potential for further concordance.

These observations should stimulate molecular work and provide important clues to the basic mechanisms involved in this crucial, if not initial, step in the multistep development of lymphohematopoietic malignancies.

ACKNOWLEDGMENTS

Supported in part by Grants CA-31024 and CA-33314 from the National Cancer Institute, National Institutes of Health, Bethesda, MD. The editorial assistance of William Hoffman is gratefully acknowledged.

REFERENCES

1. Collins, S. R., Kubonishi, I., Miyoshi, I., Groudine, M. T. Altered transcription of the c-abl oncogene in K–562 and other chronic myelogenous leukemia cells. *Science 225:* 72–74, 1984.
2. Cooper, G. M. Cellular transforming genes. *Science 217:* 801–806, 1982.

3. Cooper, G. M. Activation of cellular transforming genes in neoplasms. In: *Advances in Gene Technology: Human Genetic Disorders*, ICSU Short Reports, vol.1,1984, Proceedings of the 16th Miami Winter Symposium, pp. 2–5.

4. Croce, C. M., Erikson, J., ar-Rushdi, A., Aden, D., and Nishikura, K. Translocated c-myc oncogene of Burkitt lymphoma is transcribed in plasma cells and repressed in lympho-blastoid cells. *Proc. Natl. Acad. Sci. USA 81:* 3170–3174, 1984.

5. Das, S. K., Lau, C. C., and Pardee, A. B. Comparative analysis of caffeine and 3-amino-ben-zamide as DNA repair inhibitors in Syrian baby hamster kidney cells. *Mutation Res 131:* 71–79, 1984.

6. Han, T., Ozer, H., Sadamori, N., Emrich, L., Gomez, G. A., Henderson, E. S., Bloom, M. L., and Sandberg, A. A. Prognostic importance of cytogenetic abnormalities in patients with chronic lymphocytic leukemia. *N. Engl. J. Med. 310:* 288–292, 1984.

7. Jhanwar, S. C., Changanti, R. S. K., and Croce, C. M. *Som. Cell. Mol. Gen., 11:95–102,* 1985.

8. Jhanwar, S. C., Neel, B. G., Hayward, W. S., and Chaganti, R. S. K. Localization of c-ras oncogene family on human germ-like chromosomes. *Proc. Natl. Acad. Sci. USA 80:* 4794–4797, 1983.

9. Kaiser-McCaw, B., and Hecht, F. Ataxia-telangiectasia: Chromosomes and cancer. In: *Ataxia-telangiectasia—A Cellular and Molecular Link between Cancer, Neuropathology, and Immune Deficiency*, edited by Bridges and Harden. New York, John Wiley & Sons, 1982, pp. 243–244.

10. Leder, P., Battey, J., Lenoir, G., Moulding, C., Murphy, W., Potter, H., Stewart, T., and Taub, R. Translocations among antibody genes in human cancer. *Science 222:* 765–771, 1983.

11. Nathwani, B. N., Dixon, D. O., Jones, S. C., Hartsock, R. J., Rebuck, J. W., Byrne, G. E., Shechan, W. W., Kim, H., Coltman, C. A., and Rappaport, H. The clinical significance of the morphological subdivision of diffuse "histiocytic" lymphoma: A study of 162 patients treated by the Southwest Oncology Group. *Blood 60:* 1068–1074, 1982.

12. Neel, B., Jhanwar, S. C., Chaganti, R. S. K., and Hayward, W. S. Two human c-onc genes are located on the long arm of chromosome 8. *Proc. Natl. Acad. Sci. USA 79:* 7842–7846, 1982.

13. Sigarix, F., Berger, R., Bernheim, A., Valensi, F., Daniel, M. T., and Flandrin, G. Malignant lymphomas with band 8q24 chromosome abnormality: A morphologic continuum extending from Burkitt's to immunoblastic lymphoma. *Br. J. Haematol. 57:* 393–405, 1984.

14. Sutherland, G. R., Jacky, P. B., Baker, E., and Manuel, A. Heritable fragile sites of human chromosomes. X. New folate-sensititve fragile sites: 6p23, 9p21, 9q32, and 11q23. *Am. J. Hum. Gent. 35:* 432–437, 1983.

15. Tsujimoto, Y., Finger, L., Yunis, J. J., Nowell, P. C., and Croce, C. M. Molecular cloning of the chromosomal breakpoint of follicular lymphomas with the t(14;18) chromosome transloca-tion. *Science, 226:1097–1099,* 1985.

16. Tsujimoto, Y., Yunis, J. J., Onorato-Showe, L. R., Nowell, P. C., and Croce, C. M. Molecular cloning of the chromosomal breakpoint of B cell lymphomas and leukemias with the t(11;14) chromosome translocation, *Science 224:* 1403–1406, 1984.

17. Ueshima, Y., Rowley, J. D., Variakojis, D., Winter, J., and Gordon, L. Cytogenetic studies on patients with chronic T cell leukemia/lymphoma. *Blood 63:* 1028–1038, 1984.

18. Yunis, J. J. The chromosomal basis of human neoplasia. *Science 221:* 227–236, 1983.

19. Yunis, J. J. Recurrent chromosomal defects are found in most patients with acute non-lympho-cytic leukemia. *Cancer Genet. Cytogenet. 11:* 125–137, 1984.

20. Yunis, J. J. Fragile sites and predisposition to leukemia and lymphoma. *Cancer Genet. Cytogenet. 12:* 85–88, 1984.

21. Yunis, J. J. Genes and chromosomes in human cancer. *Prog. med. Virol. 32: 58–71,*1985.

22. Yunis, J. J., Bloomfield, C. D., and Ensrud, K. All patients with acute nonlymphocytic leuke-mias may have a chromosomal defect. *N. Engl. J. Med. 305:* 135–139, 1983.

23. Yunis, J. J., Brunning, R., Howe, R. B., and Lobell, M. High-resolution chromosomes as an independent prognostic indicator of acute non-lymphocytic leukemia. *N. Engl. J. Med. 311:* 812–818, 1984.

24. Yunis, J. J., Oken, M. M., Kaplan, M. E., Ensrud, K. M., Howe, R. B., and Theologides, A. Distinctive chromosomal abnormalities in histologic subtypes of non-Hodgkin's lymphoma. *N. Engl. J. Med. 307:* 1231–1236, 1982.

25. Yunis, J. J., Oken, M. M., Theologides, A., Howe, R. B., and Kaplan, M. E. Recurrent chromosomal defects are found in most patients with non-Hodgkin's lymphoma. *Cancer Genet. Cytogenet. 13:* 17–28, 1984.
26. Yunis, J. J., and Soreng, A. L. Constitutive fragile sites and cancer. *Science, 226: 1199–1204,* 1985.

Chapter 5

Ionizing Radiation and Neoplasia*

LUIS FELIPE FAJARDO L-G

INTRODUCTION

Among the well accepted causes of neoplasia, ionizing radiation is quite prominent. Its oncogenic role was suspected by a few pioneers in the field of radiation biology, and some evidence for its oncogenicity has been available for almost 80 years. Since then unquestionable and abundant proof, statistical and experimental, has linked radiation with multiple tumors in mammals.

Other forms of radiation (*e.g.*, ultraviolet) are also causally related to neoplasia. This review, however, refers only to the tumors associated with ionizing radiation, either electromagnetic (*i.e.*, gamma and x-rays) or particulate (alpha particles, neutrons, *etc.*).

The field of radiation oncogenesis can be compared to a sea of hypotheses, with a few solid islands of facts. Let us deal first with the facts (specific radiation-induced neoplasms, risk data, *etc.*) and then consider some of the hypotheses (possible mechanisms of radiation oncogenesis).

For the purpose of this publication, radiation doses are expressed in *rad*.† Only when rad doses are unavailable or inappropriate will other units be used: Curie (Ci), rem, Roentgen (R), Sievert (Sv), Working Level Month (WLM), *etc.* For those who wish to think in terms of Grays: 1 Gy corresponds to 100 rad. Definitions of these various units are found in standard texts.[27, 35]

GENERAL CHARACTERISTICS OF RADIATION-INDUCED TUMORS

EVIDENCE OF RADIATION INDUCTION

Clearly, radiation is the cause, or one of the major causes, of a number of human neoplasms. In other mammals the number of radiation-induced tumors is even larger, and the evidence for a causal role is better.

Claims of radiation oncogenesis for given individual neoplasms are made al-

---

*The author wishes to dedicate this chapter to the memory of Henry Seymour Kaplan (1918–1984), whose classic work on radiation murine leukemias is described in this chapter.

†rad = dose of radiation that results in the absorption of 100 ergs / g of absorbing medium. Kerma (Kinetic Energy Released in Material) = a unit of quantity that represents the kinetic energy transferred to charged particles by the uncharged particles per unit mass of the irradiated medium.

TABLE 5.1. To Be Acceptable as Radiation-Induced,
a Human Neoplasm Should Include the Following

1. Possible radiation induction	Occur in the tissue(s) exposed to radiation (for solid tumors)
	Be different from any local neoplasm present prior to radiation exposure
	Appear after a period of latency (probably more than 2 years for leukemias and 6 years for solid tumors)
	Have enough observations (cases) available to suggest a causal relation
2. Satisfactory evidence of radiation induction	Show statistically significant difference in incidence between the irradiated and a comparable control population
3. Proof of radiation induction	Show positive correlation between dose and incidence

most weekly as case reports in the clinical literature. Unfortunately, many such individual cases have a questionable or unproven relationship to radiation.

Thus, in order to use only valid data it is important to set clearly defined conditions for the acceptance of a given neoplasm as *radiation-induced*. These conditions may vary somewhat with the concepts and purpose of the investigator.

I feel that a reasonable list of conditions should be narrow enough to weed out unfounded claims but elastic enough to include associations that are promising although still unproven.[35] Based on this philosophy, I have proposed the list of conditions at three levels that appears in Table 5.1. This list of criteria and its sequence may not satisfy the opinions of either more liberal or more strict investigators.

Obviously, the Level 1 conditions are to be fulfilled by the first observers, *i.e.*, those directly engaged in patient care: clinicians, pathologists, *etc.* These conditions are often met but *do not* constitute evidence of radiation induction.

It is my view that radiation should be considered etiologically associated with a given neoplasm only when there are enough observations (cases) to establish a significant statistical difference between the irradiated population and a reasonably similar control population (Level 2). Further proof of a cause and effect relationship is the demonstration of a positive correlation between radiation dose and incidence of the neoplasm (Level 3).

Even if these conditions are met, one should be aware of the possible causes of error. The accuracy of the sources of information is of paramount importance: extensive epidemiologic work has been rendered worthless when the raw data have become questionable.

How many are "enough cases"? This is difficult to define, and it probably depends on the spontaneous incidence of a given tumor: if the neoplasm is common (*e.g.*, pulmonary squamous carcinoma), hundreds of cases may be necessary to show a relationship. If the tumor is rare (*e.g.*, liver angiosarcoma), a small number of cases might be acceptable.

There are many possible biases in the statistical analysis of these groups: The underlying disease that has led to radiotherapy, in some groups, may be inherently associated with a high risk of neoplasia independently of ionizing radiation; in general, the risk of spontaneous second neoplasms must be taken into account. The interaction of radiation with other cancer risk factors (environmental, genetic, *etc.*) must be considered when comparing various populations. If the follow-up period is not long enough, some radiation-induced neoplasms may not be recognized as such: in the A-bomb survivors the increased incidence of alimentary tract cancers was not apparent until almost 30 years of observation had been accumulated.[54] The methods used for surveillance may select certain neoplasms and ignore others. Also special diagnostic procedures may have been introduced in the irradiated populations and not in the control groups because of cost or inconvenience to the controls; this increases the ability to detect neoplasia in the determinate group but not in the control group. Lastly, we cannot ignore the remote possibility that the surveillance procedures themselves may be carcinogenic, especially when repeated over many years.

Successful radiation induction of a given neoplasm in another species is not necessarily proof that the same occurs in humans. In fact this could be misleading: for instance, radiation produces a high yield of ovarian tumors in mice, while there is no evidence that ovarian tumors can be radiation-induced in humans.

Radiation-Induced Human Tumors

By the above criteria, *satisfactory evidence* of radiation induction is available for the *human* neoplasms listed in Table 5.2. There is a longer, and growing, list of human neoplasms for which there is a *strong suggestion* of radiation induction. Most of these appear in Table 5.3. I do not claim that these lists are complete or up-to-date; these merely represent my interpretation of the literature according to the conditions set in Table 5.1.

It should be fairly obvious that known radiation accounts only for a small proportion of the cases of each of these neoplasms, *e.g.*, breast carcinoma. "It has been inferred that about 3% of the cancer burden" (deaths per year) in the United States may be attributable to radiation of various sources: 1.5–2% to natural background exposure‡; 0.5% to medical uses; 1% or less to occupational sources.[96] As will be noted below, very few (if any) neoplasms occur after very low doses of radiation; most occur after midrange exposures (*e.g.*, breast carcinoma in atom bomb survivors), and a few follow large, therapeutic doses of local radiation (*e.g.*, uterine sarcoma after pelvic irradiation). Certain tumors appear after prolonged exposures to locally deposited isotopes (*e.g.*, radium and thorium). What is common to all is a period of latency, usually of more than 2 years.

RADIATION-INDUCED TUMORS IN OTHER ANIMALS

To list here the multitude of neoplasms induced by radiation in nonhuman animal species, particularly in rodents, would be a lengthy endeavor. Some of these tumors appear in Table 5.4.

---

‡Natural background radiation has not been proven to be oncogenic. In fact, some observers claim that it is not.

TABLE 5.2. HUMAN TUMORS WITH EVIDENCE OF RADIATION INDUCTION

Neoplasm(s)	Type of Exposure
Thyroid carcinoma (usually papillary)	Atom bomb survivors[48, 56] Irradiation for benign conditions of head and neck ("thymic enlargement," tinea capitis, acne, *etc.*)[30, 45, 62, 76]
Leukemia (usually granulocytic)	Atom bomb survivors[13, 27] Irradiation for ankylosing spondylitis[27, 28] Occupational exposure[25, 59] Irradiation for "metropathia hemorrhagica"[2, 48] Thorotrast injection[79] Systemic use of ^{32}P for polycythemia vera[11, 47, 69, 77]
Breast carcinoma (same histologic types as in nonirradiated)	Atom bomb survivors[72, 124] Multiple fluoroscopies[64] Irradiation for acute postpartum mastitis[102]
Liver, various malignant neoplasms (mostly cholangio-carcinomas and angiosarcomas)	Thorotrast deposition from diagnostic procedures[27, 36, 79, 111]
Multiple myeloma	Atom bomb survivors[30, 49, 50] Occupational exposure (radium-dial painters)[30]
Bone, sarcomas	Occupational exposure (radium-dial painters)[37, 48, 90] Radium injection[48]
Soft tissue sarcomas; cavitary mesotheliomas	Thorotrast deposition from diagnostic procedures[44, 68]
Paranasal sinuses (carcinomas)	Systemic use of thorium or radium[11, 27, 37, 48, 90, 106]
Skin carcinoma (basal and squamous)	Occupational exposure[27, 125] Early radiotherapy technics[23, 27, 67]
Pulmonary carcinoma	Atom bomb survivors[9, 50, 54] Irradiation for ankylosing spondylitis[27] Uranium, fluorspar, and metal miners[27, 86, 91, 93, 123]
Esophageal carcinoma	Atom bomb survivors[54]
Gastric carcinoma	Atom bomb survivors[54]
Colonic carcinoma (except rectum)	Atom bomb survivors[27, 54] Irradiation for "metropathia hemorrhagica"[27, 104]

RISK ESTIMATES

There are several methods to determine the probability of occurrence of a given radio-induced neoplasm in a population. These are usually based on the observation of a number of cases, correlation with doses, time, *etc.*, and comparison with the spontaneous incidence of the same neoplasm.

The estimates of risk can be expressed in various ways.[27, 126] A form frequently used is to state the number of cases of the given neoplasm in *excess* of those occurring in the absence of radiation, for the same type of population: this is called the *absolute risk* model and is often expressed as the number of excess cases per certain number of individuals (*e.g.*, 1 million), per unit of time (usually 1 year), per certain dose of radiation (almost always per rad or per rem) (Figs. 5.1–5.3). As an example, the absolute risk of skin cancer (mainly,

TABLE 5.3. HUMAN TUMORS WITH POSSIBLE RADIATION INDUCTION

Neoplasm(s)	Type of Exposure
Salivary gland tumors, benign and malignant (adeno-carcinoma, mucoepidermoid carcinoma, *etc.*)[a]	Atom bomb survivors[10, 92, 112] Irradiation for benign head and neck conditions[27, 76, 99] Irradiation in childhood for tinea capitis[76]
Pharyngeal carcinoma	Irradiation for ankylosing spondylitis[27]
Parathyroid adenomas	Irradiation for benign head and neck conditions (*e.g.*, tuberculous lymphadenitis)[25, 114, 117]
Pancreatic carcinoma	Irradiation for ankylosing spondylitis[27]
Kidney (unspecified malignant tumors)[a]	Atom bomb survivors[54]
Urinary bladder (unspecified malignant tumors)[a]	Atom bomb survivors[54]
Uterine sarcomas or mixed Mullerian tumors	Radiotherapy for pelvic neoplasms[31, 83]
Brain tumors (gliomas, meningiomas, *etc.*)	Irradiation for tinea capitis[1, 27, 76, 94]
Leukemia (usually granulocytic)	Radiotherapy for some solid tumors (*e.g.*, carcinoma of cervix[48, 130] Total nodal irradiation for Hodgkin's disease[8, 48]
Various, *second*, nonlymphomatous neoplasmas	Total nodal irradiation for Hodgkin's disease[8, 48]
Lymphoma (not specified)	Irradiation for ankylosing spondylitis[27] Atom bomb survivors, uranium workers[27]
Bone, sarcomas	Radiotherapy for adjacent tumors[73, 116] Radiotherapy for Ewing's tumor (long-term survivors)[110]
Osteochondromas (cartilaginous exostoses)	Irradiation in childhood for malignant tumors (Wilms', *etc.*)[26, 107]
Various second neoplasms in childhood (bone and soft tissue sarcomas, thyroid carcinoma)	Radiotherapy for various childhood malignancies (Wilms', neuroblastoma, retinoblastoma, etc.)[60]
Malignant tumors in childhood (mainly leukemia)[a]	Diagnostic radiation exposure *in utero* [12, 48, 65, 75, 108, 109]

[a]Evidence of induction may be available.

basal and epidermoid carcinomas) among Caucasian individuals irradiated for tinea capitis (during 1940–1955) or for "thymic enlargement" (1926–1957) was 0.44 to 1.02/10[6] individuals/year/rad.[27] This risk was estimated on the basis of follow-ups varying from 10 to 49 years.[27] Absolute risk estimates for some of the important neoplasms appear in Table 5.5.

Another frequently used expression of probability is the *relative risk* model. In this model the risk is stated as a *ratio* between the incidence observed in the irradiated population and that of the nonirradiated, control population (Fig. 5.4). For instance, the relative risk of mortality from multiple myeloma for A-bomb survivors receiving 200 rad or more during the period from 1950–1978

TABLE 5.4. SOME RADIATION-INDUCED TUMORS IN NONHUMAN VERTEBRATESS[a]

Primates:	Malignant gliomas
Sheep:	Thyroid tumors
Swine:	Leukemia (myeloid), lymphoma
Dogs:	Bone sarcomas, leukemia (acute myeloid), liver tumors (benign and malignant), lymphomas, skin tumors
Guinea pigs:	Leukemia (chronic lymphatic)
Hamsters:	Pulmonary tumors
Rats:	Alimentary tract adenomas and carcinomas (gastric, enteric, and colonic), bone sarcomas, hepatomas, mammary tumors (adenocarcinoma, fibroadenoma), pancreatic islet cell tumors, pituitary adenomas, renal adenomas and carcinomas, skin tumors, thyroid tumors (papillary and follicular adenoma and carcinoma),
Mice:	Adrenal cortical adenomas; adrenal medullary chromaffin tumors; alimentary adenomas and carcinomas (gastric, enteric, and colonic); hepatomas; leukemia (myeloid); mammary adenocarcinomas, fibroadenomas, and sarcomas; multiple ovarian neoplasms; osteosarcoma; pituitary adenomas; pulmonary adenomas (often papillary); renal adenoma and carcinoma; pulmonary adenomas (often papillary); renal adenoma and carcinoma; skin papillomas; skin tumors; thymic lymphoma-leukemia, thyroid tumors
Fish:	Neuroblastoma

[a]Based on numerous publications, some of which are listed in the bibliography.

was approximately 6.5.[54] For lung and breast cancers in the same population it was 2.[54]

Alternately, the number of *observed* cases in the determinate group can be compared with the number of *expected* cases in the nonirradiated population during a given period of time. For instance, among patients treated by x-radiation for ankylosing spondylitis (Jan. 1963 follow-ups) five cases of cancer of the pharynx were observed, *vs.* 1.05 expected; thus there were 3.95 excess cases (90% confidence limits = 0.9, 9.5; $p < 0.025$).[27, 28]

For some neoplasms the risk changes considerably as a function of time after radiation exposure: *e.g.*, in the A-bomb survivors the leukemia incidence increased to a peak at approximately 7 years after exposure,[13] and then it decreased to the point that Nagasaki survivors showed no increased incidence between 1975 and 1978.[54] Therefore, the expression of risk of such neoplasms should take into account various intervals from exposure, as well as corrections for patient survival. Figure 5.5 is an illustration of this form of risk analysis.

The usefulness of the risk-per-person-rad model is that, under otherwise equal conditions, it can be applied to a range of doses. It should not be assumed, however, that dose and incidence follow a proportional (linear) relationship throughout the entire range of doses (Figs. 5.1–5.3).[126] Proportionality may be present for some tumors in the range between 50 and 500 rad. For smaller doses there is often no linear relationship, and the number of cases is so low that it has been questioned as to whether radiation is carcinogenic at all below doses of 10 rad.[121, 126] Above 500 rad the number of observations is lower, with exception of those in patients treated for malignant tumors, who receive local kilorad doses. For some tumors, at least, the incidence reaches a plateau or even decreases between 500 and 2000 rad. Because of these uncertainties in the very low and very high regions, it has been stated that the no-

TABLE 5.5. RISK ESTIMATES FOR SOME RADIATION-INDUCED NEOPLASMS

	Absolute Risk (Excess no. of Cases)	Period for the Risk Estimated Here	Population
Leukemia (granulocytic, acute and chronic)	2.24[a]	2–25 yr after exposure	A-bomb survivors (all)[27]
	4.13[a]	5–10 yr after exposure	A-bomb survivors (all)[54]
	0.44[a]	30–33 yr after exposure	A-bomb survivors (all)[54]
	0.8–1.2[a]		Anykylosing spondylitis[27]
	40[b]	Beginning 8 yr after exposure	Thorotrast patients[27]
Thyroid carcinoma (papillary > follicular)	4[a]		All groups[27]
	5.80[a]		Women[27]
	2.20[a]		Men[27]
Breast carcinoma (usual types in women)	1.89[a]	30–33 yr after exposure	A-bomb survivors[54]
	6.6–10.4[a]		American women[27]
Lung carcinoma (small cell, epidermoid, adenocarcinoma)	2.59[a]	30–33 yr after exposure	A-bomb survivors[54]
	2.8[a]	Beginning 9 yr after exp	Ankylosing spondylitis[27]
	22–45[a] (converted from WLM)		Uranium, metal, and fluorspar miners[27]
	6–47/10⁶ 10⁶ persons/year/WLM[c]		Uranium, metal, and fluorspar miners[27]
Liver neoplasms (cholangiocarcinoma and angiosarcoma principally)	260 to 300[b]	Beginning 10 yr after exposure	Thorotrast patients[27]
Benign thyroid masses (nodules or adenomas)	12[a]		All groups[27]

[a]Per 10⁶ persons/year/rad.

[b]Per 10⁶ persons/for life/rad.

[c]WLM, working level month: exposure resulting from inhalation of air with a concentration of 1 WL during 170 working hours[27] (WL, Working Level: a combination of radon daughters in 1 liter of air that ultimately will result in the emission of 130,000 MeV of potential alpha energy.[27])

threshold, linear model is not applicable to the incidence of most radiogenic tumors.[126] Webster has suggested that "a linear-quadratic relation, when fitted to the human data, provides a reasonable and conservative basis for risk estimation".[126] Examples of dose-response curves, for three neoplasms, are shown in Figures 5.1, 5.2, and 5.3.

It is important to notice that some risk estimates refer to *tumor incidence*, others to *tumor death*. In the case of acute leukemia and other rapidly fatal neoplasms, there is little difference between incidence and mortality risks. For other neoplasms there is significant difference. For instance, thyroid cancer has a long survival, and its risk is best expressed in terms of incidence: as of 1980, it was estimated to be (overall) almost 4/million/year/rad for various exposed populations.[27]

FACTORS THAT INFLUENCE RISK

Numerous variables influence the risk of radiogenic neoplasia. Among these are: (1) age at time of exposure; (2) length of observation of the population; (3) characteristics of the radiation: electromagnetic *vs.* particulate; (4) source and type of exposure (external *vs.* internal, single dose *vs.* fractionated *vs.*

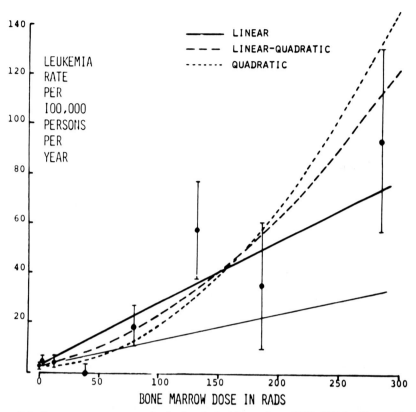

F<small>IG</small>. 5.1. Dose-response curves for leukemia incidence from 1950–1971 in Nagasaki A-bomb survivors. Age-adjusted rates are shown with SEs errors (68% confidence limits), based on data of Land[58] taken from Life Span Study sample.[51] *Lower solid line* represents slope of linear-quadratic curve at the origin (*i.e.*, at low doses). Reproduced with permission from E. W. Webster[126] and the *American Journal of Roentgenology* and the American Roentgen Ray Society (Williams & Wilkins, agent).

continuous); (5) rate of exposure; (6) dose; (7) characteristics of the population (*e.g.*, racial and environmental risk of nonradiogenic neoplasia) *etc.* Examples of these variables follow.

A<small>GE AT</small> T<small>IME OF</small> E<small>XPOSURE</small>

Incidence is affected by age at exposure. In general, it appears that the relative and absolute risks—for specific age-at-death intervals—tend to be higher for individuals exposed at a younger age, especially among the A-bomb survivors.[54, 75] The risk of leukemia among the A-bomb survivors was about three times higher for individuals who were less than 10 years of age at the time than for older individuals. Benign (and rare malignant) thyroid tumors have occurred in almost all of the victims of the heavy fallout from the Bikini test of 1954 who were less than 10 years old at the time.[75] The highest risk of radiation-induced breast cancer is for women exposed during the second decade of life.[27] Nevertheless, with the exception of leukemia—which has a shortened interval from exposure to death—radiation-induced cancers tend to appear in the same age groups of their spontaneous counterparts.[54]

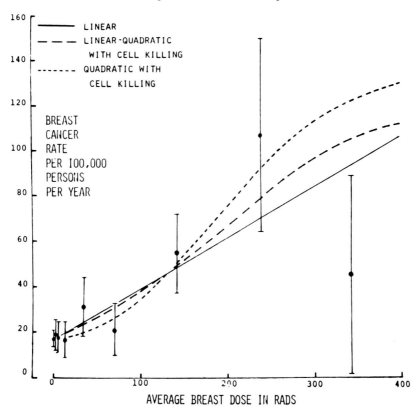

Fɪɢ. 5.2. Dose-response curves for breast cancer incidence from 1950–1974 in Nagasaki A-bomb survivors. Age-adjusted rates with SEs (68% confidence limits). Data taken from Land[58] and Tokunaga *et al.*[115] Highest dose point (586 rad) (5.86 Gy) is not shown on this plot. Reproduced with permission from E. W. Webster[126] and © *The American Journal of Roentgenology* and the American Roentgen Ray Society (Williams & Wilkins, agent).

CHARACTERISTICS OF THE RADIATION

Most studies show that radiation of high linear energy transfer (LET), such as alpha particles and neutrons, is more efficient as a carcinogen than low LET radiation (x-rays, gamma rays).[57, 120] For instance, it has been estimated that internal ^{32}P, a beta emitter, is 60 times more leukemogenic than external gamma radiation.[69] In the low-dose range, high LET radiation may be 10–20 times more oncogenic than x- or gamma radiation.[119, 120] These observations are supported by *in vitro* studies described below.[15]

There appears to be variation in the oncogenic effect of high-dose rate single exposure *vs.* fractionated exposure *vs.* low-dose rate continuous exposure. For instance, within the range of 30–300 rad, the incidence of breast carcinoma is much higher among women subjected to multiple fluoroscopies in Massachusetts (100 to 220 cases/100,000 women/year), than among A-bomb survivors who had a single exposure (30–75 cases/100,000 women/year).[27] It is unlikely that racial or environmental factors can account for such a difference. This variation, however, has not been adequately quantitated for most human tumors.

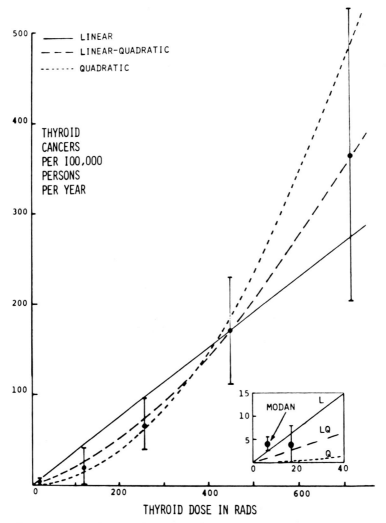

F IG. 5.3. Dose-response curves for thyroid cancer after childhood x-ray therapy to upper chest. Data from Hempelmann *et al.*[46] and Shore *et al.*[102] *Error bars* are 1 SE. Insert magnifies the relationships over the dose range 0–40 rad (0.4 Gy) and shows the point at 6.5 rad (0.065 Gy) deduced from the study by Modan *et al.*[76, 78] Reproduced with permission from E. W. Webster[126] and the *American Journal of Roentgenology* and the American Roentgen Ray Society (Williams & Wilkins, agent).

Total body exposures tend to induce certain types of neoplasms: initially, the most obvious neoplasm among the A-bomb survivors was leukemia. Currently, solid tumors (which seldom appear before an interval of 10 years) are of greater numerical significance than leukemia.[27] Those solid tumors include breast (in women), thyroid, lung, and alimentary tract carcinomas.[54] Regional or local exposures, as expected, induce neoplasms in the tissues where energy is absorbed. In this respect it is important to remember the lack of uniformity in the deposition of radionuclides, even within tissues that have high affinity for such isotopes. External radiation also can be inhomogeneous within a presumably uniform field.

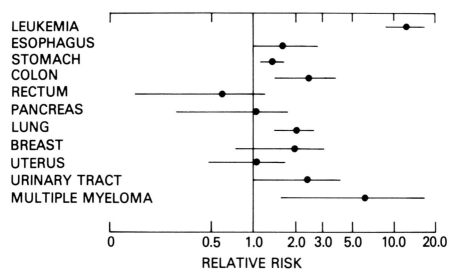

Fig. 5.4. Relative risk (and 90% confidence intervals) of *mortality* caused by neoplasms of various sites in atom bomb survivors who received at least 200 rad, as compared to the population that received 0 rad. These risk estimates are for the period of 1950 to 1978. Notice that there is no increased risk for uterus, pancreas, and rectum (although there is significant increase for the rest of the colon). This example of relative risk includes only some of the data in the original figure. Modified from H. Kato and W. J. Schull[54] and *Radiation Research*.

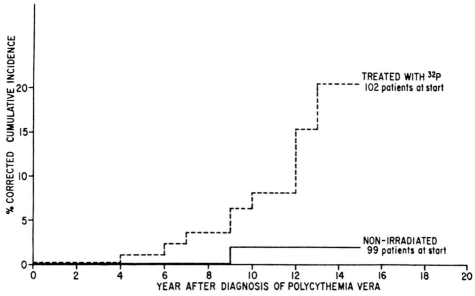

Fig. 5.5. Corrected cumulative incidence of leukemia in patients with polycythemia vera (data taken from B. Modan and A. M. Lilienfeld: *Medicine 44:* 305–344, 1965.) Correction is made for the decreasing number of patients at risk at each year after diagnosis using the method of Kaplan and Meier (J. Am. Stat. Assoc. *53:* 457, 1958). The final corrected cumulative incidence is 20% in the ^{32}P-treated patients, but only 2% in the nonirradiated patients, suggesting that about 90% of the leukemias in the ^{32}P-treated group were radiation-induced, with the other 10% due to other factors. Reproduced from *Health Physics*, Vol. 25, p. 589 by permission of the Health Physics Society and C. W. Mays.[69]

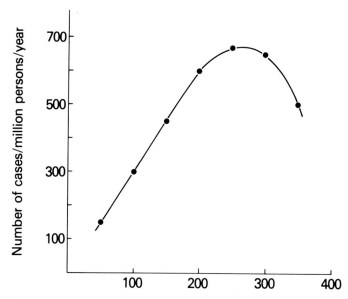

FIG. 5.6. Theoretical dose-incidence curve for a radiation-induced human neoplasm following a single total-body exposure, such as that suffered by Atom-bomb survivors. This curve assumes a relative risk of 3 additional cases/10^6 individuals/year/rad and a linear relation in the range between 50 and 200 rad. Below 50 rad the incidence is usually uncertain, and the linear relation often cannot be extrapolated.[126] Above 250 rad the incidence actually may decrease if it is assumed that high doses kill potentially neoplastic cells. There are few or no observations above 350 rad since this is the LD_{50} for total body irradiation under atomic warfare conditions.[35]

In general, for the well established group of human radiation-induced neoplasms (Table 5.2), the radiation dose has been in the intermediate range of 50 to 500 rad.[54, 75, 120, 126] It has been claimed that childhood neoplasms, especially leukemia, occur as the result of diagnostic (very low dose) radiological procedures while in utero.[65, 108] However, the induction of tumors by doses of radiation below 10 rad has been seriously questioned.[20, 22, 105, 121, 126] Neoplasms induced by local therapy for other tumors (*e.g.*, fractionated radiation, usually in the order of 3000–7000 rad) are clearly less common than those in the intermediate range[120] and, as discussed above, their relation to radiation is often very difficult to prove.[35]

These human observations fit well with the hypothesis that radiation oncogenesis requires a threshold of cell injury, beyond which the incidence of neoplastic transformation is proportional to dose, and up to a point where the number of potentially neoplastic cells killed by the radiation is equal to, or larger than, the number of neoplastically transformed cells. If this hypothesis is correct, the dose-incidence curve may have the shape illustrated in Figure 5.6.

In fact, curves reminiscent of that in Figure 5.6 have been obtained in experimental animals (Figs. 5.7 and 5.8) and in a few human neoplasms. Thyroid carcinoma, for instance, is clearly associated with *external* irradiation of 50–1500 rad, and between 100 and 500 rad it is dose dependent.[46, 84, 89, 94, 95] It is very rare after external exposures of more than 2000 rad[70] and essentially nonexistent following radioiodine treatment for hyperthyroidism, in which the

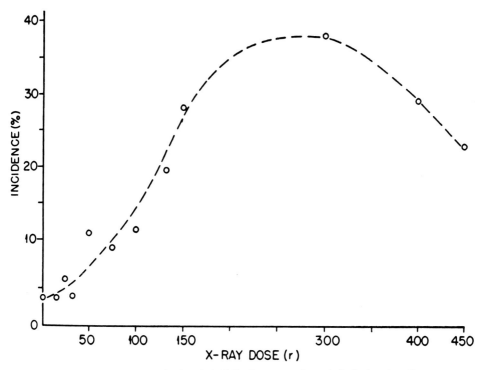

Fɪɢ. 5.7. Incidence of myeloid leukemia in RF mice exposed to whole-body x-irradiation at 5–10 weeks of age. Reproduced with permission from A. C. Upton[118] and *Cancer Research*.

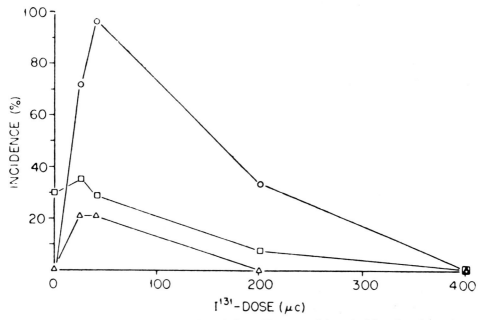

Fɪɢ. 5.8. Incidence of thyroid tumors in male Long-Evans rats injected with various doses of [131]I. Follicular adenoma(○). Alveolar carcinoma(□). Papillary and follicular carcinoma(△). Reproduced with permission from A. C. Upton[118] and *Cancer Research*.

local dose is in the order of 8000 rad[103] but can be as high as 30,000 rad. Furthermore, the incidence of neoplastic cell transformation *in vitro* (Figs. 5.9 and 5.10) may follow a type of curve similar to that of Figure 5.6.

LENGTH OF SURVEILLANCE

The importance of prolonged observation of the population at risk has been well recognized for the individuals harboring long-lived radioisotopes such as thorium dioxide: persons subjected to radiographic procedures using thorotrast as a contrast medium, prior to 1955, have shown a remarkably high incidence of liver tumors, such as cholangiocarcinomas, angiosarcomas, and hepatomas. Their risk starts 10 years later and continues for life. It is one of the highest risk coefficients for radiation carcinogenesis: 300 liver cancers/ millions/rad/per life.[27] Not until recently, however, was it appreciated that single exposures of external radiation could also produce neoplasms after a long delay: among the A-bomb survivors, increased incidence of colonic cancers was only observed 30–35 years later.[54]

The incidence of a neoplasm may also decline with time. As stated above, the overall absolute risk of leukemia among the A-bomb survivors was 1.72/mil-

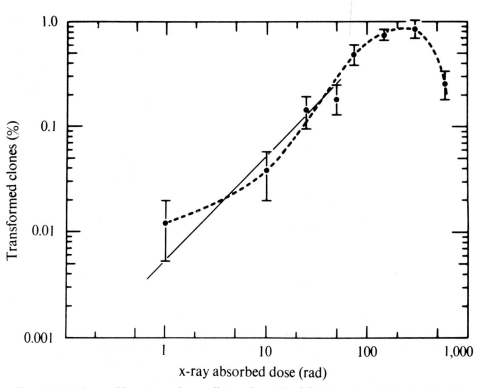

FIG. 5.9. Incidence of hamster embryo cell transformation following x-irradiation *in vitro*. The *broken line* is drawn by eye to the *mean data points*; the *solid line* has a slope of +1 and passes through the *error bars* of *each datum* point. Reprinted by permission from *Nature*, Vol. 243, pp. 450–453, Copyright(c) 1973, Macmillan Journals Limited, and C. Borek.

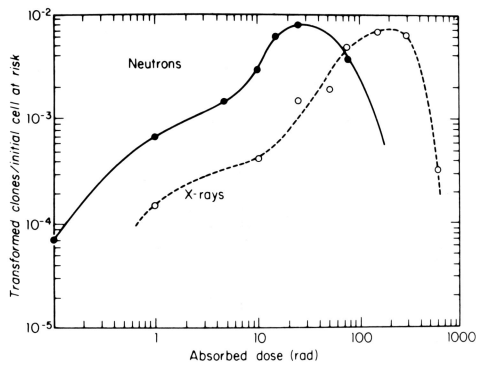

FIG. 5.10. Dose-response for *in vitro* neoplastic transformation of Golden hamster embryo cells. The number of transformed clones per initial cell at risk is plotted as a function of dose of neutrons or x-rays. Neutrons are considerably more efficient than x-rays as transforming agents in this system. Reproduced with permission from C. Borek, E. J. Hall, H. H. Rossi: *Cancer Res. 38:* 2997–3005, 1978.

lion/year/rad during the period from 1950 to 1978. This overall estimate, however, does not inform about the variation in risk related to time from exposure: the maximum incidence was 7 years after exposure (4.3/million/year/rad), and the incidence has since declined progressively; in the period from 1975 to 1978 the absolute risk was only 0.44/million/year/rad,[54] and it was only demonstrable in the Hiroshima survivors.

SEX, ETHNIC, AND GEOGRAPHIC CHARACTERISTICS

The tumors induced by radiation in humans tend to have the same sex, racial, and geographic distribution as the "spontaneous" neoplasms (in this context, tumors occurring in nonirradiated individuals). For instance, among 2215 individuals followed after receiving scalp doses of 450–850 rad (given during childhood for tinea capitis), there was an excess of carcinomas of the scalp (mainly, basal cell carcinomas) with an observed/expected ratio of 29:7.8.[27] No cancers, occurred, however, among the black patients, who comprised 25% of the group.[27] Spontaneous basal cell carcinomas of the skin are quite uncommon in blacks.

Lack of Specificity of Radiation-induced Neoplasms

As far as we know, there is no single tumor in humans that is exclusively, or even usually, produced by radiation. Furthermore, radiation-induced tumors represent only a small proportion of the total number of neoplasms occurring in a given organ or system.

In other mammals radiation produces a high yield of certain tumors. In mice, for instance, 50 rad of x-rays are sufficient to induce ovarian tumors,[119] and 87–350 R of total body exposure produce neoplasms of the ovary in almost 100% of animals so treated that survive to old age.[34] These tumors are of multiple histologic types: granulosa-cell tumor, tubular adenoma lutein-or-thecal tumors, mesothelioma, *etc.*[119] But spontaneous ovarian tumors also are common in old mice.[119]

Morphologically, the neoplasms induced by radiation are no different from those that occur in nonirradiated individuals. In some instances there is a greater proportion of a given type of neoplasm: livers exposed to decades of alpha particles from Thorotrast tend to develop cholangiocarcinomas and angiosarcomas rather than hepatomas.[35]

MECHANISMS OF RADIATION ONCOGENESIS

How does ionizing radiation generate neoplasia? Conceptually, radiation may be an *inducer,* or a *promoter,* or *both* (complete carcinogen). In fact, experimental data indicate that it may play—depending upon the neoplasm in each case—each of these roles.

Let us consider first the interaction of radiation with other oncogenic agents, then contemplate the possibility of direct carcinogenesis by ionizing radiation.

Radiation and Hormonal Regulation

The interaction of ionizing radiation with the endocrine system and/or exogenous hormones has been the subject of extensive research in the past. It is now well demonstrated that radiation may have an important, although often secondary, role in the promotion of neoplasms under hormonal control. Some examples follow.

Irradiation results in the production of mammary neoplasms in rats, often in large numbers.[100, 101] The yield of these neoplasms (mostly fibroadenomas and adenocarcinomas) can be increased by treatment with estrogen or decreased by ovariectomy.[122] Also mammotrophic pituitary tumors, which secrete prolactin, stimulate the production of such radiation-associated mammary neoplasms. The effects of hormones and radiation in the production of mammary neoplasms may be additive (or even occasionally synergistic[101]) in certain strains of rats exposed to diethylstilbestrol and x-radiation.[98, 101] Chemical carcinogens enhance this radiation effect in rats, but the interaction of these two agents with hormones appears to be different: both lactating and old rats lose responsiveness to chemical carcinogenesis, but they still develop mammary tumors in response to radiation.[101]

As indicated above, mice are extremely susceptible to induction of ovarian tumors by radiation. The tumor growth, however, is delayed many months, and it depends on stimulation by pituitary gonadotropins. In fact the shielding of one ovary, or the use of estrogen replacement therapy, inhibits the development of ovarian neoplasms.[119] A very high yield of neoplasms is obtained by irradiating the ovaries *in situ* and transplanting them intramuscularly into castrated mice.[29]

Some mouse strains with a tendency to undergo an early menopause spontaneously develop a high incidence of ovarian tumors. Therefore, the tumorigenic effect of radiation has been viewed as merely the production of an early menopause.[29, 119]

In vitro carcinogenesis is also the subject of hormonal influence: thyroid hormones (in the serum added to the medium) are essential for neoplastic transformation of normal hamster embryo fibroblasts.[15] Beta-estradiol added to the cultures enhances transformation.[15]

Pituitary tumors (thyrotropic) induced in mice by thyroid ablation with ^{131}I are examples of an *indirect* tumorigenic effect of radiation,[39] through an alteration in the hormonal feedback mechanisms.

RADIATION AND CHEMICAL CARCINOGENESIS

Evidence of interaction of these two different tumorigenic agents has been provided by *in vitro* and *in vivo* studies.

The rate of transformation of mouse embryo cells by x-rays is enhanced by exposure to the tumor promoter 12-O-tetradecanoyl-phorbol-13-acetate.[15, 55] Pretreatment of Syrian hamster cells with radiation enhances the frequency of transformations usually produced with chemical carcinogens such as benzo (*a*)pyrene.[32]

In 1942, McEndy *et al.* first showed the additive effects of methylcholanthrene and x-radiation on the induction of leukemia in mice.[71] The incidence of lymphoma and skin tumors in mice is increased by the interaction of chemical carcinogens and radiation.[119] In humans a likely candidate for this form of cooperation is pulmonary carcinoma. Both chemical carcinogens and radioactive elements occur in cigarette smoke: Radford and Hunt[85] demonstrated the presence of Polonium-210 in 1964. It appears that [210]Po and its precursor ^{210}Pb accumulate in the airways of cigarette smokers, particularly at bifurcations, delivering lifetime local doses (mainly of alpha radiation from [210]Po) in the order of 1600 rem.[66] Alpha radiation is 10–1000 times more carcinogenic than x-radiation,[129] and its contribution to bronchial oncogenesis may be quite significant. Whether or not it is as significant as that of the well-known polycyclic hydrocarbons, *N*-nitrosamines, and other chemical carcinogens known to be present in cigarette smoke is difficult to say. In fact, interaction between benzo (*a*)pyrene and [210]Po in the induction of lung cancer has been shown experimentally by Little *et al.*[63]

Radiation may not always necessarily potentiate chemical carcinogenesis.[119] In some experiments acute irradiation "consistently inhibited the oncogenic action of nitrogen mustard and urethan on the mouse lung".[81]

RADIATION AND THE IMMUNE RESPONSE

One of the oldest theories of oncogenesis is that tumors grow and kill the host because of failure of the "Immunological surveillance" (I-surveillance).

This concept initially proposed by Ehrlich in 1909[33] and developed by others[21] implies that incipient neoplasms are destroyed *in situ* by thymus-derived lymphocytes. The concept does not concern itself with the initial oncogenic mechanism(s) but only with the ability (or failure) to prevent the growth of small tumor clones, which possess antigenic characteristics different from those of the normal host cells.

It would seem appropriate, therefore, to expand this concept of radiation oncogenesis by speculating that one mechanism of radiation oncogenesis is an interference with I-surveillance, *e.g.*, by killing or altering T lymphocytes. This simplistic explanation may be incorrect.

In the first place the entire concept of I-surveillance as stated orginally is probably erroneous.[24, 80] Although cellular immune deficiency is associated in some cases with increased number of *certain* neoplasms (*e.g.*, Kaposi's sarcoma in AIDS patients), in most immunologically suppressed individuals is no increased incidence of neoplasms (nor is there in nude mice).[24] Furthermore, the immunosuppressed individuals who do develop neoplasms tend to have single, instead of multiple, tumors, as one might expect from a general failure of I-surveillance.[80] Other reasons militate against this concept. For instance, there is no increase in the incidence of neoplasms in patients afflicted by diseases such as leprosy and sarcoidosis, in whom there is significant immunosuppression.[24]

Radiation does interfere with both cellular and humoral immune responses.[4, 5] The magnitude of this effect depends upon many variables, the most important of which are total dose, the fractionation scheme and, especially, the extent of the irradiated area. In humans the greatest immune depression by radiation results from fractionated doses in the order of 4000–5000 rad, to the lymphatic tissues ("total lymphoid irradiation," as used for the treatment of lymphomas) or total body doses of 1000 rad (*e.g.*, prior to bone marrow grafts).

Total lymphatic irradiation does appear to be associated with a slightly increased incidence of neoplasms,[7, 8, 41, 48] but such tumors tend to be hematolymphoid, and, of course, they occur in individuals treated precisely for lymphomas. Furthermore, lymphoma—and other cancers—are spontaneously associated with immunologic deficiencies, independent of radiation.

The majority of radiation-induced neoplasms in humans have followed *local* doses of 50–500 rad, or *total body* doses of 50–300 rad. It is unlikely that such doses produce severe or permanent immune depression.[35] As far as I know, no evidence of significant or consistent immune deficiency has been demonstrated among the A-bomb survivors.[3]

Thus, it is unlikely that interference with immune response is an important mechanism of radiation oncogenesis, although it may play a role in some specific tumors. Even if this were the case, it would apply only to tumor *promotion* or to tumor *growth*, not to tumor *induction*. The initial mechanism(s) of cellular transformation appear to be independent of immune competence.

RADIATION AND VIRUSES

The extensive and elegant experiments of Henry S. Kaplan and collaborators in the 1950s and 1960s conclusively proved the interaction of radiation with viruses in the development of lymphatic murine leukemia.[52] Mice of the C57BL and other strains have a spontaneous, low-incidence rate of leukemia caused by viruses, which are vertically transmitted.[40, 52] Most animals harbor these latent leukemogenic viruses for life, without obvious ill effects. Exposure to radiation (or some chemical carcinogen) produced leukemias in an increased number of animals.[52] The incidence of radiation-induced leukemia was inversely proportional to age of the mice.[43] The optimal fractionation scheme was four total body exposures of 150–170 R given at weekly intervals.[43] Although the leukemia developed in the thymus, irradiation of the thymus alone did not initiate it. Furthermore, radiation leukemogenesis could be prevented by shielding the spleen or bone marrow, or by injecting isologous bone marrow after radiation.[43, 52] Thymic grafts restored the incidence of radiation leukemia in animals that had lost it by thymectomy.[53] Leukemia could be produced by injection of cell-free preparations from leukemias into isologous newborn mice or, even better, directly into the thymus of adult mice. X-radiation, given shortly after inoculation, markedly increased tumor incidence.[43] The agent was identified as an RNA tumor virus and was designated as the radiation leukemia virus (RadLV).[61] Although the yield of leukemia in irradiated mice was high (70–90%), the latent period before overt development of leukemia was long (90–200 days on the average).[43, 52, 61] Subsequently, Haran-Ghera[43] demonstrated preleukemic cells in the bone marrow of mice within 4 weeks after radiation.[43]

A large proportion of leukemias also develop in AKR mice infected with the closely related C-type RNA virus(es) discovered by Ludwik Gross[40]; these do not require radiation for a high tumor yield.[40, 52]

The mechanism of radiation oncogenesis in the lymphatic murine leukemia is poorly understood. It may be related to activation of the viruses (which has been demonstrated *in vitro*), and this in turn would produce cell transformation. Another hypothesis proposes that the cells containing the viruses normally have a repressor which restricts provirus transcription. Radiation would decrease the affinity of the repressor for the provirus, thus allowing transcription.[113] Cell division appears to be necessary for the expression of the activated provirus.[113] In either situation radiation would act as a promoter or "coleukemogenic" agent.[43]

The interaction of radiation and viruses has been considered in several other neoplasms (and in fact it may occur in many mammalian tumors), but documentation is not as extensive as in radiation murine leukemias. There is evidence of some interaction between radiation (especially from the bone-seeking nuclide strontium-90) and viruses in the development of osteosarcomas in mice.[38, 87] At least three presumably different viruses (FBJ, FBR, and RFB) have been implicated in the production of bone tumors in mice so irradiated.[87]

When there is proven cooperation between radiation and a virus in the genesis of a given tumor, a method to prevent such a tumor might be to immunize the host against the virus. This interesting approach has been used in the osteosarcoma system mentioned in the preceding paragraph. Vaccination with formalin-inactivated FBJ viruses successfully delayed the appearance of bone tumors in animals treated with ^{90}Sr.[87] Ultimately, however, the tumor incidence of vaccinated and nonvaccinated animals was not much different.

RADIATION AND HEREDITY

Radiation may increase the risk of neoplasms in individuals who have an inherited tendency to develop tumors.

In humans there are at least 40 inherited conditions associated with specific neoplasms, such as retinoblastoma.[57] There is information suggestive of risk enhancement for some of these neoplasms by ionizing radiation: several children with the hereditary multiple basal cell nevus syndrome have developed basal cell nevi concentrated in areas of prior irradiation for medulloblastoma.[74] The types of human leukemia induced by radiation are almost exclusively granulocytic, acute and chronic; both are associated with chromosomal abnormalities in a substantial number of cases[74] (see preceding chapter); this suggests interaction of a cytogenetic defect and radiation. Children irradiated for retinoblastoma, often develop orbital sarcomas in the field of therapy (as well as occasional sarcomas of bone in the unirradiated lower extremities).[74] There is also some *in vitro*, indirect evidence of increased susceptibility to radiation: for instance, fibroblasts obtained from patients with retinoblastoma and ataxia telangiectasia are more sensitive to radiation killing *in vitro*[6, 127] than those from normal individuals.

In some fish of the *Xiphophorus* genus (platyfish and swordtail), classic Mendelian techniques have demonstrated a gene responsible for the development of cancers in various tissues, including neuroblastoma.[57, 97] Under normal circumstances this gene appears to be repressed by regulating genes, which are tissue specific.[57] Radiation, and other agents (such as nitrosourea), may produce inhibition or deletion of the regulating genes, or translocation of the neoplastic gene, resulting in the development of periocular neuroblastoma[57, 97] and other neoplasms.

The interplay between genetic factors and radiation can be illustrated by a study on the incidence of mammary tumors in five genetically different strains of rats.[122] The investigators observed these groups of female rats for one year following a *uniform*, single total-body exposure of 50 rad of fission neutrons.[122] In the Sprague-Dawley and Long-Evans strains, 56% of the rats developed at least one mammary neoplasm; in the Fischer-344 and Buffalo strains the incidence was 25–29%; in the Wistar Lewis it was 5%. Among the 73 nonirradiated controls, only one tumor occurred in the same period of time. Adenocarcinomas comprised one-third of the tumors, and the rest were classified as fibroadenomas and "adenofibromas".[122] Similar observations had been made by other investigators.[101]

In this instance, it is possible that the genetic differences among these strains of rats relate to differences in hormonal levels or hormonal response, since it is known that mammary tumors are at least under estrogenic and prolactin control. (The interaction of hormones and radiation has already been discussed above.)

Additionally, there is now some evidence indicating that radiation may induce *heritable* tumors. Nomura[82] observed that x-ray doses of 36–504 rad (or urethane) given to ICR parent mice produced a dose-dependent increase in neoplasms in the progeny. Most tumors were papillary adenomas of the lung (87%) and the rest were various solid neoplasms, leukemias, *etc*.[82] To confirm this finding, male survivors of the F_1 progeny (there were many lethal abnormalities aside from tumors) were mated and their progeny examined: the F_2 and F_3 generations also showed an increase in tumors. Nomura's findings indicate a dominant pattern of inheritance, with approximately 40% penetrance.

The number of animals (2904 parents, 12,905 live born, 9645 fetuses) in this study, which took 14 years,[82] is one assurance of a solid statistical data base. The author, however, points out that this phenomenon might be characteristic of ICR mice.

Several of Nomura's observations on heritable tumors are consistent with the production of specific locus mutation by radiation.[88] It is important to reemphasize that, aside from tumors, the progeny mice developed multiple genetic abnormalities, often lethal.[82]

In vitro evidence "that DNA is the carrier of the radiation-induced transforming trait"[18] has been obtained by transfecting NIH/3T3 cells with DNA purified from x-ray-transformed mouse C3H/10T 1/2 cells.[18] The transformed cells overexpressed the oncogenes *c-abl*, *c-sis*, *cHa-ras*, and *B-lym-l*.[18]

Radiation as Inducer of Neoplasia

A considerable volume of information indicates that ionizing radiation can be a direct tumor inducer. Most of the important cellular effects of radiation occur in DNA. Therefore, it is quite possible that radiation carcinogenesis results from interaction of ionizing energy with genetic material, directly or through highly reactive radicals.

Since radiation cannot contribute additional genetic information to the cell (as viruses do), one has to postulate that the alteration of the genome would result from point mutations, or from deletions or rearrangements of the genetic material, or from a combination of these mechanisms. This could occur at the time of absorption of energy, or at the time of repair: if the usually efficient repair systems fail to reconstitute the original genetic sequences, an abnormal rearrangement might transform a normal cell into a neoplastic one.

The study of direct radiation oncogenesis has been greatly facilitated by *in vitro* techniques. It has been demonstrated that x-radiation can produce neoplastic transformation of normal mammalian cells in culture.[19] This cell transformation is shown best in fibroblast-like, diploid hamster embryo cells.[15] Human fibroblasts also can be transformed *in vitro*, but the number of transformed cells (clones) is lower than that of rodent cells for a given dose. Transformed cells have alterations in morphology (pleomorphism, *etc.*), growth pattern (increase in cell density, multilayering, *etc.*), nutrient requirements (decreased need for serum), surface components (such as glycoproteins), cytoskeleton, *etc.*[15] All of these characteristics, especially the growth pattern, make it possible to distinguish transformed cells. Some of them— such as surface changes—can be detected within 1 week after radiation.[16] Rather important is the fact that transformed cells survive much longer in continuous subcultures than the normal, eventually senescent diploid line from which they originated. In fact some become "immortal".[15] The unequivocal proof of transformation is the ability to grow as neoplasms when implanted into appropriate host animals.[15]

A series of experiments, mainly by Borek and collaborators, using *in vitro* transformation, have given important information about radiation carcinogenesis.[17] These *in vitro* studies have confirmed the *in vivo* observation that high LET radiation is more oncogenic than electromagnetic radiation (Figs. 5.9 and 5.10). This transformation is dose-dependent, and it is best demonstrated in the 10–150 rad range of single doses (Figs. 5.9 and 5.10). Beyond 300, rad transformations appear to *decrease* with dose.[15] Extrapolation to the low dose (<1 rad) range from the high dose range may be inaccurate (as it is in the human epidemiologic studies for less than 10 rad), and no extrapolation can be made from single-dose to fractionated radiation.[15]

In theory, the transformation could occur at any stage of the cell cycle, but there is information suggesting that some event(s) occurring during cell division are required for transformation.[14, 80] In fact, probably one or two divisions may be necessary to permanently establish the neoplastic state.[14, 19]

Several agents that enhance transformation have been identified: some are hormonal (beta-estradiol); others are known carcinogens, such as benzopyrene. Miscellaneous agents include pyrolysate products, the phorbol ester derivative 12-O-tetradecanoyl-phorbol 13-acetate (TPA), etc. Antipain (a protease inhibitor) also enhances transformation when added *prior* to radiation.[15] It has also been observed that thyroid hormones contained in the serum enriching the medium are essential for transformation.[15]

Conversely, several compounds inhibit transformation *in vitro*: these include analogs of vitamin A (retinoids), selenium, the free radical scavenger superoxide dismutase (SOD), catalase, and also Antipain added *after* radiation.[15]

Various end-points have been used to study the effects of initiators, promoters (cocarcinogens), and inhibitors in the process of *in vitro* transformation. These include the study of chromosomal aberrations, analysis of sister chromatid exchanges, determination of ploidy (unfortunately, most hamster and human cells remain diploid, or nearly diploid after transformation), determination of cytoskeletal changes, and evaluation of the cell surface expressions of DNA damage, some morphologic, some chemical (*e.g.*, alterations in the levels of the sodium transport enzyme Na^+/K^+ ATPase).[15]

At present, the molecular events of malignant cell transformation by radiation are unknown. Among the various chromosomal changes postulated are: damage to specific genes, gene amplification, chromosomal imbalance, and disproportional DNA replication.[15] Deletion of a regulating gene that normally represses the expression of oncogenes is one possible mechanism, already suggested by the studies in fish mentioned above.[57, 97]

Some experiments suggest that the genetic alterations in radiation oncogenesis are different from those of viral-induced transformation. For instance, the cellular oncogene *C-mos* and the *V-mos* viral oncogene have been studied in cells transformed either by a virus (Moloney murine sarcoma virus, Mo-MSV) or by radiation.[128] In the virus-transformed cells the *V-mos* sequence was integrated at new sites within the host genome, was undermethylated, and was extensively transcribed. In the radiation (or chemical carcinogen)-transformed cells, the *C-mos* sequence was not rearranged, was hypermethylated, and was transcriptionally silent.[128]

A recent experiment that may shed some light on radiation carcinogenesis was based on the fact that high molecular weight DNA from some primary tumors or from tumor cell lines can transform rodent cultured cells.[42] The investigators used DNA from mouse thymic lymphomas induced either with *N*-nitrosomethyl urea or with radiation (600 rad in four weekly fractions). Both types of tumoral DNA transformed NIH 3T3 and Rat-2 cells. The transformed cells contained extra copies of the *C-ras* gene family, but these were different for the two forms of induction: while all of the carcinogen-induced tumors activated the *N-ras* gene, the radiation-induced tumors activated the *K-ras* gene.[42] The *K-ras* gene is the cellular counterpart of the viral *ras* oncogene in the Kirsten murine sarcoma virus.[42] The transformed cells also showed increased transcription for the activated genes.

In vitro transformation studies suggest that the mechanisms of cell repair may differ from those of cell transformation.[15] Cell mutation, which can be produced by radiation, is not necessarily associated with transformation, and "transformation cannot be equated with mutagenesis".[15]

Genetic alterations occurring in a single cell, and leading to the formation of a single clone of transformed neoplastic cells, is a plausible explanation for the monoclonality of many neoplasms, but it may not explain all the known facts about carcinogenesis in general or radiation oncogenesis in particular.

CONCLUSIONS

Obviously, the most immediate practical application of the above body of information is to reduce the possibility of radiogenic cancer.

Some controllable risks have been abolished, at least in most industrialized countries. The use of radiotherapy for benign conditions such as acne or tinea capitis is no longer acceptable. Contemporary diagnostic radiology equipment has reduced to a minimum the radiation exposure to patients and operators and multiple fluoroscopies are seldom needed. Thorotrast is not used anymore. Diagnostic radiology *in utero* is avoided at all costs.

Other risks have been decreased but not eliminated. In countries with effective health programs, miners are monitored for radiation exposure (*e.g.*, from radon daughters) and allowed to work underground for only a limited number of days per year. International agreements have curtailed ground testing of nuclear weapons and most (but unfortunately not all) "atomic" countries carry out only underground testing. Most manufacturers and users of radioactive isotopes have strict codes for handling and disposal (although the control of isotopes in some developing countries is pitiful!).

Certain risks cannot be eliminated, at least at the present time. Radiation therapy, for instance, is a very valuable cancer treatment modality. Since, as indicated above, the oncogenic potential of kilorad doses is low, in the case of radiotherapy the benefits greatly outweigh the carcinogenic risks.

Although the proportion of cancer deaths attributable to man-made radiation is low (<1.5% in the USA), the prevention of even this number of tumors is worth a strong radiation-control program. Furthermore, oncogenesis is only one of the effects of radiation, and one has to consider that the burden of neoplasms and other complications would be much higher if some degree of exposure control had not existed all along in the USA.

So one corollary of our knowledge of radiation oncogenesis is prevention. What about the populations that have already acquired the risk? Our knowledge of the neoplasms that they may develop and the periods of latency permit careful monitoring of each individual known to be exposed. This should allow early therapy of tumors like carcinomas of breast, thyroid, and colon, and some sarcomas. Patients with other neoplasms obviously may not benefit, *e.g.*, acute myeloid leukemia.

The predictable and long period of latency may be used in the future more practically if one considers that factors other than radiation contribute to many "radiogenic" neoplasms. Of these factors, hormones, chemical carcinogens, and viruses might be amenable to manipulations that eliminate or render them inactive, thus decreasing the risk. For instance, as described above, vaccination against oncogenic viruses might prevent neoplasms that result from viral-radiation cooperation.

Of course, the ultimate therapy would be the modification of the genetic structure of the cells at risk. Such an approach would suppose the ability to: identify the potentially oncogenic cells; detect the abnormal genetic sequences (*i.e.*, oncogenes); delete or neutralize them. Obviously, this ideal and "futuristic" therapy would apply to neoplasia of almost any etiology, and because of the rapid advances in DNA technology, it may not be an unrealistic long-range goal.

ACKNOWLEDGMENTS

Drs. Carmia Borek (Columbia University), Errol C. Friedberg, and Jeffrey L. Sklar (Stanford University) kindly reviewed this chapter and made useful suggestions. Donna L. Buckley provided valuable secretarial assistance.

REFERENCES

1. Albert, R. E., Omran, A. R., Brauer, E. W., Dove, D. C., Cohen, N. C., Schmidt, H., Baumring, R., Morrill, S., Schultz, R., and Baer, R. L. Follow-up study of patients treated by x-ray for tinea capitis. *Am. J. Publ. Health 56:* 2114–2120, 1966.
2. Alderson, M. R., and Jackson, S. M. Long term follow-up of patients with menorrhagia treated by irradiation. *Br. J. Radiol. 44:* 295–299, 1971.
3. Anderson, R. E. V. Immunopathology (Symposium on delayed consequences of exposure to ionizing radiation. Pathology studies at the Atomic Bomb Casualty Commission, Hiroshima and Nagasaki, 1945–1970). *Hum. Pathol. 2:* 563–566, 1971.
4. Anderson, R. E. and Standefer, J. C. Radiation injury of the immune system. In: *Cytotoxic Insult to Tissue: Effects on Cell Lineages*, edited by C. S. Potten and J. H. Hendry. London, Churchill Livingstone, in press, 1981.
5. Anderson, R. E. and Warner, N. L. Ionizing radiation and the immune response. *Adv. Immunol. 24:* 215–235, 1976.
6. Arlett, C. F., and Harcourt, S. A. Survey of radiosensitivity in a variety of human cell strains. *Cancer Res. 40:* 926–932, 1980.
7. Armitage, J. O., Dick, F. R., Goeken, J. A., Foucar, M. K., and Gingrich, R. D. Second lymphoid malignant neoplasms occurring in patients treated for Hodgkin's disease. *Arch. Int. Med. 143:* 445–450, 1983.
8. Arsenau, J. C., Sponzo, R. W., Levin, D. L., Schnipper, L. E., Bonner, H., Young, R. C., Canellos, G. P., Johnson, R. E., and DeVita, V. T. Nonlymphomatous malignant tumors complicating Hodgkin's disease. *N. Engl. J. Med. 287:* 1119–1122, 1972.

9. Beebe, G. W., Kato, H., and Land, C. E. Studies on the Mortality of A-bomb survivors. VI. Mortality and radiation dose, 1950–1974. *Radiat. Res. 75:* 138–201, 1978.

10. Belsky, J. L., Tachikawa, K., Cihak, R. W., and Yamamoto, T. Salivary gland tumors in atomic bomb survivors, Hiroshima-Nagasaki, 1957 to 1970. *J.A.M.A. 219:* 864–868, 1972.

11. Berlin, N. I., and Wasserman, L. R. The association between systemically administered radioisotopes and subsequent malignant disease. *Cancer 37:* 1097–1101, 1976.

12. Bithell, J. F., and Stewart, A. M. Prenatal irradiation and childhood malignancy: A review of British data from the Oxford survey. *Br. J. Cancer 31:* 271–287, 1975.

13. Bizzozero, O. J., Johnson, K. G., and Ciocco, A. Radiation-related leukemia in Hiroshima and Nagasaki. I. Distribution, incidence and appearance time. *N. Engl. J. Med. 274:* 1095–1101, 1966.

14. Borek, C. *In vitro* transformation by low doses of x-radiation and neutrons. In: *Biology of Radiation Carcinogenesis*, edited by J. M. Yuhas, R. W. Tennant, and J. D. Regan New York, Raven Press, 1976, pp. 309–326.

15. Borek, C. Radiation oncogenesis in cell culture. *Adv. Cancer Res. 37:* 159–232, 1982.

16. Borek, C., and Fenoglio, C. M. Scanning electron microscopy of surface features of hamster embryo cells transformed in vitro by x-irradiation. *Cancer Res. 36:* 1325–1334, 1976.

17. Borek, C., Hall, E. J., and Zaider, M. X-rays may be twice as potent as gamma-rays for malignant transformation at low doses. *Nature 301:* 156–158, 1983.

18. Borek, C., Ong, A., Bresser, J., and Gillespie, D. Transforming activity of DNA of radiation transformed cells and identification of activated oncogenes in the donor cells (abstr.). *Proc. Am. Assoc. Cancer Res. 25:*100, 1984.

19. Borek, C., and Sachs, L. Cell susceptibility to transformation by x-irradiation and fixation of the transformed state. *Proc. Natl. Acad. Sci. USA 57:* 1522–1527, 1967.

20. Brent, R. L. Cancer risks following diagnostic radiation exposure (commentary). *Pediatrics 71:* 288–289, 1983.

21. Burnet, F. M. Immunological surveillance in neoplasia. *Transplant Rev. 7:* 3–68, 1971.

22. Caldwell, G. G., Kelley, D., Zack, M., Falk, H., and Heath, C. W. Mortality and cancer frequency among military nuclear test (Smoky) participants, 1957 through 1979. *J.A.M.A. 250:* 620–624, 1983.

23. Cannon, B., Randolph, J. G., and Murray, J. E. Malignant irradiation for benign conditions. *N. Engl. J. Med. 260:* 197–202, 1959.

24. Castro, J. E. An overview of tumour immunology and immunotherapy. In: *Immunological Aspects of Cancer*, edited by J. E. Castro. Baltimore, Universary Park Press, 1978, pp. 1–14.

25. Christensson, T. Hyperparathyroidism and radiation therapy. *Ann. Intern. Med. 89:* 216–217, 1978.

26. Cole, A. R. C., and Darte, J. M. Osteochondromata following irradiation in children. *Pediatrics 32:* 285–288, 1963.

27. Committee on the Biological Effects of Ionizing Radiations. *The Effects on Populations of Exposure to Low Levels of Ionizing Radiation: 1980.* National Research Council-National Academy Press, Washington, D.C., 1980, pp. 265–476.

28. Court-Brown, W. M., and Doll, R. Mortality from cancer and other causes after radiotherapy for ankylosing spondylitis. *Br. Med. J. 2:* 1327–1332, 1965.

29. Covelli, V., Di Majo, V., Bassani, B., Metalli, P., and Silini, G. Radiation-induced tumors in transplanted ovaries. *Radiat. Res. 90:* 173–187, 1982.

30. Cuzick, J. Radiation-induced myleomatosis. *N. Engl. J. Med. 304:* 204–210, 1981.

31. Czesnin, K., and Wronkowski, Z. Second malignancies of the irradiated area in patients treated for uterine cervix cancer. *Gynecol. Oncol. 6:* 309–315, 1978.

32. Di Paolo, J. A. *In-vitro* transformation: Interactions of chemical carcinogens and radiation. In: *Biology of Radiation Carcinogenesis*, edited by J. M. Yuhas, R. W. Tennant, and J. D. Regan. New York, Raven Press, 1976, pp. 335–342.

33. Ehrlich, P. (cited by Moller in Ref. 80).

34. Errera, M., and Forssberg, A. *Mechanisms in Radiobiology*, New York, Academic Press, 1960.

35. Fajardo, L. F. *Pathology of Radiation Injury* New York, Masson Publishing USA, 1982.

36. Fajardo, L. F., and Berthrong, M. Radiation injury in surgical pathology. Part I. *Am. J. Surg. Pathol. 2:*159–199, 1978.

37. Finkel, A. J., Miller, C. E., and Hasterlik, R. J. Radium induced malignant tumors in man. In: *Semi-Annual Report to the Atomic Commission of Argonne Cancer Research Hospital*, Sept. 1968, pp. 69–91.
38. Finkel, M. P., and Reilly, C. A. Observations suggesting the viral etiology of radiation-induced tumors, particularly osteogenic sarcomas. In: *Radionuclide Carcinogenesis*, Vol. 29, edited by C. L. Sanders, R. H. Busch, J. E. Ballou, and D. D. Malhum. Springfield, Va., U.S. Atomic Energy Commission Symposium Series, 1973, pp. 278–288.
39. Furth, J., Haran-Ghera, N., Curtis, H. J., and Buffett, R. F. Studies on the pathogenesis of neoplasms by ionizing radiation. I. Pituitary tumors. *Cancer Res. 19:* 550–556, 1959.
40. Gross, L. *Oncogenic Viruses, Ed. 2.* New York, Pergamon Press, 1970.
41. Grunwald, H. W., and Rasner, F. Acute myeloid leukemia following treatment of Hodgkin's disease: A review. *Cancer 50:* 676–683, 1982.
42. Guerrero, I., Calzada, P., Mayer, A., and Pellicer, A. A molecular approach to leukemogenesis: Mouse lymphomas contain an activated *c-ras* oncogene. *Proc. Natl. Acad. Sci. USA 81:* 202–205, 1984.
43. Haran-Ghera, N. Pathways in murine radiation leukemogenesis-coleukemogenesis. In: *Biology of Radiation Carcinogenesis*, edited by J. M. Yuhas, R. W. Tennant, and J. D. Regan. New York, Raven Press, 1976, pp. 245–260.
44. Hasson, J., Hartman, K. S., Milikow, E., and Mittleman, J. A. Thorotrast-induced extraskeletal osteosarcoma of the cervical region. *Cancer 36:* 1827–1833, 1975.
45. Hempelman, L. H. Risk of thyroid neoplasms after irradiation in childhood. *Science 160:* 159–163, 1968.
46. Hempelman, L. H., Hall, W. J., Phillips, M., Cooper, R. A., and Ames, W. R. Neoplasms in persons treated with x-rays in infancy. *J. Natl. Cancer Inst. 55:*519–530, 1975.
47. Hutchinson, G. B. Leukemia in patients with cancer of the cervix uteri treated with radiation—A report covering the first 5 years of an international study. *J. Natl. Cancer Inst. 40:* 951–982, 1968.
48. Hutchinson, G. B. Late neoplastic changes following medical irradiation. *Cancer 37:* 1102–1107, 1976.
49. Ichimaru, M., Ishimaru, T., Mikami, M., *et al.* Multiple myeloma among atomic bomb survivors and controls in Hiroshima and Nagasaki, 1950–1976. Hiroshima, Radiation Effects Research Foundation, Report No. 9–79, 1979, pp. 9–79.
50. Ishimaru, T., and Finch, S. C. More on radiation exposure and multiple myeloma (letter to the editor). *N. Engl. J. Med. 301:* 439–440, 1979.
51. Ishimaru, T., Otake, M., and Ichimaru, M. Dose-response relationship of neutrons and gamma rays to leukemia incidence among atomic-bomb survivors in Hiroshima and Nagasaki by type of leukemia, 1950–1971. *Radiat, Res. 77:* 377–394, 1979.
52. Kaplan, H. S. On the natural history of the murine leukemias. *Cancer Res. 27:* 1325–1340, 1967.
53. Kaplan, H. S., Carnes, W. H., Brown, M. B., and Hirsch, B. B. Indirect induction of lymphomas in irradiated mice. I. Tumor incidence and morphology in mice bearing non-irradiated thymic grafts. *Cancer Res. 16:* 422–425, 1956.
54. Kato, H., and Schull, W. J. Studies of the mortality of A-bomb survivors. 7. Mortality, 1950–1978. Part I. Cancer mortality. *Radiat. Res. 90:* 395–432, 1982.
55. Kennedy, A. R., Mondal, S., Heidelberger, C., and Little, J. B. Enhancement of x-ray transformation by 12-O-tetradecanoyl-phorbol-13-acetate in a cloned line of C3H mouse embryo cells. *Cancer Res. 38:* 439–443, 1978.
56. Key, C. R. Carcinoma of the thyroid. Symposium on delayed consequences of exposure to ionizing radiation (atomic bomb survivors). *Hum. Pathol. 2:* 521–523, 1971.
57. Kohn, H. I., and Fry, R. J. M. Radiation carcinogenesis. *N. Engl. J. Med. 310:* 504–511, 1984.
58. Land, C. E. Estimating cancer risks from low doses of ionizing radiation. *Science 209:* 1197–1203, 1980.
59. Lewis, E. B. Leukemia, multiple myeloma and aplastic anemia in American radiologists. *Science 142:* 1492–1494, 1963.
60. Li, F. P., Cassady, J. R., and Jaffe, N. Risk of second tumors in survivors of childhood cancer. *Cancer 35:* 1230–1235, 1975.

61. Lieberman, M., Kaplan, H. S., and Decleve, A. Anomalous viral expression in radiogenic lymphomas of C57BL/Ka mice. In: *Biology of Radiation Carcinogenesis*, edited by J. M. Yuhas, R. W. Tennant, and J. D. Regan. New York, Raven Press, 1976, pp. 237–244.

62. Lindsay, S., and Chaikoff, I. L. The effects of irradiation on the thyroid gland with particular references to the induction of thyroid neoplasms: A review. *Cancer Res. 24:* 1099–2017, 1964.

63. Little, J. B., Kennedy, A. R., and McGandy, R. B. Lung cancer induced in hamsters by low doses of alpha radiation from [210] Polonium. *Science 188:* 737–738, 1975.

64. MacKenzie, I. Breast cancer following multiple fluoroscopies. *Br. J. Cancer 19:* 1–8, 1965.

65. MacMahon, B. Prenatal x-ray exposure and childhood cancer. *J. Natl. Cancer Inst. 28:* 1173–1191, 1962.

66. Martell, E. A. Radioactivity in cigarette smoke (letter to the editor). *N. Engl. J. Med. 307:* 309–310, 1982.

67. Martin, H., Strong, E., and Spiro, R. H. Radiation-induced cancer of the head and neck. *Cancer 25:* 61–71, 1970.

68. Maurer, R., and Egloff, B. Malignant peritoneal mesothelioma after cholangiography with thorotrast. *Cancer 36:* 1381–1385, 1975.

69. Mays, C. W. Cancer induction in man from internal radioactivity. *Health Phys. 25:* 585–592, 1973.

70. McDougall, I. R., Coleman, C. N., Burke, J. S., Saunders, W., and Kaplan, H. S. Thyroid carcinoma after high-dose external radiotherapy for Hodgkin's disease. Report of three cases. *Cancer 45:* 2056–2060, 1980.

71. McEndy, D. P., Boon, M. C., and Furth, J. Induction of leukemia in mice by methylcholan-threne and x-rays. *J. Natl. Cancer Inst. 3:* 227–247, 1942.

72. McGregor, D. H., Land, C. E., Choi, K., Tokuoka, S., Liu, P. I., Wakabayashi, T., and Beebe, G. W. Breast cancer incidence among atomic bomb survivors. Hiroshima and Nagasaki, 1950–1969. *J. Natl. Cancer Inst. 59:* 799–811, 1977.

73. Meadows, A. T., Strong, I. C., Li, F. P., D'Angio, G. J., Schweisguth, O., Freeman, A. I., Jenkin, R. D. T., Morris-Jones, P., and Nesbit, M. E. Bone sarcoma as a second malignant neoplasm in children: Influence of radiation and genetic predisposition. *Cancer 46:* 2603–2606, 1980.

74. Miller, R. W. The feature in common among persons at high risk of leukemia. In: *Biology of Radiation Carcinogenesis*, edited by J. M. Yuhas, R. W. Tennant, and J. D. Regan. New York, Raven Press, 1976, pp. 45–50.

75. Miller, R. W. Radiation effects: Highlights of a meeting. *J. Pediatr. 101:* 887–888, 1982.

76. Modan, B., Baidatz, D., Mart, H., Steinitz, R., and Levin, S. G. Radiation-induced head and neck tumors. *Lancet 1:* 277–279, 1974.

77. Modan, B., and Lilienfield, A. M. Leukemogenic effect of ionizing-irradiation treatment in polycythemia. *Lancet 2:* 439–441, 1964.

78. Modan, B., Ron, E., and Werner, A. Thyroid cancer following scalp irradiation. *Radiology 123:* 741–744, 1977.

79. Mole, R. H. The radiobiological significance of the studies with [224]Ra and thorotrast (surveys in Denmark, Portugal and Germany). *Health Phys. 35:* 167–174, 1978.

80. Moller, G. and Moller, E. Immunological surveillance against neoplasia. In: *Immunological Aspects of Cancer*, edited by J. E. Castro. Baltimore, University Park Press, 1978, pp. 206–217.

81. Mori-Chavez, P., Upton, A. C., Salazar, M., and Conklin, J. W. Influence of altitude on late effects of radiation in RF/Un mice: Observations on survival time, blood changes, body weight and incidence of neoplasms. *Cancer Res. 30:* 913–928, 1970.

82. Nomura, T. Parental exposure to x-rays and chemicals induces heritable tumours and anomalies in mice. *Nature 296:* 575–577, 1982.

83. Norris, H. J., and Taylor, H. D. Postirradiation sarcomas of the uterus. *Obstet. Gynecol. 26:* 689–694, 1965.

84. Pillay, R., Graham-Pole, J., Miraldi, F., Yulish, B., Newman, A., and Libman, J. Diagnostic x-irradiation as a possible etiologic agent in thyroid neoplasms of childhood. *J. Pediatr. 101:* 566–568, 1982.

85. Radford, E. P., and Hunt, R. Polonium-210: A volatile radioelement in cigarettes. *Science 143:* 247–249, 1964.
86. Radford, E. P., and St. Clair Renard, K. G. Lung cancer in Swedish iron miners exposed to low doses of radon daughters. *N. Engl. J. Med. 310:* 1485–1494, 1984.
87. Reif, A. E., and Triest, W. E. Vaccination against ^{90}Strontium-induced bone tumors. *J. Natl. Cancer Inst. 71:* 545–552, 1983.
88. Roberts, P. B. Heritable cancer and radiation risks. *Health Phys. 45:* 798–801, 1983.
89. Ron, E., and Modan, B. Benign and malignant thyroid neoplasms after childhood irradiation for tinea capitis. *J. Natl. Cancer Inst. 65:* 7–11, 1980.
90. Rowland, R. E., Stehney, A. F., and Lucas, H. F. Dose-response relationships for female radium dial workers. *Radiat. Res. 76:* 368–383, 1978.
91. Saccomanno, G., Archer, V. E., Auerbach, O., Kuschner, M., Saunders, R. P., and Klein, M. G. Histologic types of lung cancer among uranium miners. *Cancer 27:* 515–523, 1971.
92. Sagan, L. Salivary gland tumors in atomic bomb survivors. (letter to the editor). *J.A.M.A. 220:* 7238, 1972.
93. Samet, J. M., Kutvirt, D. M., Waxweiler, R. J., and Key, C. R. Uranium mining and lung cancer in Navajo men. *N. Engl. J. Med. 310:* 1481–1484, 1984.
94. Sandler, D. P., Comstock, G. W., and Matanoski, G. M. Neoplasms following childhood radium irradiation of the nasopharynx. *J. Natl. Cancer Inst. 68:* 3–8, 1982.
95. Schneider, A. B., Fabus, M. J., Strachura, M. E., Arnold, J., Arnold, M. J., and Frohman, L. A. Incidence, prevalence and characteristics of radiation-induced thyroid tumors. *Am. J. Med. 64:* 243–252, 1978.
96. Schottenfeld, D. Radiation as a risk factor in the natural history of colorectal cancer (editorial). *Gastroenterology 84:* 186–187, 1983.
97. Schwab, M., Kollinger, G., Haas, J., Ahuja, M. R., Abdo, S., Anders, A., and Anders, F. Genetic basis of susceptibility for neuroblastoma following treatment with *N*-methyl-*N*-nitrosourea and x-rays in *Xiphophorus. Cancer Res. 39:* 519–526, 1979.
98. Segaloff, A., and Maxfield, W. S. The synergism between radiation and estrogen in the production of mammary cancer in the rat. *Cancer Res. 31:* 166–168, 1971.
99. Sener, S. F., and Scanlon, E. F. Irradiation induced salivary gland neoplasia. *Ann. Surg. 191:* 304–306, 1980.
100. Shellabarger, C. J. Radiation carcinogenesis: Laboratory studies. *Cancer 37:* 1090–1096, 1976.
101. Shellabarger, C. J. Modifying factors in rat mammary gland carcinogenesis. In: *Biology of Radiation Carcinogenesis*, edited by J. M. Yuhas, R. W. Tennant, and J. D. Regan. New York, Raven Press, 1976, pp. 31–43.
102. Shore, R. E., Hempelmann, L. H., Kowaluk, E., Mansur, P. S., Pasternack, B. S., Albert, R. E., and Haughie, G. E. Breast neoplasms in women treated with x-rays for acute post partum mastitis. *J. Natl. Cancer Inst. 59:* 813–822, 1977.
103. Silver, S. *Radioactive Nuclides in Medicine and Biology.* Philadelphia, Lea and Febiger, 1968, p. 165.
104. Smith, P. G., and Doll, R. Late effects of x-irradiation in patients treated for metropathia hemorrhagica. *Br. J. Radiol. 49:* 224–232, 1976.
105. Spengler, R. F., Cook, D. H., Clarke, E. A., Olley, P. M., and Newman, A. M. Cancer mortality following cardiac catherization: A preliminary followup study on 4891 irradiated children. *Pediatrics 71:* 235–239, 1982.
106. Spiess, H., and Mays, C. W. Bone cancers induced by radium-224 (Th X) in children and adults. *Health Phys. 19:* 713–729, 1970.
107. Spjut, H. J., Dorfman, H. D., Fechner, R. D., and Ackerman, L. V. *Tumors of Bone and Cartilage.* In: *Atlas of Tumor Pathology*, (Fasc. 5). Washington, D.C., Armed Forces Institute of Pathology, 1971, pp. 65–193.
108. Stewart, A., and Kneale, G. W. Radiation dose effects in relation to obstetric x-rays and childhood cancers. *Lancet 1:* 1185–1188, 1970.

109. Stewart, A., Webb, J., and Hewitt, D. A survey of childhood malignancies. *Br. Med. J. 1:* 1495–1508, 1958.

110. Strong, L. C., Herson, J., Osborne, B. M., and Wataru, W. S. Risk of radiation-related subsequent malignant tumors in survivors of Ewing's sarcoma. *J. Natl. Cancer Inst. 62:* 1401–1408, 1979.

111. Swarm, R. L. Late effects following the medical uses of colloidal thorium dioxide. In: *Medical Radionuclides—Radiation Dose and Effects*, edited by R. J. Cloutier, C. L. Edwards, and W. S. Snyder. AEC Symposium Series No. 20, 1970, pp. 387–398.

112. Takeichi, N., Hirose, F., Yamamoto, H., Ezaki, H., and Fujikura, T. Salivary gland tumors in atomic bomb survivors, Hiroshima, Japan. II. Pathologic study and supplementary epidemiologic study and supplementary epidemiologic observations. *Cancer 52:* 377–385, 1983.

113. Tennant, R. W., Otten, J. A., Quarles, J. M., Yang, W-K., and Brown, A. Cellular factors that regulate radiation activation and restriction of mouse leukemia viruses. In: *Biology of Radiation Carcinogenesis* edited by J. M. Yuhas, R. W. Tennant, and J. D. Regan. New York, Raven Press, 1976, pp. 227–235.

114. Tisell, L. E., Hansson, G., Lindberg, S., and Ragnhult, I. Hyperparathyroidism in persons treated with x-rays for tuberculous cervical adenitis. *Cancer 40:* 846–854, 1977.

115. Tokunaga, M., Norman, J. E., Asano, M., Tokuoka, S., Ezaki, H., Nishimori, I., and Tsuji, Y. Malignant breast tumors among atomic bomb survivors, Hiroshima and Nagasaki, 1950–1974. *J. Natl. Cancer Inst. 62:* 1347–1359, 1979.

116. Tountas, A. A., Fornasier, V. L., Harwood, A. R., and Leung, P. M. K. Postirradiation sarcoma of bone: A perspective. *Cancer 43:* 182–187, 1979.

117. Triggs, S. M., and Williams, E. D. Irradiation of the thyroid as a cause of parathyroid adenoma. *Lancet 1:* 593–594, 1977.

118. Upton, A. C. The dose-response relation in γ-radiation-induced cancer. *Cancer Res. 21:* 717–729, 1961.

119. Upton, A. C. Radiation and carcinogenesis. *An Acad. Bras. Cienc. 39:* 129–161, 1967.

120. Upton, A. C. Radiation carcinogenesis. *Front. Radiat. Ther. Oncol. 6:* 470–478, 1972.

121. Upton, A. C. The biological effects of low-level ionizing radiation. *Sci. Am. 246:* 41–49, 1982.

122. Vogel, H. H., and Turner, J. E. Genetic component in rat mammary carcinogenesis. *Radiat. Res. 89:* 264–273, 1982.

123. Wagoner, J. K., Archer, V. E., Lundin, F. E., Jr., *et al.* Radiation as the cause of lung cancer among uranium miners. *N. Engl. J. Med. 273:* 181–188, 1965.

124. Wanebo, C. K., Johnson, K. G., Sato, K., *et al.* Breast cancer after exposure to atomic bombings of Hiroshima and Nagasaki. *N. Engl. J. Med. 279:* 667–671, 1968.

125. Warren, S. Radiation effects on the skin. In: *The Skin*, edited by E. B. Helwig, and F. K. Mostofi. Baltimore, Williams & Wilkins, 1971, pp. 261–278.

126. Webster, E. W. On the question of cancer induction by small x-ray doses. Garland Lecture. *A.J.R. 137:* 647–666, 1981.

127. Weichselbaum, R. W., Nove, J., and Little, J. B. X-ray sensitivity of fifty human diploid fibroblast cell strains from patients with characterized genetic disorders. *Cancer Res. 40:* 920–925, 1980.

128. Weinstein, I. B., Gattoni-Celli S., Kischmeier, P., and Dina D. The possible role of cellular genes related to retroviruses in the process of chemical and radiation carcinogenesis. In: *Primary and Tertiary Structure of Nucleic Acids and Cancer Research*, edited by M. Miwa *et al.* Japan Sci. Soc. Press, Tokyo, 1982, pp. 139–151.

129. Winters, T. H., and DiFranza, J. R. Radioactivity in cigarette smoke (letters to the editor). *N. Engl. J. Med. 306:* 364–365, 1982, and *307:* 312–313, 1982.

130. Zippin, C., Bailar, J. C., Kohn, H. I., Lum, D., and Eisenberg, H. Radiation therapy for cervical cancer—Late effects on life span and on leukemia incidence. *Cancer 28:* 937–942, 1971.

Chapter 6

Papillomaviruses and Neoplasia in Man

MARVIN A. LUTZNER

HISTORICAL ASPECTS

Papillomaviruses have played an important role historically in our understanding of virus-induced neoplasias in man. The first human tumor known to
be transmitted by a virus was the papillomavirus-induced benign skin wart
discovered by Ciuffo[9] in 1907, 4 years prior to Rous' Nobel prize-winning discovery that malignant sarcomas in chickens were transferable by a filterable
agent.[87] Papillomavirus and warts played another key role in the chain of
events when Shope[94] discovered that skin papillomas of the wild cottontail
rabbit were caused by a filterable agent, followed by Rous' discovery 2 years
later that these papillomas in rabbits often degenerated into squamous cell
cancers.[88] This was the initial demonstration of the role of an oncogenic virus in
mammals. Then, Rous[89] in 1938 demonstrated viral-chemical cocarcinogenesis
for the first time in this same rabbit model.

EARLY PAPILLOMAVIRUS BIOLOGY

Early electron microscopic and biochemical studies in the 1950s and 1960s
were performed most commonly on virus obtained from plantar warts since
relatively large amounts of virus particles could be obtained from these lesions. The papillomavirus, a member of the papovavirus group, was found to be
55 nm in diameter and composed of a protein shell or capsid with 72 capsomeres,[43] and a DNA-containing nucleoid with a molecular weight of 5×10^6
daltons, representing about 8000 base pairs (Figs. 6.1 and 6.2)).[12] This DNA
was found to exist in a double-stranded, covalently closed, supercoiled configuration (form I), an open circular form (form II), and a linear form (form III)
(Fig. 6.3).[12] More recent evidence has shown that the DNA in this virus exists
as beaded filaments or "minichromosomes" composed of DNA strands, interconnecting regions of folded DNA surrounding host cell histones (nucleosome-
like structures) (Fig. 6.4)[23] and compacted into the virus nucleoid.

UNITARIAN THEORY

The unitarian concept that all kinds of warts were caused by the same virus
was founded primarily on observations that extracts from one type of wart,

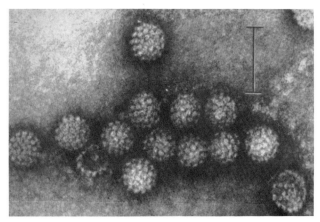

FIG. 6.1. Papillomavirus particles extracted and purified from a human wart and visualized by electron microscopy using the negative-staining technique.[43] The icosahedral particles are 55 nm in diameter and are encapsulated by 72 cylindrical protein capsomeres. One particle is ruptured, and the internal cavity which contains the DNA nucleoid can be seen. Marker represents 1 μm. (Courtesy of O. Croissant.)

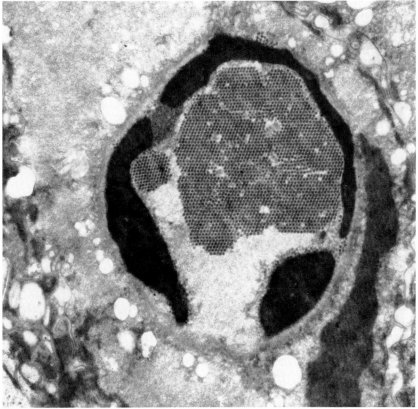

FIG. 6.2. Transmission electron microscopic visualization of a keratinocyte in the upper layers of a human wart. The nucleus contains papillomavirus-like particles in a crystalloid-array. Electron-dense marginated chromatin is seen.

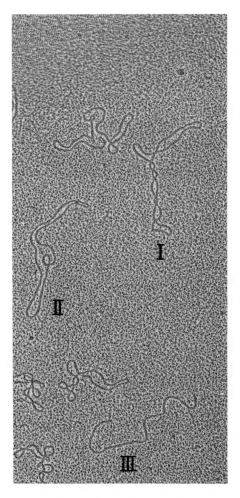

FIG. 6.3. Three forms of papillomavirus DNA visualized by electron microscopy after spreading on a molecular film and shadowing with a palladium-platinum mixture.[12] These are the superhelical form *I*, probably a "minichromosome," as shown in Figure 6.4, which has been stripped of its nucleosomes by chemical and physical handling; the closed circular form *II* results from nicking, strand relaxation, and untwisting of form *I*; and the linear form *III* results from nicking of both strands of the double-stranded DNA. (Courtesy of O. Croissant.)

FIG. 6.4. Papillomavirus genome as carried by double-stranded DNA visualized by the method described in Figure 6.3, but with special handling.[23] It appears as a "minichromosome" structure composed of a filament of DNA interconnecting "nucleosome" regions composed of folded DNA surrounding host cell histones. (Courtesy of O. Croissant.)

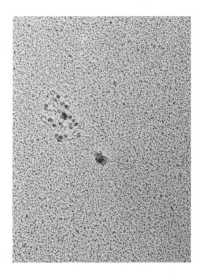

such as genital condylomas, would produce ordinary skin warts when inoculated into other skin sites. These observations led to the conclusion, in 1967, that the clinical type of lesion was determined by the local conditions at the site of infection and not by the virus.[90]

ESTABLISHMENT OF THE PLURALITY OF PAPILLOMAVIRUSES AND THEIR CLASSIFICATION

Although many attempts have been made, no one yet has developed a successful tissue culture system for the propagation of papillomaviruses, a factor which has slowed progress in the field. These viruses seem to be fastidious, requiring a well-differentiated epithelial cell for replication and assembly.[96] Fortunately, viral DNA can now be cloned in bacteria by recombinant DNA techniques, and this new source of viral DNA has been a major investigative aid.[32] With the use of these cloned DNAs and other new techniques developed in the 1970s, the unitarian theory could be further explored. Let us look at some of these new methods.

Immunocytologic techniques have demonstrated that antibodies directed against full virions are type specific and, when conjugated with fluorescein, can be used on cryostat sections to identify structural antigens of different papillomavirus types (Figs. 6.5 and 6.6).[73, 74] Specific monoclonal antibodies are also being developed for this purpose.[86] Antibodies directed against alkali or detergent disrupted virions,[70] rather than being type specific, were found to be group specific,[42, 70] evidence for a polypeptide conserved in all papillomaviruses tested to date. When these antibodies are used with a peroxidase-antiperoxidase marker, they can detect antigens present in all papillomaviruses, regardless of type or species, even in routinely fixed and embedded warts (Fig. 6.7).[42] This technique serves as a useful screening test for the presence of papillomaviruses in lesions such as laryngeal papillomas[48, 50] and genital condylomas,[47, 67] in which virus particles are sparse and difficult to locate by other histologic techniques.

New biochemical techniques have also been developed. Viral DNA can be extracted from lesions and examined by agarose gel electrophoresis and ethidium bromide staining. Papillomaviruses have a recognizable migration position. When papillomavirus DNAs are digested with a battery of restriction endonucleases which can recognize and incise DNA at particular short base-pair sequences, characteristic fingerprint patterns can be established for the papillomavirus DNAs (Fig. 6.5A and B).[28, 72-74] Furthermore, when the DNA fragments on the gel are transferred to nitrocellulose membranes (Southern blots), hybridization with radio-labeled probes of known papillomavirus DNAs can be used to determine homology under stringent conditions, an even more sensitive and specific method for typing papillomaviruses (Figs. 6.8 and 6.9).[37, 44, 45, 72] If less stringent conditions are used, this method can serve as a screening procedure for papillomavirus sequences of unknown types such as was done for laryngeal papillomas.[50] Using these methods, classification criteria for papillomavirus types were established according to the extent of DNA homology[11]; two different types share less than 50% homology. Subtypes or variants are defined by differences in the restriction enzyme cleavage patterns of their DNA, but with homology exceeding 50%.

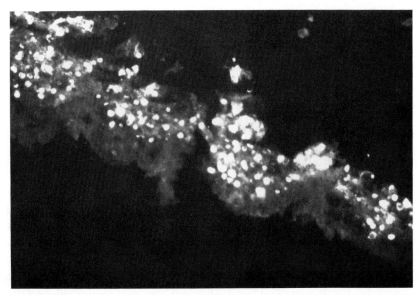

FIG. 6.5. *Immunofluorescence microscopy* performed on an acetone-fixed cryostat section of a portion of a biopsy of a macular lesion from a patient with epidermodysplasia verruciformis (EV). Note the specific fluorescent staining (white) nuclei of keratinocytes restricted to upper epidermal layers. This specimen was stained for specific structural antigens of EV HPVs using an indirect method employing anti-EV HPV guinea pig antisera followed by fluorescein-labeled anti-guinea pig IgG, rabbit IgG.[73, 74] This patient's lesions were known to be infected with HPV-8.(Courtesy of G. Orth.)

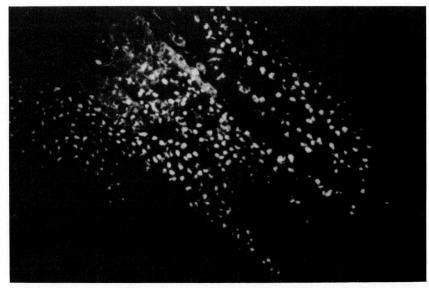

FIG. 6.6. Detection of HPV-2 structural antigen in a common wart using a direct method with flourescein-labeled anti-HPV-2 guinea pig antisera. (Courtesy of G. Orth.)

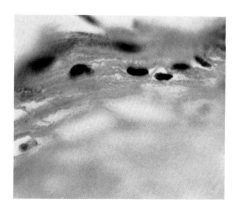

FIG. 6.7. Peroxidase-antiperoxidase-stained, paraffin-embedded section of a focal epithelial hyperplasia lip lesion using cross-reacting "group, " detergent-disrupted bovine papillomavirus 1 (BPV-1) anti-rabbit serum.[42, 70] Black nuclei indicate the presence of papillomavirus "group" antigen (counterstained with hematoxylin).

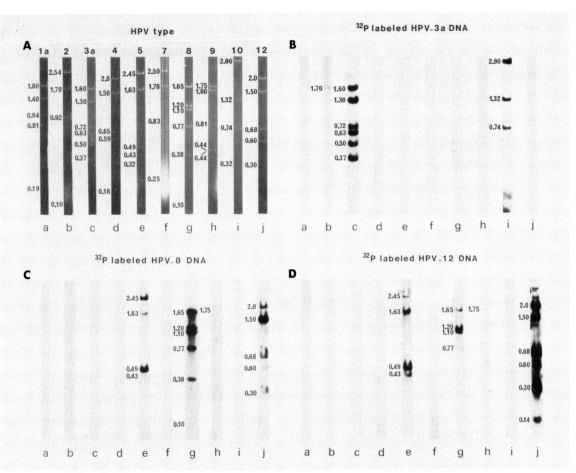

FIG. 6.8. DNA sequence homology among HPV genomes as indicated by blot hybridization experiments.[44, 45] Series A shows restriction endonuclease cleavage patterns of a variety of HPVs electrophoresed in vertical 1.2% agarose slab gels and stained with ethidium bromide. Fragments on this gel were denatured, transferred to a Gene Screen hybridization transfer membrane, and hybridized with ^{32}P-labeled HPV-3a DNA, HPV-8 DNA, and HPV-12 DNA, in series B, C, and D, respectively. Molecular weights of the DNA fragments are indicated on the left of the lanes. This establishes the restriction endonuclease patterns of these HPV DNAs and shows homology between HPV-3 and HPV-10 and homology between HPV-5, HPV-8, and HPV-12. (Courtesy of G. Orth.)

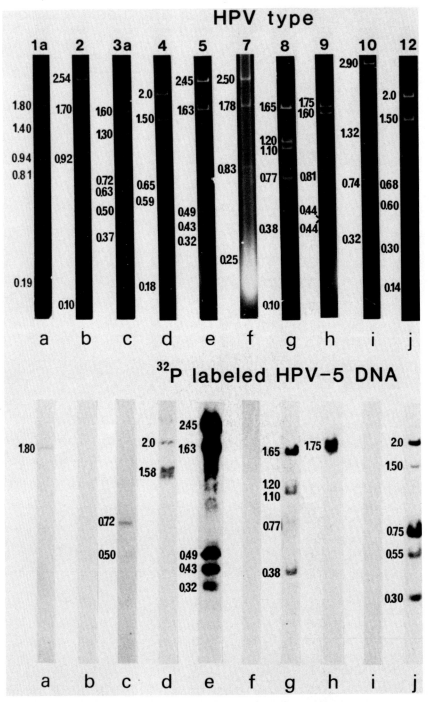

FIG. 6.9. Upper series shows the restriction endonuclease patterns by gel electrophoresis of a number of HPVs as shown in the *A* portion of Figure 6.8. The *lower series* shows by blot hybridization the homologies between HPV-5, HPV-8, HPV-9, and HPV-12 using ^{32}P-labeled HPV-5 DNA as probe. (Courtesy of G. Orth.)

TABLE 6.1. TWENTY-FOUR HUMAN PAPILLOMAVIRUS TYPES (HPVs) AND ASSOCIATED WARTS AND CANCERS

HPV Type	Type of Wart	HPV Type	Type of Cancer
1	Deep, painful plantar warts		None
2, 4, 7	Common skin warts, HPV-7 most common on hands of butchers		None
3, 10	Flat skin warts; sometimes seen in epidermodysplasia verruciformis (EV) patients	3	None
		10	EV skin cancer
5, 8, 9, 12, 14, 15, 17 19-24	Benign EV lesions	5, 8, 14	EV skin cancer
		5	Skin cancer in immuno-suppressed renal transplant patient
6, 11	Condylomas (genital warts) Laryngeal papillomas	6, 11	Buschke-Lowenstein verrucous carcinoma
		11	Rare cervical cancer
13	Focal epithelial hyperplasia (Heck's disease)		None
16	Atypical, "dysplastic" condylomas of uterine cervix Bowenoid papulosis	16	Squamous cell carcinoma of cervix Bowen's skin cancer
18		18	Squamous cell carcinoma of cervix

Using all of these techniques it has now been determined that the unitarian theory was incorrect and that there are at least 24 different papillomaviruses associated with different types of warts (Table 6.1).[59, 60] Eight of the 24 appear to play an oncogenic role. But, before considering these important 8 papillomaviruses, let us look at information known about the others since this may offer clues to mechanisms of oncogenesis.

PAPILLOMAVIRUS-INDUCED BENIGN DISEASES

Acanthosis and hyperplasia are histopathologic phenomena common to most papillomavirus-induced epithelial lesions, and these most certainly result from stimulatory effects of early papillomavirus gene products on the basal cell population. *In situ* hybridization studies[71] have shown no evidence for viral DNA production in the basal layer of the epidermis; viral DNA production seems to begin in the mid and upper spinous layer (Fig. 6.10), and final virus assembly resulting from late viral gene-induced capsid production occurs in the granular layer, as evidenced by electron microscopy.

Almost all of the papillomavirus types discovered by these techniques seem to be associated with lesions that exhibit characteristic histopathologic and cytologic features,[39, 53, 59, 60] Human papillomavirus type 1 (HPV-1) is associated with deep, solitary, painful plantar warts (Fig. 6.11). Infected keratinocytes of the granular layer fill with giant, polyangular, keratohyaline-like granules (Figs. 6.12 and 6.13). HPV-2 is found associated with common warts that may

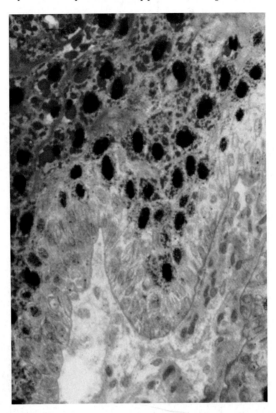

FIG. 6.10. Light optical micrograph of a section through a plantar wart. *In situ* hybridization was performed using an *in vitro* ³H-labeled human papillomavirus one (HPV-1) DNA probe.[71] The nuclei appearing black contain large amounts of HPV-1 DNA, indicating vegetative viral synthesis. Cells in the basal layer of the epidermis and dermal fibroblasts have no detectable viral DNA. Large moderately electron-dense cytoplasmic inclusions typical of plantar warts can be seen in the upper layers. (Courtesy of O. Croissant.)

be located on any skin surface (Fig. 6.14), in mosaic plantar warts (Fig. 6.15), and warts of the hard palate (Fig. 6.16).[63] Cells in the granular layer show "composite" keratohyaline-like granules (Fig. 6.17), best visualized by electron microscopy (Fig. 6.18).[53] HPV-3 and 10 are associated with flat warts most commonly located on the face and back of the hands (Fig. 6.19). The characteristic cytopathic finding is a perinuclear empty space, with keratohyaline granules and tonofilaments pushed to the cell periphery (Fig. 6.20), giving rise to the so-called "owl-eyed" cell (Fig. 6.21). HPV-4 is associated with hand warts, particularly those on hands that are dome shaped (Fig. 6.22).[39] Giant, crescentic, tonofilament-containing masses may be found, usually in a juxtanuclear position (Figs. 6.23–6.26).[62] HPV-7 also is associated with common warts, to date found exclusively on the hands of butchers.[75] HPV-13[77] is associated with focal epithelial hyperplasia,[2] a disease of the oral mucosa (Fig. 6.27) occurring in 30% of Greenland eskimos,[81] 3% of American Indians,[2] and rarely in the rest of the world's population. Microscopically the lesions show a peculiar "Bronze Age axe" architecture (Fig. 6.28) and a peculiar "mitosoid" cytological feature

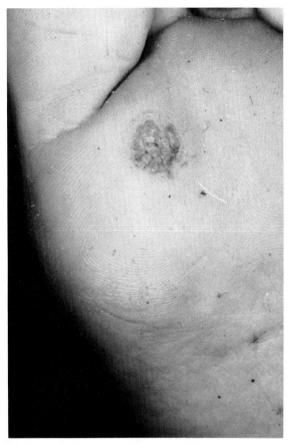

FIG. 6.11. A painful, deep, plantar wart infected with HPV-1.

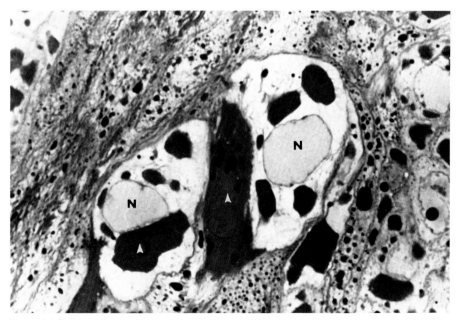

FIG. 6.12. Light microscope section through a plantar wart infected with HPV-1 showing the typical cytologic changes particularly noticeable in the granular layer as illustrated here. Nuclei (N) are filled with homogeneous inclusions which on electron microscopy are viral crystalloids; cytoplasm is electron-lucid and contains large electron-dense bodies (arrows) which may be ovoid, or irregular, often with polyangular shapes.

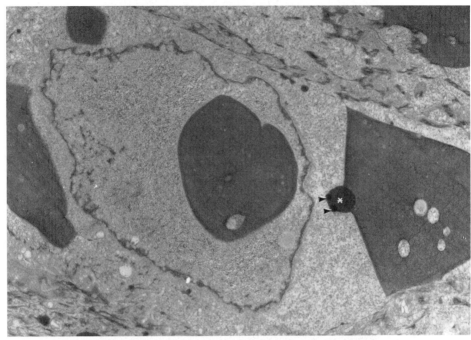

FIG. 6.13. Electron microscope section through the granular layer of a plantar wart infected with HPV-1. The nucleus is filled with papilloma-virus particles arranged in paracrystalline arrays, or in a dispersed state. A large rounded granule appears in the nucleus. The cytoplasm contains giant, angular bodies; the one on the right has an electron-dense rounded granule embedded along its left side (*) which itself contains two smaller rounded, even more dense granules on its left border (*arrows*).

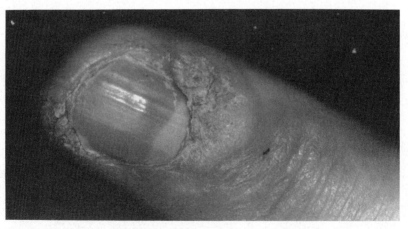

FIG. 6.14. Periungual warts, probably HPV-2-induced, on the finger of a patient with a deficiency of his cell-mediated immune system.

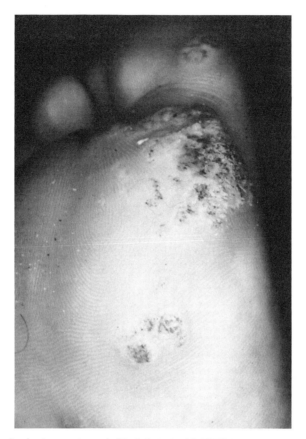

FIG. 6.15. Mosaic plantar warts probably infected with HPV-2.

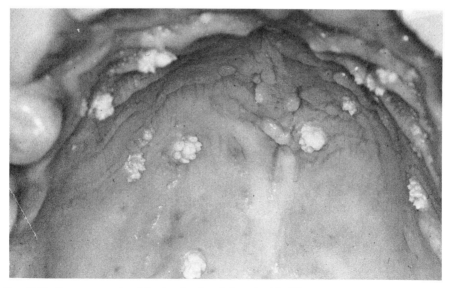

FIG. 6.16. Common warts of the hard palate infected with HPV-2.[63]

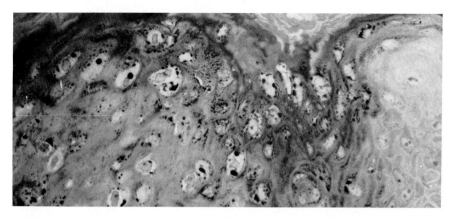

FIG. 6.17. Light microscope section of a common wart infected with HPV-2. The basal cell layer is hyperplastic. Cells of the granular layer are enlarged and have clear cytoplasm with both normal-sized and enlarged keratohyaline granules.

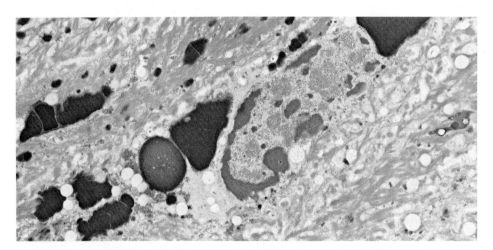

FIG. 6.18. Electron micrograph of a cell of the granular layer of an HPV-2-induced common wart. The nucleus has multiple clusters of papillomavirus-like particles in crystalloid-arrays and dense marginated chromatin. The cytoplasm has normal-appearing tonofilament bundles and large keratohyaline-like granules. These "composite" granules are compartmentalized and may exhibit different electron-densities.[63]

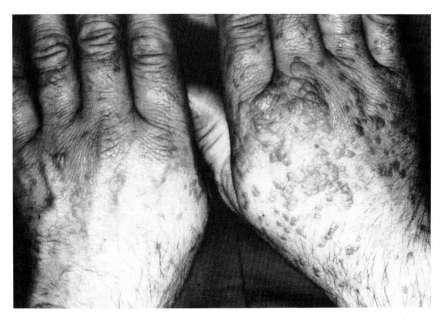

FIG. 6.19. HPV-3-induced flat warts on the back of the hands of an immunosuppressed renal allograft recipient. (Courtesy of M-F. Ducasse.)

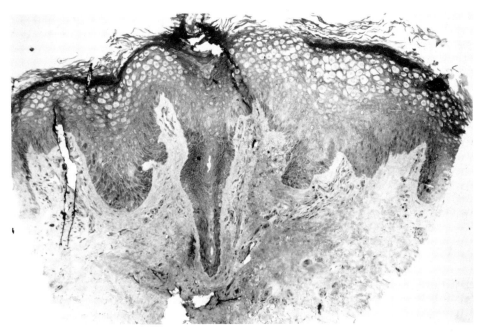

FIG. 6.20. Light micrograph of a flat wart infected with HPV-3. Note the characteristic "basket-weave" pattern of the stratum corneum, and the "owl-eyed" cells of the upper epidermis. These cells have centrally placed nuclei surrounded by clear cytoplasm.

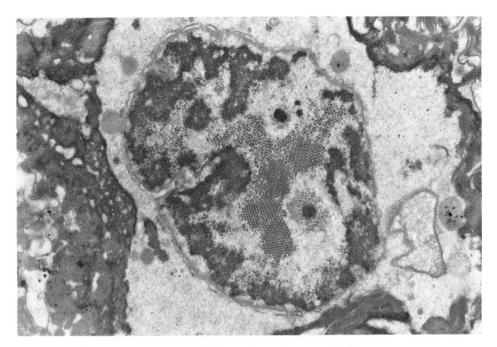

FIG. 6.21. Electron micrograph of an HPV-3-induced flat wart. This keratinocyte of the granular layer demonstrates papillomavirus-like particles both dispersed and in crystalloid arrays. Dense chromatin may be seen. The cytoplasm surrounding the nucleus is empty except for some finely granular material and mitochondrial remnants. Tonofilament bundles and some amorphous material are clustered at the cell periphery.

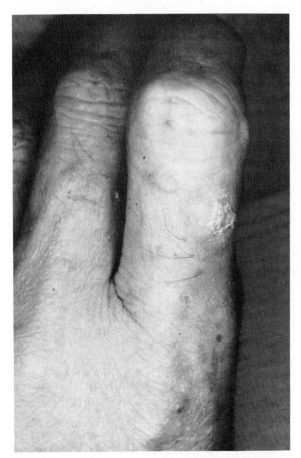

FIG. 6.22. Rounded wart probably HPV-4-induced, on the finger of an immunosuppressed renal allograft recipient.[62]

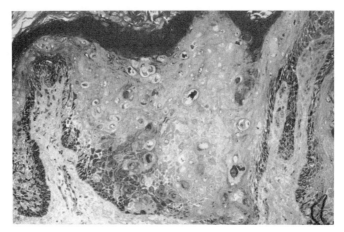

FIG. 6.23. Light micrograph of the lesion shown in Figure 6.22, probably HPV-4-induced. There is hyperkeratosis, acanthosis, papillomatosis; the basal cell layer is hyperplastic. Note the bizarre cells throughout the epidermis with large, crescentic cytoplasmic masses.[62]

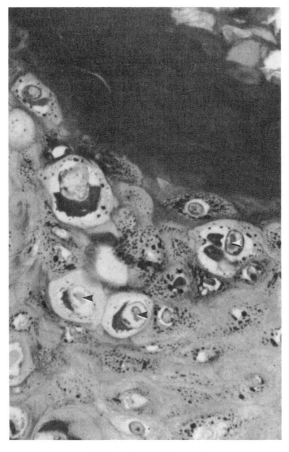

FIG. 6.24. Higher magnification light micrograph showing more detail of the bizarre keratinocytes. Note the juxtanuclear crescentic masses and round nuclear inclusions (*arrows*).[62]

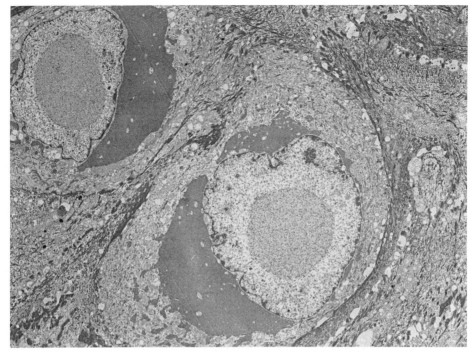

FIG. 6.25. Electron micrograph of this same lesion showing the juxtanuclear crescentic masses in two keratinocytes of the squamous cell layer. Within each nucleus is a round mass which on even higher magnification was seen to contain papillomavirus-like particles embedded in a filamentous matrix.[62]

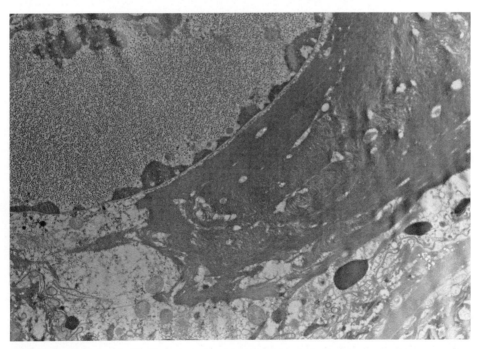

FIG. 6.26. Higher magnification electron micrograph showing the juxtanuclear crescent composed of tonofilamentous-like material and a nucleus filled with dispersed papillomavirus-like particles.[62]

(Fig. 6.29).[82] Papillomavirus-like particles are sparse in this disease (Fig. 6.30).[63, 83] A similar disease has been reported in a colony of chimpanzees (Fig. 6.31).[35]

ROLE OF HUMAN PAPILLOMAVIRUSES IN NEOPLASIA

Evidence for virus-induced malignancies in man has been achieved for the herpesvirus (Epstein-Barr)-induced Burkitt's lymphoma[22] and nasopharyngeal carcinoma[33]; hepatitis B virus-induced hepatocellular carcinoma[4]; human T-cell retrovirus (HTLV)-induced T-cell lympholeukemia[80]; and now for papilloma virus-induced skin and mucosal squamous cell cancers.[5, 13, 19, 26, 27, 29, 30, 38, 60, 61, 64, 72, 76, 78, 100, 102] Let us now explore the papillomavirus story in detail.

Although a role for papillomavirus in squamous cell cancers of the skin and mucosa of man had been suspected for some time,[1, 101] the first demonstration of the presence of a papillomavirus in such cancers came in 1980 when Orth *et al.*[72] detected human papillomavirus (HPV) type 5 DNA in squamous cell carcinomas developing in patients with the rare familial disease epidermodyplasia verruciformis (EV).[58] More recently, HPV-8[60, 79], 14[60] DNA, and HPV-10 DNA[30] have been found in EV cancers. EV is a rare familial disease characterized by the onset in early childhood of long-lasting and widespread benign macular and papular lesions (Figs. 6.32 and 6.33) which, after an average interval of 20 years, may degenerate into *in situ* and then invasive squamous cell carcinoma, especially in sun-exposed skin (Figs. 6.34*A* and *B*–6.38).[58, 60] Benign lesions have a specific, recognizable histologic and cytologic pattern (Figs. 6.39–6.43), whereas the *in situ* and invasive squamous cell cancers have the usual histologic features of such lesions (Figs. 6.44 and 6.45). Papillomavirus-like particles can be identified in benign lesions by microscopy (Fig. 6.42), but not in malignant lesions[1]; only HPV DNA is found in the latter.[72] An EV patient may have benign lesions infected by multiple HPVs of the specific types of HPV-3, 5, 8, 9, 10, 12, 14, 15, 17, 19, 20, 21, 22, 23, and 24[44, 45, 60, 72, 78, 79] whereas only types of HPV-5,8,10,14 DNA[30, 60, 72, 76] have thus far been found in cancers. HPV-5 DNA has also been found in a metastatic squamous cell cancer in an EV patient.[76] Ninety percent of EV patients have been found to have a depressed cell-mediated immune system (CMI).[39, 58] Since immunosuppressed renal allograft recipients had been observed to have an increased incidence of warts and skin cancers, especially in sun-exposed skin,[46] HPV-5 DNA was searched for in lesions from such patients (Figs. 6.46–6.50) and was found in benign and cancerous lesions.[61, 64]

That the immunosuppression of the cell-mediated immune system in EV and in organ recipients might indeed by playing a cofactor role for papillomavirus oncogenesis is supported by the observation that cattle feeding on bracken fern (a plant containing both immunosuppressive and carcinogenic agents) acquire multiple alimentary tract papillomas and carcinomas[41] associated with bovine papillomavirus type 4.[7]

Furthermore, the observation that skin cancers in renal allograft recipients and EV patients arise almost exclusively in sun-exposed skin[46, 58, 60] and are rare in EV patients with black skin,[40, 60] whose intense pigmentation protects against ultraviolet penetration, combined with the observation that the frequency of skin cancer in organ recipients is proportional not only to the duration of immunosuppression but also to the duration of sunlight exposure,[6, 31] suggests that ultraviolet (UV) light may also serve as a cofactor for oncogenesis. Further support for the cofactor role of papillomavirus and sunlight comes from the observation that papillomavirus has been found in ocular tumors of cattle exposed to the sun,[25] in cancers arising in the skin of sheep not protected by wool or pigmentation,[98] and in solar keratoses in man.[95] Still another cofactor role of sunlight exposure might be the further immunosuppression in these patients by UV light, since it is known that exposure of man to solarium UV can temporarily depress CMI[34] and that UV light can enhance suppressor T lymphocytes in mice rendering them unable to reject UV-induced tumors.[24]

The next major findings in support of papillomavirus-induced squamous cell cancers involved study of these malignancies in the genital mucosa and came primarily from the work of zur Hausen's group and others.[5, 13, 19, 26, 27, 29, 30, 38, 65-68, 93, 100-102] It had been suspected from clinical and histologic observations that certain verrucous genital condylomas[55, 100] and atypical flat condylomas of the cervix[65, 66] were prime candidates for condyloma and subsequent malignant transformation. It had also been observed that juvenile laryngeal papillomas following treatment with x-irradiation were susceptible to degeneration into squamous cell cancer.[84] In 1982 it was found that HPV-6 and HPV-11 infected both laryngeal papillomas (Fig. 6.51)[29, 68] and genital condylomas (Figs. 6.52–6.54) including those of the uterine cervix (Figs. 6.55–6.59).[26, 27, 29, 100] HPV-6 DNA[27] was found in giant condylomas of Buschke-Lowenstein verrucous carcinomas which grow rapidly inward, severely impairing underlying

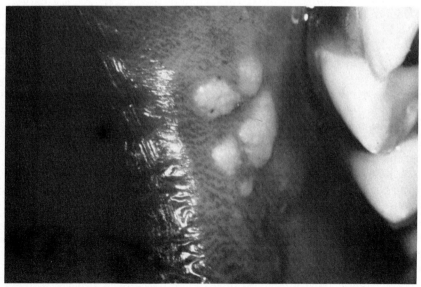

Fig. 6.27. Typical lesions of probably HPV-13-induced focal epithelial hyperplasia (FEH) in an Algerian boy.[63]

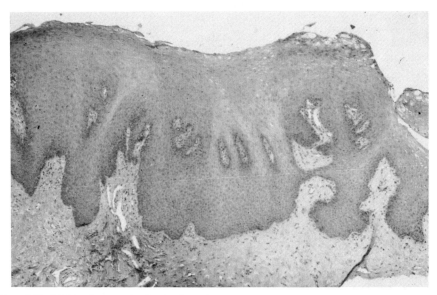

FIG. 6.28. Light micrograph of a focal epithelial hyperplasia (FEH) lesion showing acanthosis and horizontal branching of the rete ridges, the so-called "Bronze Age axe" sign.[63]

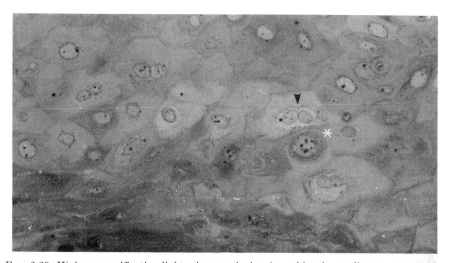

FIG. 6.29. Higher magnification light micrograph showing a binuclear cell (*arrow*). Note dense nuclear granules, especially marked in one cell (*), simulating mitosis, so-called "mitosoid" degeneration.[63]

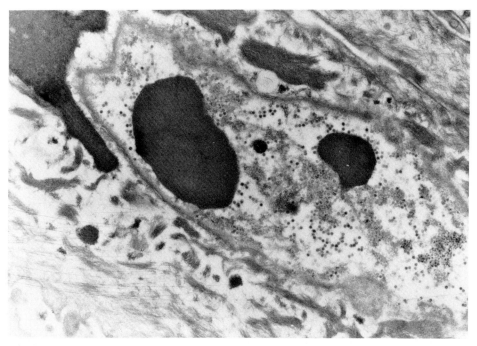

Fig. 6.30. Electron micrograph of a focal epithelial hyperplasia (FEH) lesion showing papillomavirus-like particles, sparsely dispersed throughout the nucleus. Electron-dense nuclear granules may be chromatin.[63]

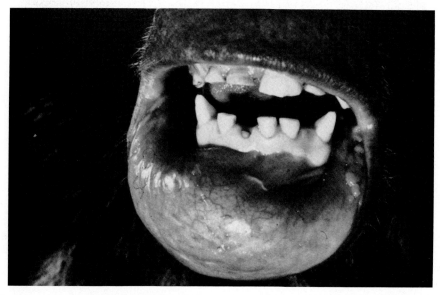

Fig. 6.31. Focal epithelial hyperplasia (FEH)-like lesions on the lips of a chimpanzee. (Reproduced with permission from C. F. Hollander and M. Van Noord.[35])

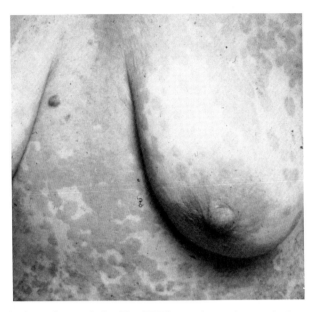

FIG. 6.32. Pityriasis (tenia) versicolor-like (PV-like) scaly patches on the breast and trunk of a patient with epidermodysplasia verruciformis (EV), infected with an EV HPV. (Courtesy of R. Caputo.)

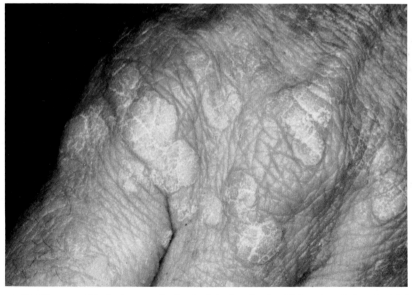

FIG. 6.33. Flat wart-like lesions on the back of the hands of an EV patient infected with HPV-5. (Courtesy of C. Blanchet-Bardon.)

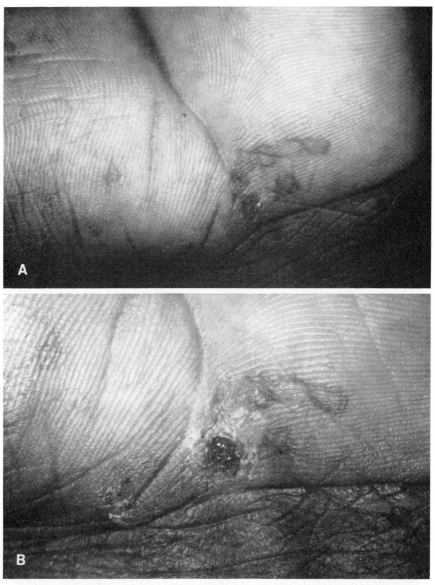

Fig. 6.34. (*A* and *B*) The palm of an EV patient showing a cluster of five macular lesions. The same patient's palm 18 months later. A fungating squamous cell carcinoma has developed at the site of one of the macules. This patient was infected with HPV-8. Reprinted with permission from M. A. Lutzner *et al.*[60] *J. Invest. Dermatol.* 83 (Suppl. 1):18s–21s, © 1984, Williams & Wilkins, Baltimore.

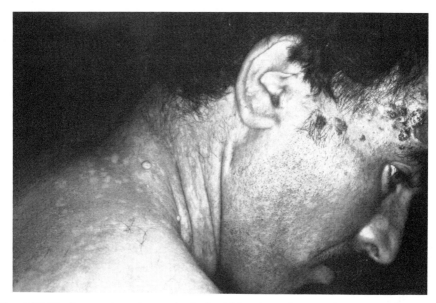

FIG. 6.35. The face, neck, and upper back of an EV patient, showing a large ulcerated squamous cell carcinoma of the forehead, pigmented Bowenoid plaques on his forehead, temple, and pre-auricular regions, and scaly depigmented benign PV-like macules on his back. This patient's benign lesions were found infected with HPV-5, and HPV-5 DNA was found in two of his cancers. (Courtesy of C. Blanchet-Bardon.)

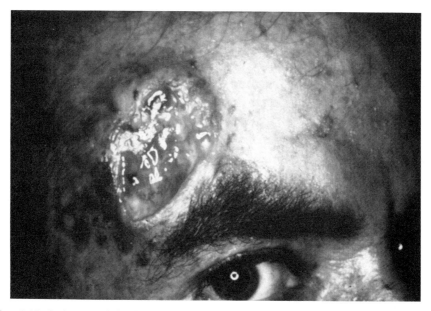

FIG. 6.36. A close-up of the forehead of the patient of Figure 6.35, showing in more detail the ulcerated squamous cell carcinoma of the forehead, the surrounding pigmented Bowenoid plaques, and additional Bowenoid plaques under his eye and on his nose. (Courtesy of C. Blanchet-Bardon.)

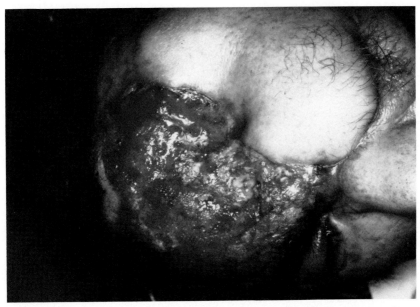

Fɪɢ. 6.37. The face of an EV patient showing a massive invasive squamous cell carcinoma resistant to both surgical intervention and chemotherapy and worsened by radiotherapy. Sinuses are invaded. Temporary improvement was achieved by systemic and intralesional alpha-interferon therapy, but the patient died of his disease. His benign PV-like lesions were found to be infected with HPV-14, and HPV-14 DNA was found in his cancer. (Courtesy of C. Blanchet-Bardon.)

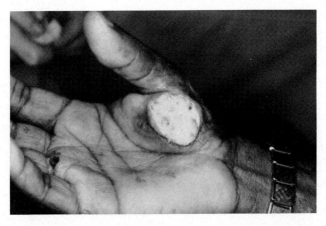

Fɪɢ. 6.38. The other palm of the patient illustrated in Figure 6.34. A large, fungating, invasive squamous cell carcinoma is seen on his thenar eminence, worsened by radiotherapy. Another smaller squamous cell carcinoma is seen at the base of his fourth finger, and brown scaly benign macules are seen on his palms and fingers. The large palmar cancer was found to harbor HPV-14 DNA. (Courtesy of C. Blanchet-Bardon.)

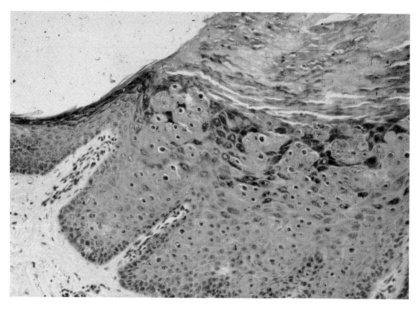

FIG. 6.39. Light micrograph of a benign EV lesion of the patient of Figure 6.32 showing its appearance in a plastic-embedded, methylene blue-basic fuchsin-stained section. Again note the hyper- and parakeratosis, and the nests of pale-staining clear cells extending almost to the basal cell layer. Note that the cytoplasm is pale-staining but not empty. (Courtesy of R. Caputo.)

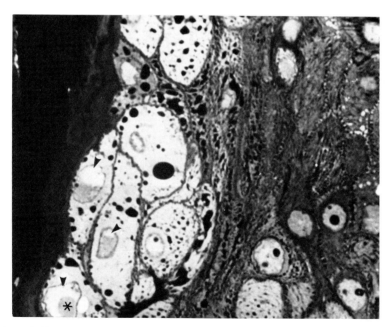

FIG. 6.40. A higher magnification light micrograph of a benign EV lesion, showing that the enlarged pale-staining cells in the granular layer have rounded keratohyaline granules, and that their nuclei may have clear spaces (*arrows*) and inclusions (*).

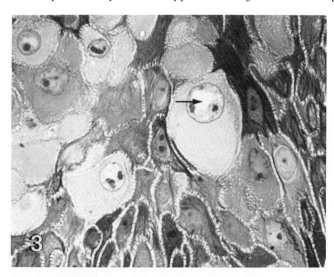

FIG. 6.41. A high magnification light micrograph of a benign EV lesion showing detail of a characteristic pale-staining cell (*arrow*). This cell has a nuclear clear space and cytoplasmic homogeneous pale-staining material surrounded at its periphery by what could be remaining tonofilaments.

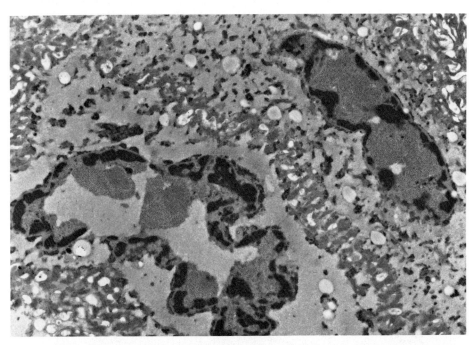

FIG. 6.42. *Electron micrograph* of a benign EV lesion showing two cells of the stratum spinosum. The nucleus of the cell to the right is completely filled with papillomavirus-like particles, but the one to the left has paracrystalline clusters of virus particles separated by typical nuclear pale-staining spaces. The cytoplasm of this latter cell is also replaced by pale-staining material. Both nuclei have dense, marginated chromatin.

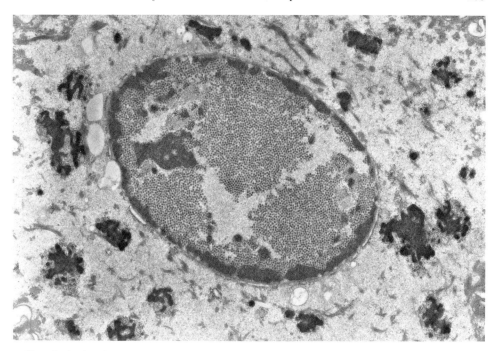

FIG. 6.43. Another high mignification electron micrograph of a benign EV lesion showing, in addition to the features described in Figure 6.41, medusa-shaped bodies in the cytoplasm.

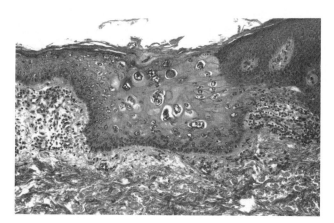

FIG. 6.44. Light micrograph of a Bowenoid *in situ* carcinoma from an EV patient. Nuclei are hyperchromatic and bizarre in shape.

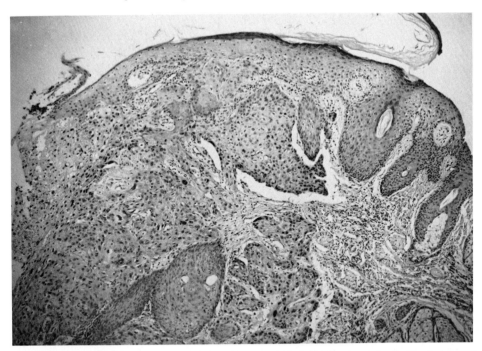

FIG. 6.45. Light micrograph of an invasive squamous cell carcinoma from the forehead of an EV patient. The dermis is almost completely replaced by nests and islands of squamous cells. The overlying epidermis is invading downward. Nuclei of invading cells in the dermis are large and hyperchromatic.

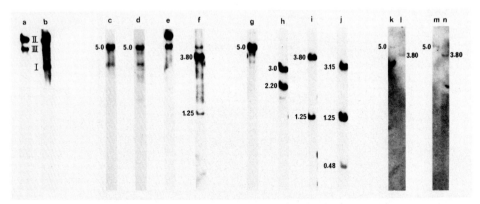

FIG. 6.46. Detection of HPV-5 DNA in benign, PV-like lesions and skin cancers of an immunosuppressed renal allograft recipient using the Southern blot technique.[64] Lane *a* contains uncleaved DNA extracted from the patient's benign lesions, and Lanes *c–f* contain this DNA cleaved with SacI, BamHI, EcoRI, and PstI endonucleases, respectively. Lane *b* contains uncleaved DNA extracted from benign lesions of an HPV-5-infected EV patient, and Lanes *g–j* contain this DNA cleaved with the same four restriction endonucleases as above. Lanes *k* and *l* contain DNA from the renal allograft recipient's *in situ* cancer cleaved with BamHI and PstI, respectively, while Lanes *m* and *n* contain DNA from the patient's invasive carcinoma cleaved with the same two restriction endonucleases. *Arabic numerals* indicate molecular weights of fragments in megadaltons; *roman numerals* indicate DNA form I (circular, supercoiled molecules), form II (circular, relaxed molecules), and form III (linear molecules).

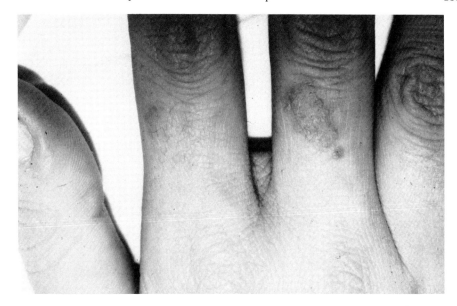

FIG. 6.47. Back of the fingers of another immunosuppressed renal allograft recipient with multiple warty lesions. A warty plaque is shown on the middle finger, an isolated papule at its lower pole, and a smaller papule on the second finger. There are distinct papules at the border of the larger plaque, giving it a circinate appearance.

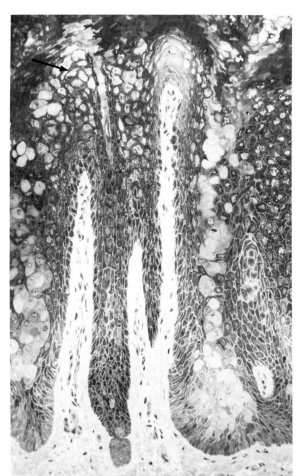

FIG. 6.48. Light micrograph of portion of the large plaque of Figure 6.47. This lesion exhibits acanthosis and papillomatosis and is not as "flat" as the usual benign EV lesion; however, note the two columns of characteristic enlarged pale-staining cells, the histologic "hallmark" of an EV-HPV infection. Note also, high in the epidermis, nests of cells *arrow*) with the characteristic histologic features of HPV-3- or HPV -10-infected flat warts, small cells with empty perinuclear cytoplasm and cytoplasmic contents pushed to the cell periphery.

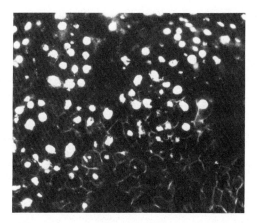

FIG. 6.49. *Immunofluorescence microscopy* performed on acetone-fixed cryostat sections of portion of the biopsy of the large plaque illustrated in Figure 6.47 which had been frozen in liquid nitrogen. Note the specific fluorescent staining of the rounded, large nuclei of cells within one of the columns of pale-staining cells shown in Figures 6.48. This section has been stained for specific structural antigens of EV-HPVs using an indirect method employing anti-EV-HPV guinea pig antisera followed by fluorescein-labeled anti-guinea pig IgG, rabbit IgG. Attempts at staining with anti-HPV-3 antisera were negative.

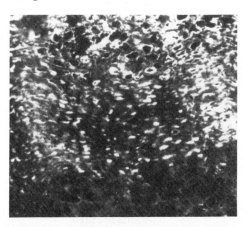

FIG. 6.50. Immunofluorescence microscopy performed by the same method described in Figure 6.6 on an adjacent cryostat section, except that it has been stained for specific structural antigen HPV-3. Note specific fluorescent staining within typical ovoid nuclei of a nest of cells with the histologic features of HPV-3 or HPV-10-infected cells. Attempts at staining these nuclei with EV-HPV antisera were negative.

structures (Fig. 6.60).[55] Next, HPV-11 DNA was found in several cervical squamous cell cancers.[29] Most importantly, it has recently been discovered that HPV-16[19] and/or HPV-18 DNA[5] can be found in 90% of cervical cancers so far explored.[26, 102] Furthermore, there seems to be a strong correlation between severe dysplasia (abnormal mitotic figures) in cervical mucosa and the presence of HPV-16 DNA[13] strongly supporting a role for HPV in squamous cell carcinoma of the cervix. HPV-16 DNA has also been recently found in lesions of Bowenoid papulosis (Figs. 6.61 and 6.62), [38] genital papules which histologically appear to be cancer *in situ* but clinically behave in a benign fashion, [99] and in a few Bowen's cancers of genital and nongenital skin.[38] Because of the apparent sexual transmission of genital condylomas, it has been suggested that lesions of Bowenoid papulosis may serve as a "resevoir" for virus spread of HPV-16.[26] A practical method for detecting HPV-16 or HPV-18 DNA on cervical smears or biopsies of colposcopically suspicious cervical lesions would be most useful for the physician.[26]

RECENT ADVANCES IN MOLECULAR BIOLOGY OF PAPILLOMAVIRUSES

Useful information about the biology of these papillomaviruses has come from the study of cells in culture which have been transformed by bovine papillomaviruses[20, 21, 36, 37, 49, 51, 54, 56, 57, 69, 91-93, 97] and from the sequence analysis of cloned papillomavirus DNAs.[8, 10, 14-16, 21, 36, 37, 92, 93] It has been shown that unlike other oncogenic viruses, papillomavirus DNA does not insert into host cell DNA but remains episomal,[54] except perhaps for HPV-18[19,] that only 69% of the viral genome is required for transformation,[10, 21, 56, 69] that only one of the DNA strands codes for proteins,[14, 15] and that transcripts indicate the active coding for 10 proteins (Fig. 6.63), E1–8, which is the transforming region, and L1–2, the region involved with vegetative or viral-assembly functions, the latter two expressed only in productively infected warts.[21] The E1 region appears responsible for papillomavirus DNA remaining episomal[57] and shows some homology with polyomavirus large T protein.[10] Data for the four papillomaviruses sequenced to date indicates a surprising homology among these viruses.[8, 14, 15, 93]

The actual mechanisms of papillomavirus cancer induction or cell transformation are not known, but E2 appears to be a most important transforming protein[56, 69] as does transcriptional enhancer elements.[92] The reader is referred to the chapter on oncogenes by Tomasi in this volume. It has been recently reported that there is homology between the *c-mos* ocogene protein product and a portion of the E2-encoded polypeptide of the cottontail rabbit papillomavirus.[16] Also it has been shown that mouse skin cancers induced *in vivo* by chemical carcinogens have a transforming Harvey-*ras* oncogene.[3] Perhaps of interest is some recent evidence that transforming proteins derived from DNA tumor viruses may be captured by retroviruses and transferred to cells in culture which then become transformed, suggesting a common mechanism for oncogenesis by both RNA and DNA tumor viruses.[18] Further, the long delay between the onset of benign lesions and cancer appearance in EV patients suggests a multistep process, and again recent evidence has shown that *onc* genes can work in groups,[52] and that DNA tumor virus gene products may work in concert with *onc* genes,[17] opening many speculative pathways for papillomavirus oncogenesis. Also, there is a recent report that human skin cells can be made neoplastic in culture by the combined action of an adeno 12-SV40 hybrid virus and the Kirsten murine sarcoma virus. This cell line is immortalized, transformed as determined by tumor formation in nude mice, and apparently is highly differentiated, suggesting it may be a useful tool for papillomavirus culture.[85]

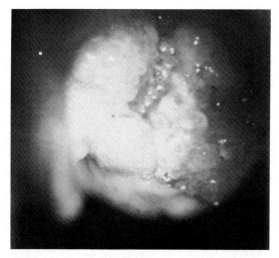

FIG. 6.51. Laryngeal papillomas, probably HPV-6 or HPV-11-induced, visualized through a laryngoscope. The papillomatous growths are obscuring the vocal cords of this child.

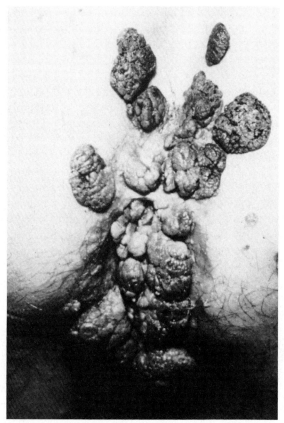

FIG. 6.52. A large cluster of perianal condylomas.

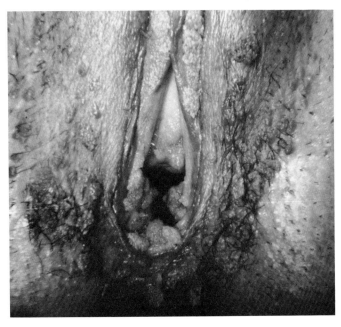

FIG. 6.53. HPV-6-induced multiple condylomas of the perineum, labia majora, labia minora, introitus, and vaginal mucosa which developed in a woman on combined chemotherapy for a chronic leukemia.

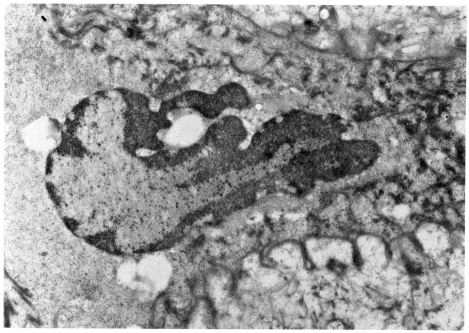

FIG. 6.54. Electron micrograph of a section from a biopsy of one of the perineal condylomas of Figure 6.53. The nucleus of this cell contains a small number of dispersed papillomavirus-like particles.

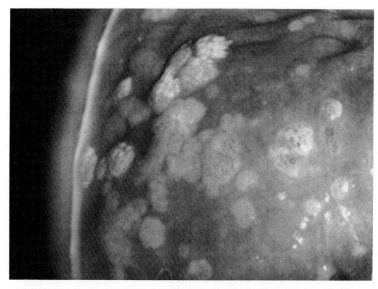

FIG. 6.55. Multiple condylomas, probably HPV-6- or HPV-11-induced, of the uterine cervix of a young woman visualized through a colposcope. Some lesions are flat, and others are raised. Some have a smooth surface, and others have a verrucous surface. (Courtesy of A. Meisels.)

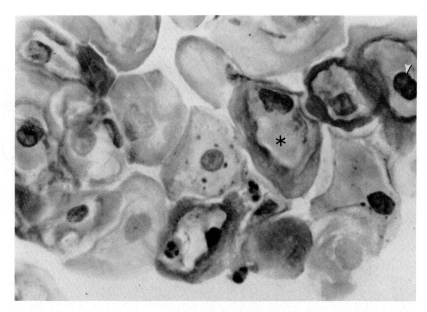

FIG. 6.56. Light micrograph of a Papanicolau smear taken from a woman with a cervical condyloma. So-called "koilocytes, " typical for condylomas can be seen. They may be binucleated (*arrow*) and have a "spooned-out" or pale-staining perinuclear cytoplasm (*). Cytoplasmic contents are compressed to the cell periphery. (Courtesy of A. Meisels.)

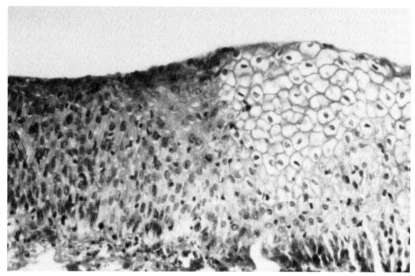

Fig. 6.57. (*A*) Light micrograph of a section through a flat "atypical" cervical condyloma. To the *right* the cervial mucosa is replaced by "koilocytes, " typical of a cervical condyloma; to the left there is an abrupt transition to dysplasia. (Courtesy of A. Meisels.)

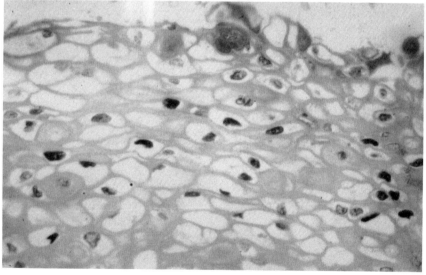

Fig. 6.57*B*. A flat cervical condyloma stained by the peroxidase-antiperoxidase marker, "group" antigen technique illustrated in Figure 6.7, showing darkly stained nuclei of "koilocytes" indicating the presence of papillomavirus antigen.

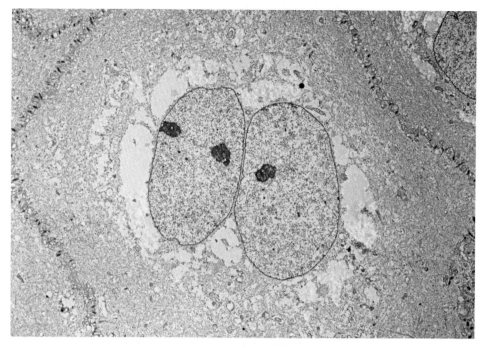

FIG. 6.58. Electron micrograph from a section taken from the biopsy of a cervical condyloma. This is a "koilocyte." It is binucleate and exhibits a perinuclear clear space. Sparse papillomavirus-like particles are not possible to discern at this low magnification.

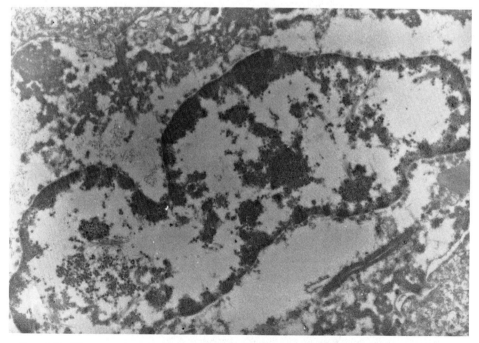

FIG. 6.59. Electron micrograph of a "koilocyte" in a cervical condyloma. Sparse and disperse papillomavirus-like particles can be seen. The nucleus is mostly empty, except for marginated chromatin. The perinuclear cytoplasm is almost empty. Some tonofilament bundles can be seen at the cell periphery.

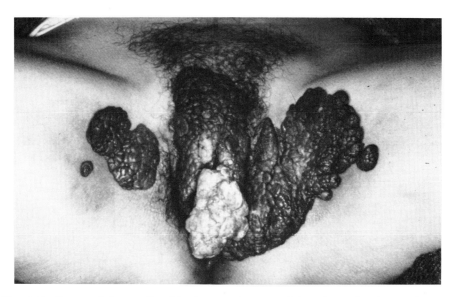

FIG. 6.60. Giant condyloma or Buschke-Lowenstein tumor of the vulva and perineum of a young woman. HPV-6 DNA was found in this verrucous carcinoma, which is multicentric and, for the most part, heavily pigmented. (Courtesy of Dr. Masse.)

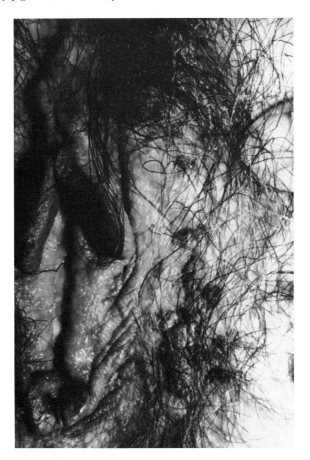

FIG. 6.61. Multicentric pigmented papules of the perineal skin of a young woman. Some papules also appear on the labia majora. These are lesions of Bowenoid papulosis, probably HPV-16-induced. (Courtesy of M-F. Ducasse.)

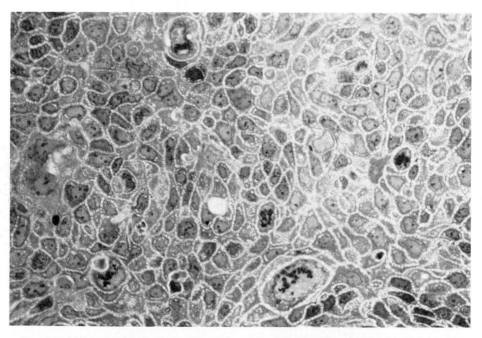

F<small>IG</small>. 6.62 Light micrograph of one of the lesions biopsied from patient of Figure 6.61. There are features of Bowen's *in situ* carcinoma as characterized by hyperchromatic nuclei, abnormal mitotic figures, and loss of cell polarity.

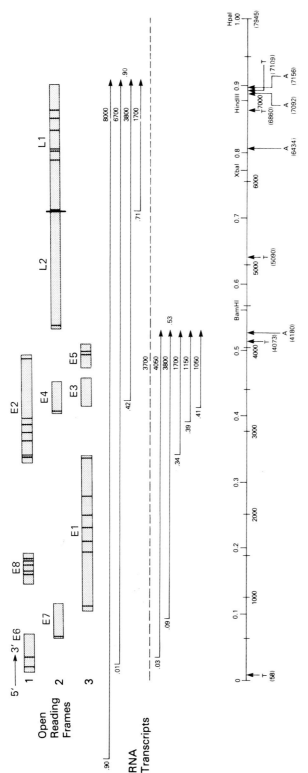

Fig. 6.63. Transcriptional and translational map of BPV-1 DNA. The full molecule (7945 base pairs) of BPV-1 DNA opened at the unique *HpaI* site is marked off in bases and map units at the bottom of the figure. Potential polyadenylation recognition sites (*A*) and potential TATAAA and TATATA promoter elements (*T*) are indicated. The bodies of the BPV-1-specific-polyadenylated RNA transcripts and their sizes in bases are drawn immediately above. The horizontal *dashed bars* represent the open reading frames and, therefore, the potential regions encoding BPV-1-specific proteins in each of the three reading frames. The *vertical black lines* indicate on the open reading frames the positions of in frame translational initiation codon ATG. Open reading frames within the transforming region have been designated E1 to E8. The two open reading frames within the 31% region not essential for transformation, L1 and L2, are partitioned by a single stop codon. (Courtesy of P. Howley.)

An unexpected byproduct of papillomavirus research has been the use of papillomavirus DNA as a cloning vector in eukaryotic cells. The ability of this DNA to remain extrachromosomal and to transform eukaryotic cells allows it to serve as a "shuttle" vector between bacterial and mouse cells producing a number of potentially useful proteins.[36, 91]

Finally, 8 of the 24 described papillomaviruses thus far appear to have an oncogenic potential, and these papillomaviruses join the Epstein-Barr, hepatitis B, and HTLV viruses as role players in human neoplasia.

ACKNOWLEDGMENTS

This work was supported in part by the Lique Nationale Française Contre le Cancer and the Phillipe Foundation.

REFERENCES

1. Aaronson, C. M., and Lutzner, M. A. Epidermodysplasia verruciformis and epidermoid carcinoma. Electron microscopic observations. *J.A.M.A. 201:* 775–777, 1967.

2. Archard, H., Heck, J., and Stanley, H. Focal epithelial hyperplasia: An unusual oral mucosal lesion found in Indian children. *Oral Surg. 20:* 201–212, 1965.

3. Balmain, A., and Pragnell, I. B. Mouse skin carcinomas induced *in vivo* by chemical carcinogens have a transforming Harvey-*ras* oncogene. *Nature 303:* 72–74, 1983.

4. Blumberg, B. S., and London, W. T. Hepatitis B virus and primary hepatocellular carcinoma: Relationship of "icrons" to cancer. *Cold Spring Harbor Conf. Cell Proliferation. 7:* 401–421, 1980.

5. Boshart, M., Gissmann, L., Ikenberg, H., Uleinheinz, A., Scheurlen, W., and zur Hausen, H. A new type of papillomavirus DNA: Its presence in genital cancer biopsies and in cell lines derived from cervical cancer. *EMBO J. 3:* 1151–1157, 1984.

6. Boyle, J., Briggs, J. D., MacKie, R. M., Junor, B. J. R., and Aitchison, T. C. Cancer, warts, and sunshine in renal transplant patients. A case-control study. *Lancet i:* 702–705, 1984.

7. Campo, M. S., Moar, M. H., Jarrett, W. F. H., and Laird, H. M. A new papillomavirus associated with alimentary cancer in cattle. *Nature 286:* 180–182, 1980.

8. Chen, E. Y., Howley, P. M., Levinson, A. D., and Seeburg, P. H. The primary structure and genetic organization of the bovine papillomavirus type 1 genome. *Nature 299:* 529–534, 1982.

9. Ciuffo, G. Innesto positivo con filtrato di verruca volgare. *G. Ital. Mal. Venereol. 48:* 12–17, 1907.

10. Clertant, P., and Seif, I. A common function for polyoma virus large-T and papillomavirus E1 proteins? *Nature 311:* 276–279, 1984.

11. Coggin, J. R., and zur Hausen, H. Workshop on papillomaviruses and cancer. *Cancer Res. 39:* 545–546, 1979.

12. Crawford, L. V. A study of human papilloma virus DNA. *J. Mol. Biol. 13:* 362–372, 1965.

13. Crum, C. P., Ikenberg, H., Richart, R. M., and Gissmann, L. Human papillomavirus type 16 and early cervical neoplasia. *N. Engl. J. Med. 310:* 880–883, 1984.

14. Danos, O., Giri, I., Thierry, F., and Yaniv, M. Papillomavirus genomes: Sequences and consequences. *J. Invest. Dermatol. 83* (Suppl.):7s–11s, 1984.

15. Danos, O., Katinka M., and Yaniv, M. Human papillomavirus 1a DNA sequence: A novel type of genome organization. *EMBO J. 1:* 231–236, 1982.

16. Danos, O., and Yaniv, M. An homologous domain between the c-*mos* gene product and a papillomavirus polypeptide with putative role in cellular transformation. In: *Cold Spring Harbor Conferences on Cell Proliferation and Cancer. 12. The Cancer Cell. Oncogenes and Viral Genes*, in press, 1985.

17. Donner, P., Greiser-Wilke, K., and Moelling, K. Nuclear localization and DNA binding of the transforming gene product of avian myelomatosis virus. *Nature 296:* 262–266, 1982.

18. Donoghue, D. J., Anderson, C., Hunter, T., and Kaplan, P. L. Transmission of the polyoma virus middle T gene as the oncogene of a murine retrovirus. *Nature 308:* 748–750, 1984.

19. Durst, M., Gissmann, L., Ikenberg, H., and zur Hausen, H. A papillomavirus from a cervical carcinoma and its prevalence in cancer biopsy samples from different geographic regions. *Proc. Natl. Acad. Sci. USA 80:* 3812–3815, 1983.

20. Dvoretzky, I., Shober, R., and Lowy, D. Focus assay in mouse cells for bovine papillomavirus. *Virology 103:* 369–375, 1980.

21. Engel, L. W., Heilman, C. A., and Howley, P. M. Transcriptional organization of bovine papillomavirus type 1. *J. Virol. 47:* 516–528, 1983.

22. Epstein, M. A. An assessment of the possible role of viruses in the aetiology of Burkitt's lymphoma. *Prog. Exp. Tumor Res. 21:* 72–99, 1978.

23. Favre, M., Breitburd, F., Croissant, O., and Orth, G. Chromatin-like structures obtained after alkaline disruption of bovine and human papillomaviruses. *J. Virol. 21:* 1205–1209, 1977.

24. Fisher, M. S., and Kripke, M. L. Systematic alteration induced in mice by ultraviolet light irradiation and its relationship to ultraviolet carcinogenesis. *Proc. Natl. Acad. Sci. USA 74:* 1688–1692, 1977.

25. Ford, J. N., Jennings, P. A., Spradbrow, P. B., and Francis, J. Evidence for papillomaviruses in ocular lesions in cattle. *Res. Vet. Sci. 32:* 257–259, 1982.

26. Gissmann, L., Boshart, M., Durst, M., Ikenberg, H., Wagner, D., and zur Hausen, H. Presence of human papillomavirus in genital tumors. *J. Invest. Dermatol. 83*(Suppl.):26s–28s, 1984.

27. Gissmann, L., de Villiers, E-M., and zur Hausen, H. Analyses of human genital warts (condylomata acuminata) and other genital tumors for human papillomaviruses type 6 DNA. *Int. J. Cancer 29:* 143–146, 1982.

28. Gissmann, L., Pfister, H., and zur Hausen, H. Human papillomaviruses (HPV): Characterization of four different isolates. *Virology 76:* 569–580, 1977.

29. Gissmann, L., Wolnik, L., Ikenberg, H., Koldovsky, U., Schnurch, H. G., and zur Hausen, H. Human papillomavirus type 6 and 11 DNA sequences in genital and laryngeal papillomas and in some cervical cancers. *Proc. Natl. Acad. Sci. USA 80:* 560–563, 1983.

30. Green, M., Brackmann, K. H., Sanders, P. R., Loewenstein, P. M., Freel, J. H., Eisinger, M., and Switlyk, S. A. Isolation of a human papillomavirus from a patient with epidermodysplasia verruciformis: Presence of related viral DNA genomes in human urogenital tumors. *Proc. Natl. Acad. Sci. USA 79:* 4437–4441, 1982.

31. Hardie, I. R., Strong, R. W., Harley, C. J., Woodruff, P. W. H., and Clunie, G. J. A. Skin cancer in Caucasian renal allograft recipients living in a subtropical climate. *Surgery 87:* 177–183, 1980.

32. Heilman, C. A., Law, M. F., Israel, M. A., and Howley, P. M. Cloning of human papilloma virus genomic DNA and analysis of homologous polypeptide sequences. *J. Virol. 36:* 395–407, 1980.

33. Henle, G., Henle, W., and Ho, H. Antibodies to Epstein-Barr virus in naso-pharyngeal carcinoma, other head and neck neoplasms, and control groups. *J. Natl. Cancer Inst. 44:* 225–231, 1970.

34. Hersey, P., Hasic, E., Edwards, A., Bradley, M., Haran, G., and McCarthy, W. H. Immunological effects of solarium exposure. *Lancet i:* 545–548, 1983.

35. Hollander, C. F., and Van Noord, M. Focal epithelial hyperplasia: A virus-induced oral mucosal lesion in the chimpanzee. *Oral Surg. 33:* 220–226, 1972.

36. Howley, P. M. The molecular biology of papillomavirus transformation. *Am. J. Pathol. 113:* 414–421, 1983.

37. Howley, P. M., Law, M-F., Heilman, C., Engel, L., Alonso, M. C., Lancaster, W. D., Israel, M. A., and Lowy, D. R. Molecular characterization of papilloma virus genomes. *Cold Spring Harbor Conf. Cell Prolif. 7:* 233–247, 1980.

38. Ikenberg, H., Gissmann, L., Gross, G., Grussendorf-Conen, E-L., and zur Hausen, H. Human papillomavirus type-16-related DNA in genital Bowen's disease and in Bowenoid papulosis. *Int. J. Cancer 32:* 563–566, 1983.

39. Jablonska, S., Orth, G., and Lutzner, M. A. Immunopathology of papillomavirus-induced tumors in different tissues. *Springer Semin. Immunopathol. 5:* 33–62, 1982.

40. Jacyk, W. K., and Subbuswamy, S. G. Epidermodysplasia in Nigerians. *Dermatologica 159:* 256–265, 1983.

41. Jarrett, W. F. H., McNiel, P. E., Grimshaw, W. T. R., Selman, I. E., and McIntyre, W. I. M. High incidence of cattle cancer with a possible interaction between an environmental carcinogen and a papilloma virus. *Nature 274:* 215–217, 1978.

42. Jenson, A. B., Rosenthal, J. R., Olson, C., Pass, F., Lancaster, W. D., and Shah, K. Immunological relatedness of papillomavirus and human papillomaviruses from different species. *J. Natl. Cancer Inst. 64:* 495–500, 1980.

43. Klug, A., and Finch, J. T. Structure of viruses of the papilloma-polyoma type. I. Human wart virus. *J. Mol. Biol. 11:* 403–423, 1965.

44. Kremsdorf, D., Jablonska, S., Favre, M., and Orth, G. Biochemical characterization of two types of human papillomaviruses associated with epidermodysplasia verruciformis. *J. Virol. 43:* 436–447, 1982.

45. Kremsdorf, D., Jablonska, S., Favre, M., and Orth, G. Human papillomaviruses associated with epidermodysplasia verruciformis. II. Molecular cloning and biochemical characterization of human papillomavirus 3a, 8, 10, and 12 genomes. *J. Virol. 48:* 340–351, 1983.

46. Koranda, F. C., Dehmel, E. M., Kahn, G., and Penn, I. Cutaneous complications of immunosuppressed renal homograft recipients. *J.A.M.A. 229:* 419–424, 1974.

47. Kurman, R. J., Shah, K. H., Lancaster, W. D., and Jenson, A. B. Immunoperoxidase localization of papillomaviruses antigens in cervical dysplasia and vulvar condylomas. *Am. J. Obstet. Gynecol. 140:* 931–935, 1981.

48. Lack, E. E., Jenson, A. B., Smith, H. G., Healy, G. B., Pass, F., and Vawter, C. F. Immunoperoxidase localization of human papillomavirus in laryngeal papilloma. *Intervirology 14:* 148–154, 1980.

49. Lancaster, W. D. Apparent lack of integration of bovine papilloma virus DNA in virus-induced equine and bovine tumors and virus-transformed mouse cells. *Virology 108:* 251–255, 1981.

50. Lancaster, W. D., and Jenson, A. B. Evidence for papillomavirus genus specific antigens and DNA in laryngeal papillomas. *Intervirology 15:* 204–212, 1981.

51. Lancaster, W. D., and Olson, C. Animal papillomaviruses. *Microbiol. Rev. 46:* 191–207, 1982.

52. Land, H., Parada, L. F., and Weinberg, R. A. Cellular oncogenes and multistep carcinogenesis. *Science 222:* 771–778, 1983.

53. Laurent, R., Kienzler, J. L., Croissant, O., and Orth, G. Two anatomo-clinical types of warts with plantar localization: Specific cytopathogenic effects of papillomavirus type 1 (HPV1) and type 2 (HPV2). *Arch. Dermatol. Res. 274:* 101–111, 1982.

53A. Laurent, R., Coume-Marquet, J. L., Kienzler, J. L., Lambert, D., and Agache, P. Comparative electron microscopy of clear cells in epidermodysplasia verruciformis and flat warts. *Arch. Dermatol. Res. 263:* 1–12, 1978.

54. Law, M-F., Lowy, D. R., Dvoretzky, I., and Howley, P. M. Mouse cells transformed by bovine papillomavirus contain only extrachromosomal viral DNA sequences. *Proc. Natl. Acad. Sci. USA 78:* 2727–2731, 1981.

55. Lowenstein, L. Carcinoma-like condylomata accuminata of the penis. *Med. Clin. North Am. 23:* 789–795, 1939.

56. Lowy, D. R., Dvoretzky, I., Shober, R., Law M-F., Engel, L., and Howley, P. M. *In vitro* tumorigenic transformation by a defined sub-genomic fragment of bovine papilloma virus DNA. *Nature 287:* 72–74, 1980.

57. Lusky, M., and Botchan, M. Characterization of the bovine papillomavirus plasmid maintenance sequences. *Cell 36:* 391–401, 1984.

58. Lutzner, M. A. Epidermodysplasia verruciformis. An autosomal recessive disease characterized by viral warts and skin cancer. A model for viral oncogenesis. *Bull. Cancer* (Paris) *65:* 169–182, 1978.

59. Lutzner, M. A. The human papillomaviruses. A review. *Arch. Dermatol. 119:* 631–635, 1983.

60. Lutzner, M. A., Blanchet-Bardon, C., and Orth, G. Clinical observations, virologic studies and treatment trials in patients with epidermodysplasia verruciformis, a disease induced by specific human papillomaviruses. *J. Invest. Dermatol. 83:* (Suppl.): 18s–25s, 1984.

61. Lutzner, M. A., Croissant, O., Ducasse, M-F., Kreis, H., Crosnier, J., and Orth, G. A potentially oncogenic human papillomavirus (HPV-5) found in two renal allograft recipients. *J. Invest. Dermatol. 75:* 353–356, 1980.

62. Lutzner, M. A., Croissant, O., Ducasse, M-F., Kreis, H., Crosnier, J., and Orth, G. An unusual wart-like skin lesion found in a renal allograft recipient. *Arch. Dermatol. 117:* 43–46, 1981.

63. Lutzner, M. A., Kuffer, R., Blanchet-Bardon, C., and Croissant, O. Different papillomaviruses as the causes of oral warts. *Arch. Dermatol. 118:* 393–399, 1982.

64. Lutzner, M. A., Orth, G., Dutronquay, V., Ducasse, M-F., Kreis, H., and Crosnier, J. Detection of human papillomavirus type 5 DNA in skin cancers of an immunosuppressed renal allograft recipient. *Lancet ii:* 422–424, 1983.

65. Meisels, A., and Fortin, R. Condylomatous lesions of the cervix and vagina. I. Cytological patterns. *Acta Cytol. (Baltimore) 20:* 505–509, 1976.

66. Meisels, A., Roy, M., Fortier, M., Morin, C., Casas-Cordero, M., Shah, K. V., and Turgeon, H. Human papillomavirus infection of the cervix. The atypical condylomata. *Acta Cytol. (Baltimore) 25:* 7–16, 1981.

67. Morin, C., Braun, L., Casas-Cordero, M., Shah, K. V., Roy, M., Fortier, M., and Meisels, A. Confirmation of the papillomavirus etiology of condylomatous cervix lesions by the peroxidase-antiperoxidase technique. *J. Natl. Cancer Inst. 66:* 831–835, 1981.

68. Mounts, P., Shah, K. V., and Kashima, H. Viral etiology of juvenile papillomas and adult-onset squamous papilloma of the larynx. *Proc. Natl. Acad. Sci. USA 79:* 5425–5429, 1982.

69. Nakabayashi, Y., Dvoretzky, I., Chattopadhyay, S. K., and Lowy, D. R. In vitro transformation by bovine papillomavirus. *J. Invest. Dermatol. 83*(Suppl.): 12s–17s, 1984.

70. Orth, G., Breitburd, F., and Favre, M. Evidence for antigenic determinants shared by the structural polypeptides of (Shope) rabbit papillomavirus and human papillomavirus type 1. *Virology 91:* 243–255, 1978.

71. Orth, G., Breitburd, F., Favre, M., and Croissant, O. Papillomaviruses: Possible role in human cancer. *Cold Spring Harbor Conf. on Cell Proliferation 4:* 1043–1068, 1977.

72. Orth, G., Favre, M., Breitburd, F., Croissant, O., Jablonska, S., Obalek, M., Jarzabek-Chorzelska, M., and Rzesa, G. Epidermodysplasia verruciformis: A model for the role of papilloma viruses in human cancer. *Cold Spring Harbor Conf. on Cell Proliferation 7:* 259–281, 1980.

73. Orth, G., Favre, M., and Croissant, O. Characterization of a new type of human papillomavirus that causes skin warts. *J. Virol. 24:* 108–120, 1977.

74. Orth, G., Jablonska, S., Favre, M., Croissant, O., Jarzabek-Chorzelska, M., and Rzesa, G. Characterization of two types of human papillomaviruses in lesions of epidermodysplasia verruciformis. *Proc. Natl. Acad. Sci. USA 75:* 1537–1541, 1978.

75. Orth, G., Jablonska, S., Favre, M., Croissant, O., Obalek, S., Jarzabek-Chorzelska, M., and Jibard, N. Identification of papillomaviruses in butchers' warts. *J. Invest. Dermatol. 76:* 97–102, 1981.

76. Ostrow, R. S., Bender, M., Niimura, M., Seki, T., Kawashima, M., Pass, F., and Faras, A. J. Human papillomavirus DNA in cutaneous primary and metastasized squamous cell carcinomas from patients with epidermodysplasia verruciformis. *Proc. Natl. Acad. Sci. USA 79:* 1634–1638, 1982.

77. Pfister, H., Hettich, I., Runne, U., Gissmann, L., and Chilf, G. N. Characterization of human papillomavirus type 13 from lesions of focal epithelial hyperplasia Heck. *J. Virol. 47:* 363–366, 1983.

78. Pfister, H., Gassenmaier, A., Nurnberger, F., and Stuttgen, G. HPV-5 DNA in a carcinoma of an epidermodysplasia verruciformis patient infected with various human papillomavirus types. *Cancer Res. 43:* 1436–1441, 1983.

79. Pfister, H., Nurnberger, F., Gissmann, L., and zur Hausen, H. Characterization of a human papillomavirus from epidermodysplasia verruciformis lesions of a patient from Upper-Volta. *Int. J. Cancer 27:* 645–650, 1981.

80. Poiesz, B. J., Ruscetti, F. W., Gazdar, A. F., Bunn, P. A., Minna, J. D., and Gallo, R. C. Detection and isolation of type C retrovirus particles from fresh and cultured lymphocytes of a patient with cutaneous T-cell lymphoma. *Proc. Natl. Acad. Sci. USA 77:* 7415–7419, 1980.

81. Praetorius-Clausen, F. Geographical aspects of oral focal epithelial hyperplasia. *Pathol. Microbiol. 39:* 204–213, 1979.

82. Praetorius-Clausen, F. Histopathology of focal epithelial hyperplasia. *Tandlaegeladet. 73:* 1013–1022, 1979.
83. Praetorius-Clausen, F., and Willis, J. M. Papova virus-like particles in focal epithelial hyperplasia. *Scand. J. Dent. Res. 79:* 362–365, 1971.
84. Rabbett, W. F. Juvenile laryngeal papillomatosis; Relationship of irradiation to malignant degeneration in this disease. *Otol. Rhinol. Laryngol. 74:* 1149–1163, 1965.
85. Rhim, J. S., Sanford, K. K., Einstein, P., Fujita, J., Jay, G., and Aaronson, S. A. Human epithelial cell carcinogenesis. Combined action of DNA and RNA tumor viruses producing malignant transformation of primary human epidermal keratinocytes. *Carcinog Compr Surv* 9: 57–66, 1985.
86. Roseto, A., Potheir, P., Guillemin, M-C., Perier, J., Breitburd, F., Bonneaud, N., and Orth, G. Monoclonal antibodies to the major capsid protein of human papillomavirus type 1. *J. Gen. Virol., 65:* 1319–1324, 1984.
87. Rous, P. Transmission of a malignant new growth by means of a cell-free filtrate. *J.A.M.A. 56:* 198, 1911.
88. Rous, P., and Beard, J. W. Carcinomatous changes in virus-induced papillomas of the skin of the rabbit. *Proc. Soc. Exp. Biol. Med. 32:* 578–580, 1935.
89. Rous, P., and Kidd, J. G. The carcinogenic effect of a papilloma virus on the tarred skin of rabbits. I. Description of the phenomenon. *J. Exp. Med. 67:* 399–428, 1938.
90. Rowson, K. E. H., and Mahy, B. W. J. Human papova (wart) virus. *Bacteriol. Rev. 31:* 110–131, 1967.
91. Sarver, N., Gruss, P., Law, M-F., Khoury, G., and Howley, P. M. Bovine papilloma virus deoxyribonucleic acid: Novel eukaryotic cloning vector. *Mol. Cell Biol. 1:* 486–496, 1981.
92. Sarver, N., Rabson, M. S., Yang, Y-C., Byrne, J. C., and Howley, P. M. Localization and analysis of bovine papillomavirus type 1 transforming fuctions. *J. Virol.,* in press, 1985.
93. Schwarz, E., Durst, M., Demankowski, C., Lattermann, O., Zech, R., Wolfsperger, E., Suhai, S., and zur Hausen, H. DNA sequence and genome organization of genital human papillomavirus type 6b. *EMBO J. 2:* 2341–2348, 1983.
94. Shope, R. E. Infectious papillomatosis of rabbits. *J. Exp. Med. 58:* 607–624, 1933.
95. Spradbrow, P. B., Beardmore, G. L., and Francis, J. Virions resembling papillomaviruses in hyperkeratotic lesions from sun-damaged skin. *Lancet i:* 189, 1983.
96. Taichman, L. B., Breitburd, F., Croissant, O., and Orth, G. The search for a culture system for papillomaviruses. *J. Invest. Dermatol. 83*(Suppl.): 2s–6s, 1984.
97. Thomas, M., Boiron, M., Tanzer, J., Levy, J. P., and Bernard, J. In vitro transformation of mice cells by bovine papilloma virus. *Nature 202:* 709–710, 1964.
98. Vanselow, B. A., and Spradbrow, P. B. Papillomaviruses, papillomas, and squamous cell carcinomas in sheep. *Vet. Rec. 110:* 561–562, 1982.
99. Wade, T. R., and Ackerman, A. B. Bowenoid papulosis of the penis. *Cancer 42:* 1890–1903, 1978.
100. Zachow, K. R., Ostrow, R. S., Bender, M., Watts, S., Okagaki, T., Pass, F., and Faras, A. J. Detection of human papillomavirus DNA in anogenital neoplasias. *Nature 300:* 771–773, 1982.
101. zur Hausen, H. Human papillomaviruses and their possible role in squamous cell carcinomas. *Curr. Top. Microbiol. Immunol. 78:* 1–30, 1977.
102. zur Hausen, H. Human genital cancer: Synergism between two virus infections or synergism between a virus infection and initiating events? *Lancet 2:* 1370–1372, 1982.

Chapter 7

Inhibition of Tumor Invasion by Tissue-derived Proteinase Inhibitors

KLAUS E. KUETTNER AND BENDICHT U. PAULI

INTRODUCTION

Mammalian cartilage is highly resistant to invasion by malignant tumor cells.[22,23] This resistance has been studied most thoroughly in human osteosarcoma.[5,10-12,14,15] Osteosarcoma almost always arises singly in the metaphyseal ends of long bones.[14,22,23] Generally, the tumor mass fills the marrow cavity in the metaphyseal region, replaces the cancellous bone, and extends along a broad front toward the unclosed epiphyseal growth plate, at which site it is stopped in its further extension.[11,12,15] Tumor spread through the epiphyseal cartilage occurs only in advanced stages of the disease. It generally proceeds along preexisting, nutritive, vascular channels that penetrate the epiphyseal cartilage in preadolescent humans.[26,27] This penetration of epiphyseal cartilage by osteosarcoma cells may be facilitated by microfractures, ischemic necrosis, and inflammation, secondary to loss of the structural support of underlying bone.[5,26,30] Once osteosarcoma cells have invaded the epiphyseal bone, rapid erosion of this bone occurs. Tumor cells reach up to the calcified matrix of the articular cartilage but do not penetrate the viable cartilage matrix.[11,12,15] This phenomenon of resistance of cartilage to invasion by osteosarcoma cells is not unique and can be observed in other cartilaginous tissues with other primary or metastatic tumors. For example, bronchial cartilage is relatively resistant to invasion by bronchogenic carcinoma, larnygeal cartilage to laryngeal squamous cell carcinoma, and intervertebral disc cartilage to metastatic mammary and prostatic carcinomas.[29]

In vitro, the interaction of human osteosarcoma cells with mammalian hyaline cartilage was studied in a specially designed culture system.[10-12,15,18] In this combined organ-cell culture system, osteosarcoma cells (and other types of malignant cell lines of human or animal origin) were unable to penetrate the hyaline cartilage of the rib costochondral junction and phalanges. Tumor cells reached as far into the epiphyseal cartilage as the vascular loops, to the area of the last hypertrophic chondrocyte and its calcified matrix.[10-12,15] The natural resistance of cartilage to tumor cell invasion was lost only when the hyaline cartilage used in our culture system was modified by salt extraction.[10,11,15,18] These findings suggested that hyaline cartilage contains extractable matrix components that inhibit invasion in an experimental system. Analysis of these salt-extractable substances revealed that the biological activity resided in molecules with a molecular weight of less than 50,000 daltons, and not in the macromolecular structural components of the tissues, *i.e.*, proteoglycans and collagen.[3, 6, 8, 9, 13, 18, 25] Among the isolated low-molecular-weight substances, functionally defined as anti-invasion factor (AIF), a spectrum of proteinase inhibitors was identified.[8, 9, 13, 18] Therefore, we hypothesized that these tissue-derived proteinase inhibitors may prevent proteinases, elaborated by malignant tumor cells (or host mesenchymal "helper" cells that are stimulated by tumor cells), from degrading the extracellular matrix of hyaline cartilage, and thereby may participate in the inhibition of tumor cell invasion into viable hyaline cartilage.[16, 18, 19]

PREPARATION OF ANTI-INVASION FACTOR (AIF)

The isolation procedure for the cartilage-derived anti-invasion factor (AIF), containing various proteinase inhibitors, is standard and has been described in detail by our laboratory. As previously described,[6, 18] slices of fresh hyaline cartilage prepared from nasal septa of 18-month-old bovines are extracted with 1 M NaCl (0.05 M Na-acetate, pH 5.8, 24 hours, at 4°C). The extract is decanted from the tissue, and in order to minimize nonspecific protein-protein interactions, is adjusted to 3 M NaCl by the addition of solid NaCl. Ultrafiltration of the crude cartilage extract yields two fractions: the XM-50 retentate (MW > 50,000), and, after dialysis and concentration, the UM-2 retentate, designated as anti-invasion factor (AIF) (1,000 > MW > 50,000 daltons). The XM-50 retentate contains the majority of the proteins and proteoglycans, as indicated by standard biochemical analyses (uronic acid, hexose, and hydroxyproline). In contrast, AIF contains only about 40 µg protein per gram tissue, with minimal amounts of hexuronic acid, hexose, and hydroxyproline. SDS-PAGE reveals that AIF contains seven major protein bands. The protein band with the highest molecular weight appears to be immunologically identical to albumin, which is apparently a result of its incomplete rejection by the XM-50 membrane (as indicated by the manufacturer, Amicon Corp.). The protein with the lowest molecular weight migrates between Trasylol (MW 6500) and insulin (MW 5700).

THE PROTEINASE INHIBITORY ACTIVITIES OF AIF

Crude AIF expresses inhibitory activity against a variety of proteinases from normal and neoplastic tissues (Fig. 7.1)[18]: (1) trypsin; (2) chymotrypsin; (3) elastase derived from human leukocytes; (4) collagenase derived from human skin, human leukocytes, TE-85 osteosarcoma, and metastatic AlAb mammary carcinoma cells; (5) type IV collagen (basement membrane collagen)-degrading, neutral metalloproteinase derived from metastatic murine PMT sarcoma; (6) type V collagen-degrading, neutral metalloproteinase derived from murine M-5076 reticulum cell sarcoma; and (7) cathepsin G derived from human leukocytes.

Our primary goal has been to separate the various proteinase inhibitory activities in AIF into single enzyme activities. This has been achieved for the

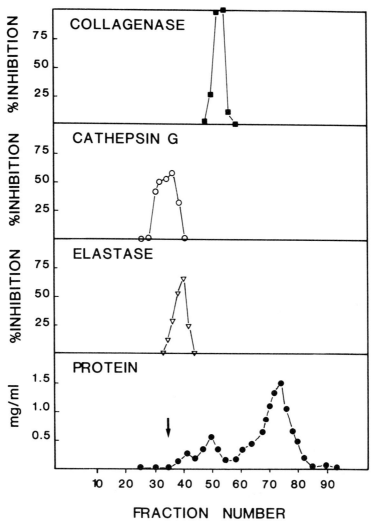

Fig. 7.1. Cartilage-derived AIF is fractioned on a Biogel P-30 column in 3 M NaCl. Fractions are analyzed for protein content (Lowry) and for inhibitory activities against collagenase, cathepsin G, and elastase.

trypsin inhibitory activity, the collagenase inhibitory activity, and the elastase inhibitory activity. Roughley *et al.*[24] also isolated a thiolproteinase inhibitory activity. The trypsin inhibitory activity has been purified by immunoadsorption techniques after separation from AIF by a trypsin-Sepharose column.

THE TRYPSIN INHIBITOR

The trypsin inhibitor in cartilage can be readily extracted by 1 M NaCl (use of dissociative solvents such as 4 M guanidinium chloride yields no further amounts). It is isolated and purified by passing AIF over an affinity column containing trypsin immobilized on Sepharose (highly purified trypsin is coupled to CNBr-activated Sepharose 4B) (Thonar *et al.*, unpublished data).

Bound inhibitor is eluted from the column with 0.3 M KCl/HCl at pH 2 (Fig. 7.2) and concentrated on a small column of CM52 (Whatman). The purified trypsin inhibitor has been found to resemble the Kunitz inhibitor (Trasylol) with respect to molecular weight (MW 6500), antigenicity, amino acid composition, and range of susceptible proteinases.[21] Susceptible proteinases are trypsin, chrymotrypsin, plasmin, proteoglycans-degrading enzymes derived from human leukocytes, and caseinolytic proteinases derived from rat bladder carcinoma (RBTCC-8).[7, 16, 18, 21, 24] The inhibitor accounts for 100% of the antitryptic activity in cartilage-derived AIF. It does not express any activity against pancreatic elastase[24] or collagenase derived from human leukocytes.

Using polyclonal rabbit anti-Trasylol antibodies in an enzyme-linked immunoabsorbent assay (ELISA) inhibition assay we have shown that (1) cartilage-derived trypsin inhibitor and Trasylol yield identical inhibition curves, and are therefore immunologically identical (Fig. 7.3); and (2) cartilage-derived trypsin inhibitor is present in AIF at concentrations ranging from 4–10 µg/ml, which corresponds to 27–66 µg/kg wet bovine nasal septum cartilage (blood serum concentration: 20 ng/ml). The rabbit anti-Trasylol antiserum used in these studies contains several types of antibodies, all of which recognize both the cartilage-derived trypsin inhibitor and the commercial Trasylol. Some of these antibodies recognize both inhibitor and inhibitor-trypsin complexes; others do not interact with the inhibitor once it is complexed. No cartilage component, even when present in excess, is able to block the specific interaction between antibody and inhibitor.

Preliminary studies of cartilage explants and chondrocyte cultures indicate that the trypsin inhibitor is not synthesized by chondrocytes. More likely, the

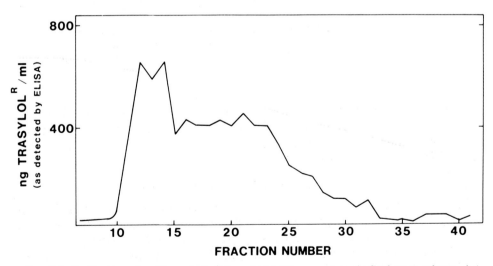

FIG. 7.2. Purification of cartilage-derived trypsin inhibitor on a trypsin-Sepharose column. A 1 M NaCl extract of bovine nasal septum cartilage (AIF) is fractionated on a trypsin-Sepharose column (trypsin is coupled to CNBr-activated Sepharose 4B), utilizing 0.3 M KCl–HCl, pH 2.0, as an elution buffer. This simple step is effective in purifying the inhibitor and separating it from the remainder of the AIF proteins. In this particular run, yields of 358 µg trypsin inhibitor/kg wet cartilage were obtained.

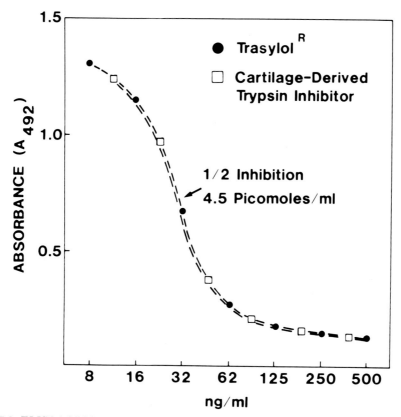

Fɪɢ. 7.3. ELISA inhibition curves for Trasylol and cartilage-derived trypsin inhibitor. A fixed amount of anti-Trasylol antibody is first allowed to interact with varying amounts of Trasylol or cartilage-derived trypsin inhibitor. One hour later, these inhibition mixtures are placed in plates coated with Trasylol and processed in an ELISA assay as described by Thonar *et. al.*[26a] Identical inhibition curves for Trasylol and cartilage-derived trypsin inhibitor, obtained by using a polyclonal anti-Trasylol antiserum, strongly suggest that the two trypsin inhibitors are antigenically identical.

inhibitor is absorbed and concentrated from blood plasma and body fluids, in which it is ubiquitously present. The polyanionic molecules of the cartilage matrix may thereby act as a "sponge" for uptake and storage of the cationic trypsin inhibitor (Fig. 7.4).[18]

THE COLLAGENASE INHIBITOR

The collagenase inhibitory activity of AIF has first been described by our laboratory[9, 13] and later purified by Roughley *et al.*[24] These investigators have been able to separate the collagenase inhibitory activity by Ultrogel AcA 54 (LKB Instruments) in 50 mM Tris/HCl, pH 7.5, containing 1 M NaCl, 5 mM CaCl₂, and 0.05% Brij 35. The collagenase inhibitory activity occurs as a single peak of about 22,000 daltons molecular weight. In a reconstituted collagen fibril assay, linear inhibition of rabbit skin collagenase and human leukocyte collagenase is observed with increasing inhibitor concentrations. No inhibition is detected against bacterial collagenase.

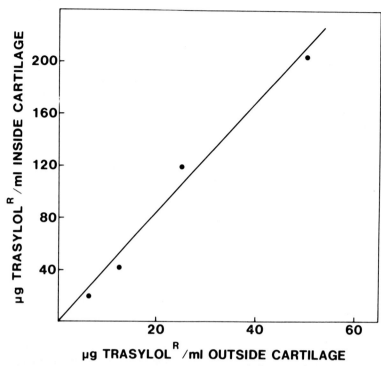

FIG. 7.4. Binding of Trasylol to cartilage matrix. Relationship between the amount of Trasylol present in the matrix of cartilage and the amount present in the solution in which the cartilage is incubated: Thin shavings of bovine nasal cartilage are incubated for 2 hours at room temperature in phosphate-buffered saline containing varying amounts of Trasylol. The shavings are rinsed for 15 minutes in large excesses of phosphate-buffered saline. The cartilage shavings are then extracted with 1 M NaCl and the Trasylol present in the extracts is quantitated by ELISA techniques. The results show that cartilage effectively binds and concentrates Trasylol from surrounding fluids. The amount bound appears to be a function of the Trasylol concentration in the surrounding fluid. The maximal amount which can be bound in this way is at least 1000-fold greater than the amount normally found in the tissue (approximately 60 ng/g wet cartilage). Once bound, the Trasylol can only be extracted by nonphysiological salt concentrations (*i.e.*, 1 M NaCl).

In our laboratory, we have reproduced the isolation and purification procedures of Roughley *et al.*[24] Although this procedure yields a single peak of enzyme activity which is reasonably well separated from other AIF proteinase inhibitory activities, we have found separation of the collagenase inhibitory activity on Biogel P-30 to be efficient. The collagenolytic activity is well separated from other proteinase inhibitory activities such as elastase and cathepsin G inhibitory activities. As estimated by SDS-PAGE, the molecular weight of our collagenase inhibitory activity is similar to that reported by Roughley *et al.*[24] The collagenase inhibitory activity is sensitive to trypsin at 37°C but is relatively resistent to heat (5 minutes at 100°C).

THE ELASTASE INHIBITOR

The elastase inhibitor has been separated from other AIF-proteinase inhibitors, utilizing a column of Bio-Gel P-30 in 3 M NaCl (Arsensis *et al.*, manuscript in preparation) (Fig. 7.5). Fractions containing elastase inhibitory activity were pooled, dialyzed, and lyophilized. The lyophilized residue was resuspended in a small volume of 0.01 M ammonium acetate, pH 7.0, and loaded onto an affinity column containing purified porcine elastase immobilized on agarose (Affi-gel 10). After washing with 0.01 M ammonium acetate, the column was eluted with a continuous gradient between 0.01 and 0.5 M ammonium acetate. The elastate inhibitor was eluted in the middle of the gradient.

The purified elastase inhibitor has an apparent molecular weight of 8000 daltons as estimated by SDS-PAGE and is trypsin and heat labile. It inhibits leukocyte elastase solubilization of a variety of substrates, including type I collagen, type IV collagen, elastin (Fig. 7.6), cartilage proteoglycans, and the synthetic elastase substrate succinyl-(alanyl)$_3$-p-nitroaniline. The inhibition is noncompetitive and irreversible. The elastase inhibitor does not inhibit trypsin, leukocyte collagenase, leukocyte cathepsin G, catheptic activity derived from rat bladder carcinoma, or any other nonelastolytic enzyme activity tested thus far.

OTHER PROTEINASE INHIBITORS

Other proteinase inhibitory activities have been isolated from AIF by Roughley *et al.*[24] and by our laboratory. These investigators have described a thiol-

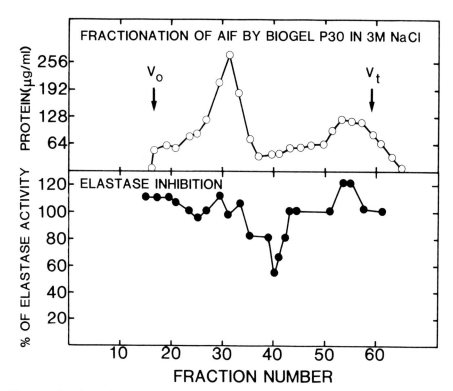

FIG. 7.5. Cartilage-derived AIF is fractionated on a Biogel P-30 column in 3 M NaCl. Fractions are analyzed for protein content (○) and inhibitory activity (●) against human leukocyte elastase (substrate = [³H]elastase). Fraction 40 contains significant elastase inhibitory activity.

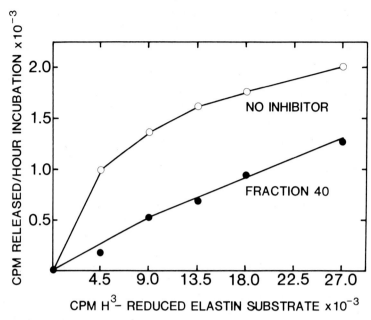

FIG. 7.6. Kinetics of elastase inhibiton. Aliquots of fraction 40 (elastase inhibitory activity) are added to increasing concentrations of [³H]elastin in the presence of a constant amount of neutrophil elastase. Assays are allowed to proceed for 3 hours at 37°C. Radioactivity that has been solubilized is plotted against substrate concentration.

proteinase inhibitor directed against cathepsin B and papain. An inhibitory activity in AIF, which is directed against cathepsin G derived from human leukocytes, has recently been detected in our laboratory. This inhibitory activity is different from the cartilage trypsin inhibitor. It has an apparent molecular weight of about 30,000 daltons.

INHIBITION OF TUMOR INVASION BY AIF PROTEINASE INHIBITORS

In vitro assay systems have been developed in our laboratory that allow for the quantitative assessment of tumor cell invasion outside the animal host and for an efficient testing of anti-invasive drugs.[15, 18] For the quantitation of invasion, these assays rely on the ability of invasive tumor cells to degrade and penetrate extracellular matrices. The degree of invasiveness is determined by (1) the depth of tumor cell invasion into a natural connective tissue substrate, using light and/or electron microscopy techniques; (2) the number of tumor cells that have penetrated a connective tissue of defined thickness; or (3) the release of radioisotopes from labeled connective tissue substrates. The systems currently in use in our laboratory are: (1) the extracted cartilage invasion assay[17, 18]; and (2) the ⁴⁵Ca-labeled fetal rat bone invasion assay.[6, 20]

The extracted cartilage invasion assay system has been previously described in detail,[17] and is therefore only briefly discussed here. In specially designed stainless steel chambers, extracted hyaline cartilage is used as growth surfaces for test tumor cells. The degree of invasiveness is measured by microscopically recording the depth of tumor cell invasion into the connective tissue substrates or by counting the number of tumor cells which totally penetrate the connective tissue substrates. For AIF testing, we used human osteosarcoma cells and human metastatic mammary carcinoma cells. These tumor cells were unable to penetrate viable cartilage during a 2-week culture period. When cartilage was devitalized by freezing and thawing, the tissue remained resistant to invasion. Cartilage, extracted with 3 M guanidine hydrochloride, however, was superficially invaded by malignant tumor cells but remained resistant to invasion by fibroblasts.[15, 18] Tumor invasion into salt-extracted cartilage was completely abolished when low concentrations of cartilage-derived AIF were added to the culture medium. This assay system has since been replaced by the more sensitive "[45]Ca-labeled fetal rat bone invasion assay."

The "[45]Ca-labeled fetal rat bone invasion assay" is a modification of that used by Raisz and Nieman[20] and Horton *et al.*[6] It employs [45]Ca-labeled fetal rat bone and test tumor cells in combined organ cell culture. Paired shafts of the radius and the ulna from 19-day-old rat fetuses, radiolabeled by injection of the mother with 250 μ Ci of [45]Ca on the previous day, are placed individually into round-bottom wells of a 96-well plate. They are incubated at 37°C in a humidified 5% CO_2/air atmosphere in 200 μl of F12/DME (1:1) growth medium, supplemented with 1 mg/ml bovine serum albumin, 1 mM L-glutamine, 100 units/ml penicillin, and 100 μg/ml streptomycin. Fresh or devitalized (repeated freezing and thawing in distilled water) bones are incubated for an initial 18-hour period, which serves to remove exchangeable [45]Ca. Varying concentrations of tumor cells are then added in growth medium with or without anti-invasive drugs. Bone shafts and tumor cells are cultured for up to 144 hours with appropriate transfer into fresh medium every 48 hours. The degree of bone resorption (osteolysis) in each culture is measured by the percent depletion of [45]Ca from radiolabeled fetal bone [100 × cpm medium/cpm medium + cpm (bone)], utilizing liquid scintillation spectrometry. The data are expressed as the mean percent of radioactivity released from four pairs of cultured bones for each test condition.   Malignant rat bladder carcinoma cells, which were previously shown to penetrate bony matrices when injected juxtafemorally into syngeneic rats, were used as test cells in this system. If tumor cells (1 x 10^6 cell/assay) were coincubated with live or dead bones, fetal rat bony matrices were destroyed by invading tumor cells, releasing approximately 65% of the total [45]Ca. Live control bones incubated without tumor cells, released 20% of the total [[45]Ca] (osteoclastic osteolysis), whereas dead bone released only 4%. These findings correlated well with data from our enzyme studies, in which extracts from malignant rat bladder carcinoma cells were shown to efficiently degrade purified matrix macromolecules (collagens of type I and type IV, proteoglycans, hyaluronic acid) and particulate collagens from rat tail tendon and anterior lens capsule (Pauli *et al.*, manuscript in preparation). Release of [45]Ca could be significantly inhibited by the addition of AIF containing the various proteinase inhibitors described above. In the presence of AIF 200 μg/ml malignant rat bladder carcinoma cells released 35% of the total [45]Ca from live bone and 10% from dead bone. These data provide evidence that the resistance of cartilage to tumor invasion is regulated at least in part by tissue-derived proteinase inhibitors.

RESISTANCE OF OTHER TISSUES TO TUMOR INVASION

Tissues which are rather resistant to invasive processes share with cartilage the property that they are devoid of an intrinsic capillary blood supply. Some of these resistant tissues are aorta, heart valves, cornea, lens, vitreous, and epithelia. Of these tissues, bovine aorta and bovine bladder epithelium have been investigated in greatest detail. Utilizing the extraction and ultrafiltration procedures that were originally developed for cartilage, Eisenstein and his associates[1-4] isolated a similar anti-invasion factor from bovine aorta. These investigators showed that the low molecular weight fraction of aortic extract contained a potent trypsin inhibitor, which also resembled the basic pancreatic trypsin inhibitor (Trasylol), as well as a collagenase inhibitor.[2] The low molecular weight fraction prepared from bovine aorta also inhibited the growth of a transplantable mammary tumor and a fibrosarcoma in mice.[4] Tumors appeared earliest and grew fastest in the control groups. They appeared later and grew more slowly in animals injected with aortic extract. In animal groups that received tumor cells suspended in medium containing the extract, tumors appeared very late and grew very slowly. The effect was greater on fibrosarcoma than on mammary tumors, perhaps because the extract had a direct growth inhibitory effect on the fibrosarcoma, at least in cell culture. Thus, aortic extract may exert its effect by inhibiting not only invasiveness but also proliferation of these tumor cells.[4]

A low molecular weight factor with bioactivities similar to those of cartilage AIF was recently isolated from bovine urinary bladder epithelium.[28] The bladder-derived AIF also contained a Trasylol-like trypsin inhibitor and a collagenase inhibitor. The inhibitory spectrum of the bladder-derived proteinase inhibitors was similar to that of the corresponding proteinase inhibitors in cartilage.

CONCLUSIONS

Invasion of malignant tumor cells into host tissues seems to be locally regulated, at least in part, by extractable low-molecular-weight components. These anti-invasive components are a spectrum of proteinase inhibitors.[15] The proteinase inhibitors are enriched in avascular tissues such as cartilage and aorta, where they seem to efficiently prevent the enzymatic degradation of extracellular matrices by malignant tumor cells and/or their host "helper cells." The applicability of proteinase inhibitors in the treatment of cancer is currently being evaluated. Results of preliminary studies, in which proteinase inhibitors are used as anti-invasive or antimetastatic drugs, are controversial, but studies have to be continued using combinations of proteinase inhibitors, rather than individual proteinase inhibitors as in the past.

ACKNOWLEDGMENTS

This work was supported by USPHS Grants CA-21566 and CA-25034 from the National Cancer Institute, and in part by Grant R-1394 from the Council for Tobacco Research-USA, Inc.

The authors wish to thank their research staffs for having contributed much of the information in this paper.

REFERENCES

1. Eisenstein, R., Goren, S. B., Schumacher, B., Choromokos, E. The inhibition of corneal vascularization with aortic extracts in rabbits. *Am. J. Ophthalmol. 88:* 1005–1012, 1979.
2. Eisenstein, R., Harper, E., Kuettner, K. E., Schumacher, B., and Matijevitch, B. Growth regulators in connective tissues. II. Evidence for the presence of several growth inhibitors in aortic extracts. *Paroi Arterielle 5:* 163–169, 1979.
3. Eisenstein, R., Keuttner, K. E., Neapolitan, C., Soble L. W., and Sorgente, N. The resistance of certain tissues to invasion. III. Cartilage extracts inhibit the growth of fibroblasts and endothelial cells in culture. *Am. J. Pathol. 81:* 337–348, 1975.
4. Eisenstein, R., Schumacher, B., Meineke, C., Matijevitch, B., and Keuttner, K. E. Growth regulators in connective tissue. Systemic administration of an aortic extract inhibits tumor growth in mice. *Am. J. Pathol. 91:* 1–10, 1978.
5. Enneking, W. F., and Kagan, A. Transepiphyseal extension of osteosarcoma: Incidence, mechanism, and implications. *Cancer 41:* 1526–1537, 1978.
6. Horton, J. E., Wezeman, F. H., and Keuttner, K. E. Inhibition of in vitro bone resorption by a cartilage-derived anti-collagenase factor. *Science 199:* 1342–1344, 1978.
7. Knight, J. A., Stephens, R. W., Bushell, G. R., Ghosh, P., and Taylor T. K. F. Neutral protease inhibitors from human intervertebral disc and femoral head articular cartilage. *Biochim. Biophys. Acta 584:* 304–310, 1979.
8. Kuettner, K. E., Harper, E. J., and Eisenstein, R. Protease inhibitors in cartilage. *Arthritis Rheum. 20:* 3124–3129, 1977.
9. Kuettner, K. E., Hiti, J., Eisenstein, R., and Harper E. Collagenase inhibition by cationic proteins derived from cartilage and aorta. *Biochem. Biophys. Res. Commun. 72:* 40–46, 1976.
10. Kuettner, K. E., and Pauli, B. U. Resistance of cartilage to normal and neoplastic invasion. Proceedings: mechanisms of localized bone loss. *Calcif Tissue Res. Abstr.* (Suppl): 251–278, 1979.
11. Kuettner, K. E., and Pauli, B. U. Resistance of cartilage to invasion. In: *Bone Metastasis,* edited by L. Weiss and H. A. Gilbert. Boston, G. K. Halls, 1981, pp. 131–165.
12. Kuettner, K. E., Pauli, B. U., and Soble, L. Morphological studies on the resistance of cartilage to invasion by osteosarcoma cells in vitro and in vivo. *Cancer Res. 38:* 227–287, 1978.
13. Kuettner, K. E., Soble, L. W., Croxen, R. I., Marczynska, B., Hiti, J., Harper, E. Tumor cell collagenase and its inhibition by a cartilage-derived protease inhibitor. *Science 196:* 653–654, 1977.
14. McKenna, R. J., Schwinn, C. P., Soong, K. Y., and Higginbotham, N. Sarcomata of the osteogenic series (osteosarcoma, fibrosarcoma, chondrosarcoma, paraosteal osteogenic sarcoma and sarcomata) arising in abnormal bone. An analysis of 552 cases. *J. Bone Join Surg. 48a:* 1–26, 1966.
15. Pauli, B. U., and Keuttner, K. E. The regulation of invasion by cartilage-derived anti-invasion factor. In: Liotta LA, Hart IR, eds. *Tumor Invasion and Metastasis,* edited by L. A. Liotta and I. R. Hart. The Hague, Martinus Nijhoff, 1982, pp. 267–290.
16. Pauli, B. U., and Kuettner, K. E. Tumor invasion and its local regulation. *Urology 23:* 18–28, 1984.
17. Pauli, B. U., and Memoli, V. A., and Kuettner, K. E. In vitro determination of tumor invasiveness using extracted hyaline cartilage. *Cancer Res. 41:* 2084–2091, 1981.
18. Pauli, B. U., Memoli, V. A., and Kuettner, K. E. Regulation of tumor invasion by cartilage-derived anti-invasion factor in vitro. *J. Natl. Cancer Inst. 67:* 65–73, 1981.
19. Pauli, B. U., Schwartz, D. E., Thonar, E. J. M., and Kuettner, K. E. Tumor invasion and host extracellular matrix. *Cancer Metab Rev. 2:* 129–152, 1983.
20. Raisz, L. G., and Niemann, I. Effects of phosphate, calcium, and magnesium on bone resorption and hormonal responses in tissue culture. *Endocrinology 85:* 446–452, 1969.
21. Rifkin, D. R., and Crowe, R. M. Isolation of proteinase inhibitor from tissues resistant to tumor invasion. *Hoppe-Seylers Z. Physiol. Chem. 358:* 1525–1531, 1977.
22. Robbins, S. L., Cotran, R. S., and Kumar, V. Pathologic basis of disease, 3rd ed. Philadelphia, W. B. Saunders, 1984, pp. 1337–1340.

23. Rosai, J. Tumors and tumor-like conditions of bone. In: *Pathology,* 7th ed., vol. 2. St. Louis, C. W. Mosby, 1977, pp. 1978–2014.

24. Roughley, P. J., Murphy, G., Barrett, A. J. Proteinase inhibitors of bovine nasal cartilage. *Biochem. J., 169:* 721–724, 1978.

25. Sorgente, N., Kuettner, K. E., Soble, L. W., and Eisenstein, R. The resistance of certain tissues to invasion. II. Evidence of extractable factors in cartilage which inhibit invasion by vascularized mesenchyme. *Lab. Invest. 32:* 217–222, 1975.

26. Spira, E., and Farin, I. The vascular supply to the epiphyseal plate under normal and pathologic conditions. *Acta Orthop. Scand. 38:* 1–22, 1967.

26a. Thonar, E. J–M., Kimura, J. H., Hascall, V. C., Poole, A. R. Enzyme-linked Immunosorbent Assay Analyses of the hyaluronate-binding region and the link protein of proteoglycan aggregate. *J. Biol. Chem. 257:* 14173–14180, 1982.

27. Trueta, J., and Morgan, J. D. The vascular contribution to osteogenesis. *J. Bone Joint Surg. 42B:* 97–109, 1960.

28. Waxler, B. Kuettner, K. E., and Pauli, B. U. The resistance of epithelia to vascularization: Proteinase and endothelial cell growth inhibitory activities in urinary bladder epithelium. *Tissue Cell 14:* 657–667, 1982.

29. Willis, R. A. *The Spread of Tumors in the Human Body.* London, Butterworths, 1952.

30. Young, M. H. Changes in the growth cartilage resulting from ischemic necrosis of the metaphysis. *J. Pathol. Bacteriol. 85:* 481–488, 1963.

Chapter 8

Tumor Invasion and Metastasis

LANCE A. LIOTTA and C. N. RAO

Metastasis is the major cause of therapeutic failure in patients with solid tumors. Surgery, chemotherapy, and radiotherapy can now cure approximately 50% of patients harboring a malignant tumor. The remaining patients succumb to the direct effect of the metastases or to complications (such as immunosuppression and coagulation disorders) resulting from metastasis treatment. Metastases are frequently multiple, in dispersed anatomic locations, and contain heterogenous cell populations. These factors hinder the clinical detection and treatment of metastases.[8, 13, 25, 35]

The histopathology of a tumor frequently does not accurately predict its aggressive behavior. This is particularly true for common cancers such as breast carcinoma and colon carcinoma. A major challenge to cancer scientists is therefore the development of improved methods to: (a) estimate the metastatic propensity of a patient's individual tumor; (b) detect clinically occult micrometastases; (c) prevent local invasion; and (d) treat established metastases in dispersed anatomic locations. This can be accomplished through a program of research leading to an understanding of the fundamental biochemical and genetic mechanisms of cancer invasion and metastasis.

The hope is that such research will uncover specific biochemical factors to be used as the basis for diagnosis and therapy strategies. A rapidly developing area of research is the interaction of the metastatic tumor cell with the extracellular matrix (ECM). Interaction with the ECM is required at many stages in the metastatic cascade. Specific receptors and enzymes are hypothesized to be involved. These results are currently being investigated for diagnostic usefulness in humans and experimental therapies in animals.

COMPLEXITY OF TUMOR INVASION AND METASTASES

Primary tumor invasion of adjacent tissue beds and neovascularization are early steps in a complex process which results in metastasis establishment and growth. Tumor cells at the invasion front penetrate host tissue barriers and gain access to vascular and lymphatic channels. Invasion of lymphatics may take place predominantly at the tumor borders since the internal regions of tumors lack a lymphatic supply.[8, 13, 19, 25]

Invasion of vessels can take place within the tumor mass or at the interface with the host stroma.[17] The defective nature of newly formed tumor vessels may facilitate intravasation by tumor cells. Once the tumor cells enter the lumen of the vascular or lymphatic channel they are dislodged and travel in the circulation as single cells or clumps.[10, 17, 18] The rate of shedding of tumor cells into the venous or lymphatic drainage is related to a variety of factors including tumor type, tumor size, anatomic location, tumor vascularity, tumor trauma, and individual properties of tumor cell subpopulations. Tumor cells traveling in the circulation must be able to evade host defenses such as macrophages and NK cells,[7, 8, 9] survive the mechanical trauma of the blood flow, and arrest in the capillary bed of the target organ. The mechanisms influencing intravascular arrest include mechanical wedging of tumor cell clumps, entrapment with platelets and fibrin, attachment to endothelial surfaces, and interaction with exposed subendothelial basement membranes.[8, 25, 26, 36]

The arrested tumor cells must invade through the vascular wall to enter the organ parenchyma. The route of migration is between endothelial cell junctions in most systems studied to date.[11, 26, 45] Alternative routes involve active destruction of the endothelial cell or stimulated retraction of the endothelial cells adjacent to the arrested tumor cell. Once the tumor cell has crossed the endothelium, it must next traverse the continuous basement membrane (BM). The BM is an insoluble continuous structure which constitutes the major structural integrity of the capillary.[24, 44] Traversal of the BM takes place within 4–12 hours and proceeds in three steps. The first step is tumor cell attachment which is not usually associated with the formation of a junctional complex. The next step is local dissolution and fragmentation of the BM at the point of tumor cell contact. The tumor cell next extrudes a pseudopodium through the defect in the BM; this is soon followed by the whole cell.[1] Superficially this route of migration closely resembles the movement of leukocytes through the vascular wall. In fact, some chemotactic factors which influence the extravasation of leukocytes also attract tumor cells.[40] In most cases tumor cell extravasation is an active phenomenon. However, rarely a tumor cell embolus can grow within the vessel and burst it.[36, 45]

Once the tumor cell has extravasated it must possess the ability to grow in a foreign "soil" different from its tissue of origin. This could mean that the colony-forming cell may respond to alternative growth factors or can generate autocrine growth factors. To be successful the metastatic tumor cell must traverse all of the above steps. It is understandable, therefore, that the metastatic process is highly inefficient.

In order to approach the complex metastatic process, investigators have focused on one step at a time. The reasoning is that if progression through any necessary step in the metastatic cascade is blocked, then metastases will be prevented. Our laboratory has concentrated on the biochemical interactions of the tumor cell with the basement membrane (BM). The BM appears to play a crucial role in the progression of invasive tumors, invasion across tissue boundaries, and vascular invasion.

DEFECTIVE BASEMENT MEMBRANES ASSOCIATED WITH MALIGNANT TUMORS

The basement membrane (BM) defines the borders of tissue compartments, acts as a selective macromolecular filter, provides a scaffolding for tissue architecture, and plays a role in cell attachment and morphogenesis.[44] Tumor cells invading nerve, muscle, epithelium, mesothelium, or endothelium must traverse the BM.[19] Normal epithelium is anchored to a continous BM secreted and assembled by the epithelial cells. General and widespread changes occur in the BM during the transition from benign to invasive carcinomas.[4, 5, 19, 27, 33] Benign proliferative disorders of the epithelium are all characterized by a continuous BM separating the epithelium from the stroma. This is the case even in nonmalignant disorders with epithelial disorganization such as pancreatitis, fibroadenomas of the breast, or sclerosing adenosis. In contrast, invasive carcinomas consistently lack a formed BM around actively invading tumor cells. In certain zones of well-differentiated carcinomas partial BM formation can be noted. However, even in these locations the basement membrane is usually abnormal because it is discontinuous, fragmented, or focally reduplicated.

Defective BM organization in malignant tumors may be due to decreased synthesis, decreased assembly of secreted BM components, or increased turnover by proteases. Certain normal parenchymal cells and benign epithelial neoplasms may require a continuous BM for anchorage and growth. Invasive tumors may lack such a requirement. Immunohistochemical staining for BM can have significant applications in surgical pathology. The loss of BM can be used to distinguish true microinvasion from a tangential cut of the gland or duct. In cases of severe dysplasia or adenosis which mimic carcinoma, staining for BM can verify the benign nature of the lesion.

ROLE OF LAMININ IN TUMOR CELL INVASION OF THE EXTRACELLULAR MATRIX

A three-step hypothesis describes the sequence of biochemical events during tumor cell invasion of the extracellular matrix. The first step is tumor cell attachment which may be mediated through specific cell surface receptors which interact with components of the ECM. These receptors may recognize the glycoprotein, collagenous, or proteoglycan components of the matrix. The attached tumor cell next secretes hydrolytic enzymes which can locally degrade components of the matrix including the attachment glycoproteins.[14, 19, 20, 34] Matrix lysis by these enzymes most likely takes place close to the tumor cell surface. The third step is tumor cell locomotion into the region of the matrix modified by proteolysis. Continued invasion may take place by cyclic repetition of these three steps.

Laminin, a glycoprotein of basement membranes,[42] may play an important role in the interaction of tumor cells with the basement membrane. Laminin regulates a variety of biologic phenomenon, including cell attachment, growth, morphology, and cell migration.[22, 23, 39, 42] The multiple biologic properties of this molecule may relate to its large size and multidomain structure.[6, 29, 31, 38, 41] Laminin is a cross-shaped molecule with three short arms (36 nm) and one long arm (75 nm). All four arms have globular end regions. The intersection of the short arms contains numerous disulfide bonds and is relatively protease resistant.[6, 15, 28-31] The carbohydrate composition of the globular end regions of the molecule are different from the rod-shaped regions.[29] The long arm of laminin contains a heparin binding site.[32, 41] One or more globular end regions of the short arms promote cell spreading and also bind to type IV collagen.[15, 29] Laminin also stimulates neurite outgrowth.[22] The protease resistant central region of laminin molecule binds to a specific cell surface receptor for laminin.[3, 31, 38]

Normal and neoplastic cells contain high affinity cell surface binding sites for laminin.[3, 12, 16, 21, 28, 31, 38] Our laboratory found that laminin would bind via a specific receptor to suspended or attached cells (Fig. 8.1). Using increasing concentrations of labeled laminin, the binding is saturable with a high proportion of specific to nonspecific binding, using 100-fold excess unlabeled laminin as a competitor. The binding occurs with a high affinity constant (nanomolar range), and 10,000–100,000 binding sites per cell. Scatchard analysis is linear (Fig. 8.1). Laminin receptors can be measured on living cells or isolated plasma membranes from cells or whole breast carcinoma tissue.[2] The laminin receptor can be isolated by laminin affinity chromatography.[12, 28, 37, 43] It has a molecular weight of slightly less than 70 kilodaltons, and the isolated receptor retains the ability to bind laminin but not fibronectin. A laminin receptor with a similar molecular weight and binding coefficient has been confirmed by at least three scientific groups.[12, 28, 43]

In order to study mechanisms regulating the expression and function of the laminin receptor, we developed a library of monoclonal antibodies (mAbs) against the purified laminin receptor extracted from human breast carcinoma plasma membranes. Two antibodies (LR1 and LR2) were found to differ in their effects on laminin binding to the receptor.[16] By solid phase radioimmunoassay LR1 and LR2 bound with equal titer to the purified receptor.[16] Using immunoblotting, both LR1 and LR2 recognize a single 67 kilodalton component among all the proteins extracted from the membranes of breast carcinoma tissue. The antibodies also bound with equal titer to isolated microsomal membranes or living breast carcinoma cells. No binding to serum components was evident. When added together with labeled ligand, mAb LR1 produced a dose-dependent inhibition of specific laminin binding to human breast carcinoma cells. In contrast mAb LR2 had no effect on laminin binding.[16] The differential effect of the two antilaminin receptor antibodies on laminin binding was confirmed by immunohistology (Fig. 8.2). Both antibodies coated the cell surface of MCF-7 breast carcinoma cells. However, when the cells were exposed to exogenous laminin, mAb LR1 but not LR2 inhibited laminin binding to the cell surface. The two classes of antibodies may therefore recognize different structural domains on the receptor molecule. Much information is lacking concerning the biology, regulation, and structure of the laminin receptor. mAb LR1 will inhibit the attachment of breast carcinoma cells to the surface of whole human amnion basement membrane (Togo *et al.*, submitted for publication).

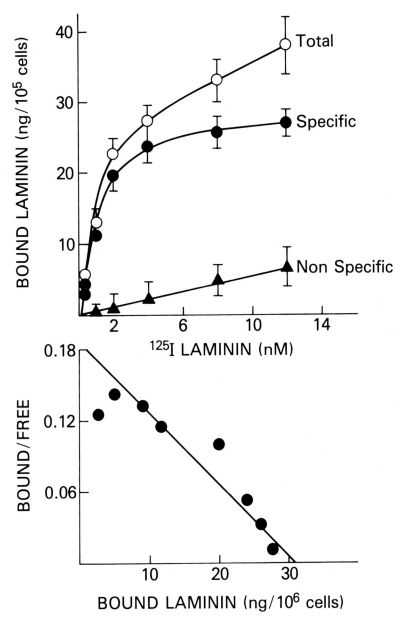

FIG. 8.1. Binding of laminin to human breast carcinoma plasma membranes and MCF-7 breast carcinoma cells. *(Top)* Saturation curve of specific binding to suspended MCF-7 5A9 breast carcinoma cells. Incubations were performed at 25°C for 40 minutes. Results expressed are the mean ± S.D. of five separate binding assays. Specific binding (●)represents the difference between binding in the absence (○) and the presence (▲) of 100-fold excess unlabeled laminin. *(Bottom)* Scatchard plot of the specific binding data for the MCF-7 cells was linear ($r = 0.90$), yielding a Kd = 1.75 nM and a B_{max} = 31 ng laminin bound per 10^6 cells (approximately 50,000 binding sites per cell).

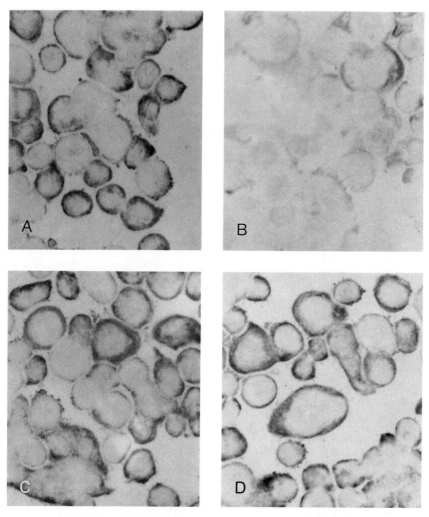

Fɪɢ. 8.2 Immunoperoxidase detection of monoclonal antilaminin receptor antibody binding to MCF-7 human breast carcinoma cells. The ethylene diamine tetraacetic acid (EDTA)-removed cells were cytocentrifuged onto BSA-coated glass slides. Incubations with mAb LR1 (*A* and *B*) or mAb LR2 (*C* and *D*) were conducted at 1/100 dilution for 1 hour. The effect of the mAbs on binding of laminin to MCF-7 cells were also studied by incubating 10 nM of laminin with the antibodies. Bound antibodies or laminin were detected by the immunoperoxidase method. Original magnification, × 4000. *(A)* mAb LR1 alone; pronounced cell surface binding. *(B)* Laminin binding in the presence of mAb LR1; inhibition of laminin binding detected by rabbit antilaminin antibodies. *(C)* mAb LR2 alone; pronounced cell surface binding. *(D)* Laminin binding in the presence of mAb LR2; a significant amount of cell surface bound laminin is present.

Laminin receptors may be altered in degree of occupancy or in absolute number in human carcinomas. Breast carcinoma and colon carcinoma tissue contain a higher number of exposed (unoccupied) receptors compared to benign breast tissue.[2, 19] This may be the indirect result of basement membrane loss in the carcinomas. The carcinoma cell may also be defective in the processing or internalization of the receptor. The laminin receptors of normal epithelium may be polarized at the basal surface and occupied with laminin in the basement membrane. In contrast, the laminin receptors on invading carcinoma cells may be distributed over the entire surface of the cell. They may be unoccupied because of the loss of formed basement membrane associated with the invading cells (Fig. 8.3).[18, 19] Using animal models, the laminin receptor can be shown to play a role in hematogenous metastases.[3, 37, 43] Tumor cells selected for the ability to attach via laminin produced 10-fold more metastases follow-

A. Benign Breast Epithelium

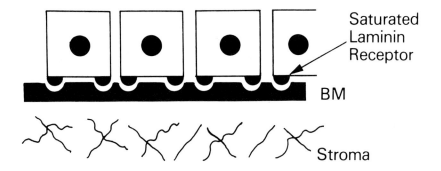

B. Invasive Breast Carcinoma

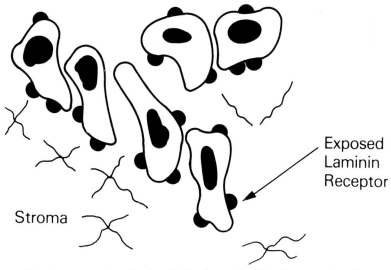

FIG. 8.3. Matrix receptor hypothesis. *(A)* Benign epithelial cells are anchored to a continuous basement membrane. The cell surface laminin receptors are polarized at the basal surface and occupied by laminin in the basement membrane. *(B)* The invading tumor cells lack a formed continuous basement membrane. They may possess increased numbers of unoccupied laminin receptors distributed over the entire cell surface.

ing intravenous injection.[37] Whole laminin bound to the tumor cell surface will stimulate hematogenous metastases.[3, 37, 43] Treating the cells with the receptor binding fragment of laminin markedly inhibits or abolishes metastases in a nontoxic fashion.[3] The laminin receptor can therefore stimulate hematogenous metastases by at least two mechanisms. The unoccupied receptor can be used by the cell to bind directly to host laminin. If the receptor is occupied with laminin, the cell can utilize the laminin as an attachment bridge through the globular end regions.[3] The fragment of laminin which binds to the receptor, but lacks the globular end regions, inhibits both of these mechanisms.[3]

Measurement of laminin receptors in human carcinoma tissue may provide additional information relating to metastatic potential.[2] As shown in Figure 8.4 preliminary studies indicate that highly metastatic human breast tumors have an increased number of unoccupied laminin receptors compared to less metastatic or benign tumors. In these studies the tumors were matched for size and cellularity. Those tumors with a higher level of exposed receptors were associated with a greater number of lymph node metastases. The most pronounced increase in receptor content was observed for tumors with more than two lymph node metastases, compared to tumors with no metastases.

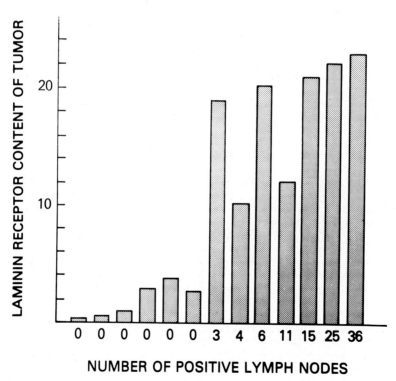

FIG. 8.4. Relationship between exposed laminin receptors in human breast cancer mastectomy specimens and the number of axillary lymph node metastases in the same specimen. Tumors were matched for size and cellularity. Specific laminin binding was compared after 100-fold excess cold laminin competition and matched for protein content. The units are nanograms of specifically bound laminin per microgram protein.

These results await confirmation in a larger ongoing series. Nevertheless, we can speculate that the measurement of laminin receptors directly or through the use of immunohistology may offer an additional parameter which can contribute to predicting the aggressive behavior of an individual patient's carcinoma.

REFERENCES

1. Babai, F. Etude ultrastructural sur la pathogeniee de l'inbasion du muscle strie' par dees tumeurs transplantables. *J. Ultrastruct. Res. 56:* 287–297, 1976.
2. Barsky, S. H., Rao, C. N., Hyams, D., and Liotta, L. A. Characterization of a laminin receptor from human breast carcinoma tissue. Breast Cancer Res. Treatment, 4: 181–188, 1984.
3. Barsky, S. H., Rao, C. N., Williams, J. E., and Liotta, L. A. Domains of laminin which alter metastases in a murine model. *J. Clin. Invest. 74:* 843–848, 1984.
4. Barsky, S. H., Siegal, G., Jannotta, F., Liotta, L. A. Loss of basement membrane components by invasive tumors but not by their benign counterparts. *Lab. Invest. 49:* 140–148, 1983.
5. Burtin, P., Chavanel, G., Foidart, J. M., and Martin, E. Antigens of basement membrane in the peritumoral stroma in human colon adenocarcinomas: An immunofluorescence study. *Int. J. Cancer 30:* 13–18, 1982.
6. Engel, J., Odermatt, E., Engel, A., Madri, J. A., Furthmayr, H., Rohde, H., and Timpl, R. Shapes, domain organization and flexibility of laminin and fibronectin, two multifunctional proteins of the extra cellular matrix. *Mol. Biol. 150:* 97–108, 1981.
7. Fidler, I. J. Inhibition of pulmonary metastasis by intravenous injection of specifically activated macrophages. *Cancer Res. 34:* 1074–1078, 1974.
8. Fidler, I. J., Gersten, D. M. and Hart, I. R. The biology of cancer invasion and metastasis. *Adv. Cancer Res. 28:* 149–160, 1978.
9. Frost, P., and Kerbal, R. S. Immunology of metastasis. Can the immune response cope with dissemination tumor? *Cancer Metastasis Rev. 2:* 239–256, 1983.
10. Glaves, D. Correlation between circulating cancer cells and incidence of metastases. *Br. J. Cancer 48:* 665–673, 1983.
11. Kramer, R. H., Gonzalez, R., and Nicolson, G. L. Metastatic tumor cells adhere preferentially to the extracellular matrix underlying vascular endothelial cells. *Int. J. Cancer 26:* 639–642, 1980.
12. Lesot, H., Kuhl, U., and Vondermark, K. Isolation of a laminin-binding protein from muscle cell membranes. *EMBO J. 2:* 861–870, 1983.
13. Liotta, L. A. Mechanisms of cancer invasion and metastases. In: *Progress in Oncology*, edited by Devita, Hellam, and Rosenberg, vol. 1. Philadelphia, J. B. Lippincott, 1985, pp. 28–41.
14. Liotta, L. A., Abe, S., Gehron, P., and Martin, G. R. Preferential digestion of basement membrane collagen by an enzyme derived from a metastatic murine tumor. *Proc. Natl. Acad. Sci. USA 76:* 2268–2276, 1979.
15. Liotta, L. A., Goldfarb, R. H., Brundage, R., Siegal, G. P., Terranova, V., and Garbisa, S. Effect of plasminogen activator (urokinase), plasmin, and thrombin on glycoprotein and collagenous components of basement membrane. *Cancer Res. 41:* 4629–4635, 1981.
16. Liotta, L. A., Horan Hand, P., Rao, C. N., Bryant, G., Barsky, S. H., and Schlom, J. Monoclonal antibodies to the human laminin receptor recognize distinct structural domains. *Exp. Cell. Res.*, *156:* 117–126, 1985.
17. Liotta, L. A., Kleinerman, J., and Saidel, G. M. Quantitative relationships of intravascular tumor cells, tumor vessels and pulmonary metastases following tumor implantation. *Cancer Res. 34:* 977–1004, 1974.
18. Liotta, L. A., Kleinerman, J., and Saidel, G. M. The significance of hematogenous tumor cell clumps in the metastatic process. *Cancer Res. 36:* 889–894, 1975.
19. Liotta, L. A., Rao, C. N., and Barsky, S. H. Tumor invasion and the extracellular matrix. *Lab. Invest. 49:* 636–649, 1983.
20. Liotta, L. A., Thorgeirsson, U. P., and Garbisa, S. Role of collagenases in tumor cell invasion. *Cancer Metastasis Rev. 1:* 277–297, 1982.
21. Malinoff, H., and Wicha, M. S. Isolation of a cell surface receptor protein for laminin from murine fibrosarcoma cells. *J. Cell Biol. 96:* 1475–1480, 1983.

22. Manthorpe, M., Engvall, E., Ruoslahti, E., Longo, F. M., Davis, G. E., and Varon, S. Laminin promotes neuritic regeneration from cultured peripheral and central neurons. *J. Cell Biol. 97:* 1882–1890, 1983.

23. McCarthy, J., Palmard, S., and Furcht, L. Migration by heptotaxis of a Schwann cell tumor line to the basement membrane glycoprotein laminin. *J. Cell Biol. 97:* 772–777, 1983.

24. Murphy, M. E., and Johnson, P. C. Possible contribution of basement membrane to the structural rigidity of blood capillaries. *Microvasc. Res. 9:* 242–245, 1975.

25. Nicolson, G. L. Cancer metastasis: Organ colonization and the cell surface properties of malignant cells. *Biochem. Biophys. Acta 695:* 113–120, 1982.

26. Nicolson, G. L. Metastatic tumor cell attachment and invasion assay utilizing vascular endothelial cell monolayers. *J. Histochem. Cytochem. 30:* 214–220, 1982.

27. Ozzello, L. The behavior of basement membranes in intraductal carcinoma of the breast. *Am. J. Pathol. 35:* 887–891, 1959.

28. Rao, C. N., Barsky, S. H., Terranova, V. P., and Liotta, L. A. Isolation of a tumor cell laminin receptor. *Biochem. Biophys. Res. Commun. 111:* 804–808, 1983.

29. Rao, C. N., Goldstein, I. J., and Liotta, L. A. Lectin binding domains on laminin. *Arch. Biochem. Biophys. 227:* 118–124, 1983.

30. Rao, C. N., Margulies, I. M. K., Goldfarb, R. H., Madri, J. A., Woodley, D. T., and Liotta, L. A. Differential proteolytic susceptibility of laminin alpha and beta subunits. *Arch. Biochem. Biophys. 219:* 65–72, 1982.

31. Rao, C. N., Margulies, I. M. K., Tralka, T. S., Terranova, V. P., Madri, J. A., and Liotta, L. A. Isolation of a subunit of laminin and its role in molecular structure and tumor cell attachment. *J. Biol. Chem. 257:* 9740–9750, 1982.

32. Sakashita, S., Engvall, E., and Ruoslahti, E. Basement membrane glycoprotein laminin binds to heparin. *FEBS Lett. 116:* 243–250, 1980.

33. Siegal, G. P., Barsky, S. H., Terranova, V. P., and Liotta, L. A. Stages of neoplastic transformation of human breast tissue as monitored by dissolution of basement membrane components. *Invasion Metastasis 1:* 54–65, 1981.

34. Strauli, P. Proteinases and tumor invasion. In *Proteinases and Tumor Invasion,* Monograph Series of the European Organization for Research on Treatment of Cancer, edited by P. M. Strauli, A. J. Barrett, A. Baici. vol. 6. New York, Raven Press, 1980, p. 215.

35. Sugarbaker, E. V., Weingard, D. N., and Roseman, J. M. Observations on cancer metastases. In *Cancer Invasion and Metastases,* edited by L. A. Liotta and I. R. Hart. Boston, Martinus Nijhoff, 1982, pp. 427–465.

36. Tarin, D., and Price, J. E. Influence of microenvironment and vascular anatomy on "metastatic" colonization potential of mammary tumors. *Cancer Res. 41:* 3604–3609, 1981.

37. Terranova, V. P., Liotta, L. A., Russo, R. G., and Martin, G. R. Role of laminin in the attachment and metastasis of murine tumor cells. *Cancer Res. 42:* 2265–2273, 1982.

38. Terranova, V. P., Rao, C. N., Kalebic, T., Margulies, I. M. K., and Liotta L. A. Laminin receptor on human breast carcinoma cells. *Proc. Natl. Acad. Sci. USA 80:* 444–451, 1983.

39. Terranova, V. P., Rohrbach, D. H., and Martin, G. R.: Role of laminin in the attachment of PAM 212 (epithelial) cells to basement membrane collagen. *Cell 22:* 719–726, 1980.

40. Thorgeirsson, U. P., Liotta, L. A., Kalebic, T., Margulies, I. M. K., Thomas, K., Rios-Candelore, M., and Russo, R. G. Effect of natural protease inhibitors and a chemoattractant on tumor cell invasion in vitro. *J. Natl. Cancer Inst. 69:* 1049–1057, 1982.

41. Timpl, R., Johansson, S., VanDelden, V., Oberbaumer, I., and Hook, M. Characterization of protease-resistant fragments of laminin mediating attachment and spreading of rat hepatocytes. *J. Biol. Chem. 258:* 8922–8928, 1983.

42. Timpl, R., Rhode, H., Robey, P. G., Rennard, S. I., Foidart, J. M., and Martin, G. R. Laminin: A glycoprotein from basement membranes. *J. Biol. Chem. 254:* 9933–9941, 1979.

43. Varani, J., Lovett, E. J., McCoy, J. P., Shibata, S., Maddox, D., Goldstein, I., and Wicha, M. Differential expression of a laminin like substance by high and low metastatic tumor cells. *Am. J. Pathol. 111:* 27–34, 1983.

44. Vracko, R. Basal lamina scaffold: Anatomy and significance for maintenance of orderly tissue structures. *Am. J. Pathol. 77:* 313, 1974.

45. Wallace, A. C., Chew, E., and Jones, D. S. The arrest and extravasation of cancer cells in the lung. In *Pulmonary Metastasis,* edited by L. Weiss, H. A. Gilbert, vol. 3. Boston, G. K. Hall, 1978, pp. 26–32.

Chapter 9

Monoclonal Antibodies in the Detection and Treatment of Breast Cancer Micrometastases

A. MUNRO NEVILLE, P. MONAGHAN, R. A. J. McILHINNEY,
B. GUSTERSON, AND R. C. COOMBES

Advances in the classification and detection as well as fundamental understanding of human tumors have been hampered for a long time by the lack of suitable probes of their structural and functional properties. The advent of immunocytochemical methods over the past two to three decades has done much to remedy this situation and is currently heralding a new era in functional pathology.

Polyclonal antisera, generally raised to known tissue components or products, *e.g.*, hormones, enzymes, *etc.*, served as the initial probes whose location at a cellular level was mostly detected with fluorescent conjugates. The more recent introduction of peroxidase—or alkaline phosphatase—conjugated antibodies as the end point–indices has enabled this approach to be extended with reliability to formalin-fixed paraffin-embedded tissues and to the electron microscope. Good histological detail and accurate localization can be achieved.

The recently developed methodology enabling the generation of monoclonal antibodies, both of rodent[28] and human origin,[38] has provided novel reagents and new insights into protean aspects of oncology. While such reagents to well characterized substances may come to replace conventional antisera, their greatest potential lies in outlining previously unrecognized and uncharacterized cell surface and cytoplasmic components of both normal and neoplastic cells. Such reagents should have major biological, pathological, and clinical value.

Initially, most of the newly derived monoclonal antibodies were directed towards normal and neoplastic lymphoreticular cells.[30] These have proved to be of important lineage and differentiation markers while also having therapeutic significance. Now, monoclonal antibodies with relevance to the study of solid tumors are being derived with similar interesting specificities and potential usefulness. Many have now been described and are the subject of a recent excellent review.

IMMUNE PROBES AND THE HUMAN BREAST

A wide range of polyclonal and monoclonal antibody probes with varying specificities for different aspects of normal and neoplastic breast cell structure and function are now available and can be used at the light and electron microscope level.[21, 29] Examples of some moieties now detectable in this manner or of antibodies with different specificities are depicted in Table 9.1. No probe with breast tumor specificity has been described.

LINEAGE SPECIFICITY

The normal human breast duct and lobuloalveolar system consists of two dominant cell types—epithelial cells which line the lumina and myoepithelial cells which form a peripheral ring of cells around the ducts and which abut onto the outer limiting basement membrane. The ectodermal origin of the breast ductal system is reflected by the intermediate filament protein expression by normal breast cells, with keratin being present in the epithelial and, to a lesser extent, myoepithelial cells.[24, 37]

CELL SPECIFICITY

Several immunological probes have become available which delineate the different cell types of the resting normal breast. Myosin is preferentially expressed in the cytoplasm of myoepithelial cells (Fig. 9.1). A monoclonal antibody, LICR-LON-23.10, detects a cell surface component only possessed by myoepithelial cells (Fig. 9.2).[23] The use of monoclonal antibodies (*vide supra*) to cytokeratins reveals that morphologically identical epithelial cells may express different keratins by a phenomenon which may also be relevant to the structural or functional maturation of such cells. Recent data suggests that tissue polypeptide antigen (TPA) is a keratin-related material.[6]

MATURATION ANTIGENS

Many different groups of workers have described rodent monoclonal antibodies with specificity for breast epithelial cell membranes.[3, 12, 18, 19, 25, 45, 46] The

TABLE 9.1. SOME PROBES WITH DIFFERING SPECIFICITIES FOR NORMAL AND NEOPLASTIC HUMAN BREAST CELLS[a]

Specificity	Components	Antibodies
Lineage	Keratins	
Cell		
Epithelial	Keratins (TPA)	Cell surface directed monoclonal antibodies
Myoepithelial	Myosin (keratin)	LICR-LON-23.10
Maturation		
Epithelial	Milk proteins Steroid receptors T-antigen CEA Enzymes Placental proteins	Cell surface directed monoclonal antibodies LICR-LON-E36
Myoepithelial	Laminin Collagen IV	

[a]Reproduced with permission from A. M. Neville and B. A. Gusterson.

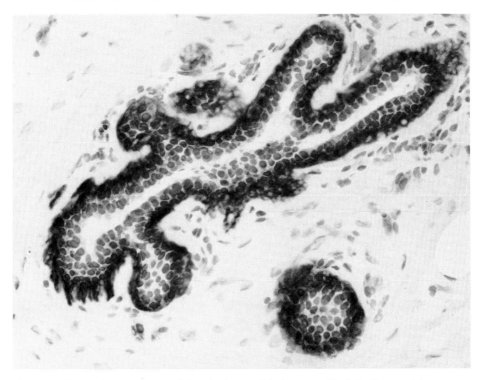

FIG. 9.1. Human breast. A normal duct is shown with the myoepithelial cells containing myosin as shown by use of an antimyosin antibody and the alkaline phosphatase technique. Original magnification, × 500.

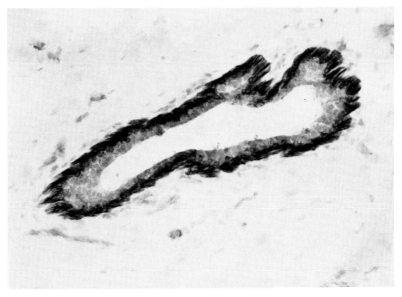

FIG. 9.2. Human breast. A normal duct is shown stained with LICR-LON-23.10. The myoepithelial cell membrane expresses the epitope. The epithelial cells and stroma are negative. Original magnification, × 260.

starting material has varied and includes primary and metastatic tumors, cell lines, or membrane preparations. Many of these antibodies are directed towards carbohydrate epitopes carried by cell surface glycoproteins and glycolipids. Such probes may, in some instances, detect antigens with structural epithelial specificity. Others directed towards the cell surface are better considered to be delineating the maturation or differentiation status of certain breast cells.[7] Further biochemical and biological studies are needed to clarify their significance.

These cell surface-directed antibodies reveal a fascinating degree of heterogeneity of the normal breast cell littoral population.[15] Such cells have similar morphological and ultrastructural appearances, whether or not they express the epitopes being detected by the individual probes (Figs. 9.3 and 9.4). Several studies have proved that this phenomenon is not an artifact of tissue preparation. The phenomenon in the breast is not cell-cycle related. Following single cell cloning of normal breast cells in monolayer culture, epitopes not originally expressed by the cell may subsequently arise. The molecular nature of this change requires to be elucidated but may represent a differentiation response to particular environmental stimuli; a similar heterogeneity can be discerned in human breast carcinomas (Fig. 9.5).

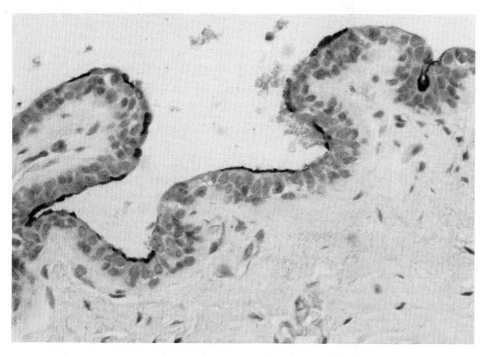

Fig. 9.3. Human breast. A normal breast duct stained with a monoclonal antibody, LICR-LON-M8, to demonstrate the heterogeneity of epitope expression by morphologically similar cells. Original magnification, × 680.

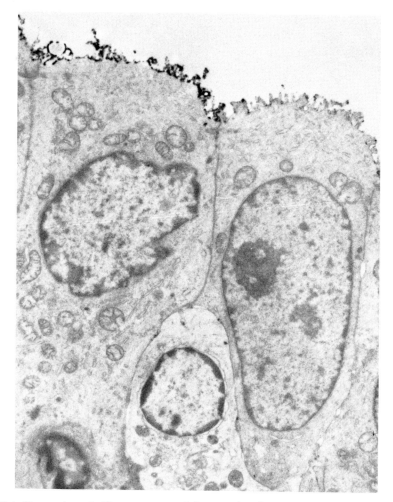

FIG. 9.4. Human breast. The same normal duct at the electron microscope level shows the LICR-LON-M8 epitope being expressed by the luminal face of one cell but not its neighbor. Both cells appear similar ultrastructurally. Original magnification, × 9000.

CHANGES IN BREAST DISEASE INCLUDING CARCINOMAS

Experimental studies have shown that the normal fully differentiated myoepithelial cell is the main source of basement membrane components, such as laminin and collagen IV.[49,50]

In benign breast diseases, immunocytochemical techniques show that the basement membrane is intact with myoepithelial cells surrounding such lesions. With the evolution of *in situ* carcinomas, while the basement membrane still forms a continuum, the myoepithelial cells become attenuated and fewer in number. With the evolution of foci of invasion, the basement membrane becomes defective, and myoepithelial cells, *i.e.*, fully differentiated myosin or

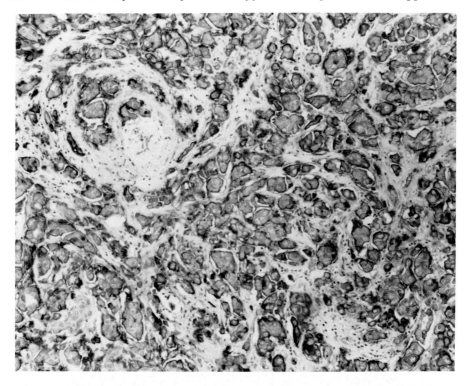

F<small>IG</small>. 9.5. Human breast carcinoma. An infiltrating breast carcinoma has been stained with LICR-LON-M8 and shows membrane and cytoplasmic staining. Heterogeneity of expression of the epitope is discernible. Original magnification, × 100.

23.10-positive cells, are no longer demonstrable.[16,24] Epithelial-directed antibodies continue to stain such carcinoma cells, albeit heterogeneously in many cases (Fig. 9.5).

Such a change may be an important factor in the invasive process, playing a role "pari passu" with degradative enzyme systems.[31] Nonetheless, this is not an all-or-none phenomenon in that in some well-differentiated cancers, basement membrane or myoepithelial cells may be demonstrable focally. Rarely, an invasive tumor with the appearance of a "lobular carcinoma" may be found when myoepithelial cells appear to be the dominant cell type.[39]

Other monoclonal antibodies, directed principally towards cytoplasmic constituents, may give some indication of the degree of differentiation of a particular breast carcinoma. These include probes for the estrogen receptor, of therapeutic and prognostic significance; secretory component, a constituent whose synthesis may be controlled by estrogen; placental proteins and estrogen-metabolizing enzymes (Table 9.1).[1,2,20,26,27] While the epithelial cells are the source of milk proteins such as alpha-lactalbumin during lactation, current data suggest that such moeities are not synthesised by breast cancers.[4] One exception may be juvenile secretory breast carcinomas.[10]

From time to time, carcinoid tumors have been recorded as being of breast origin.[47] Their site of evolution in the breast has been somewhat of a mystery.

Recently, a monoclonal antibody, LICR-LON-E,[36] has delineated a small number of cells in the normal duct as containing neurosecretory-type granules. Such expression has been noted in ~30% of invasive duct cancers (Fig. 9.6).[36]

TUMOR DETECTION

Many studies have been effected in an attempt to evolve better methods for the detection of metastatic disease. Biochemical indices measured in the blood and/or urine have proved to be successful for tumors of germ cell, colonic and prostatic origin, and lymphoreticular diseases. Similar approaches in breast cancer have delineated several marker substances whose levels are raised in the blood and/or urine in overt metastatic disease, *e.g.*, plasma carcinoembryonic antigen (CEA), alkaline phosphatase, gamma-glutamyl transpeptidase, and urinary hydroxproline.[8] However, when sequential studies are conducted, the lead time between becoming biochemically malignant (*i.e.*, pathologically elevated tumor marker levels) and the detection of metastases by other clinical and radiographic methods is short, of the order of 3–4 months.[8] Consequently, various workers have sought alternative methods.

RADIOIMMUNOLOCALIZATION

Using polyclonal antibodies labelled with different isotopes of iodine, several groups have demonstrated that external scanning procedures can localize

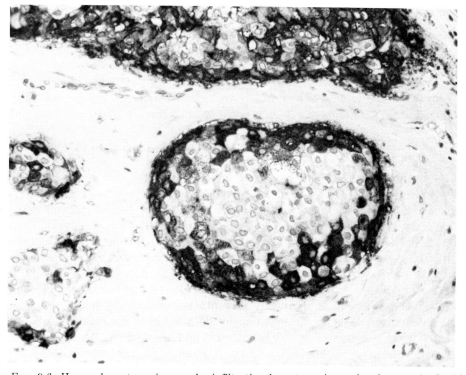

FIG. 9.6. Human breast carcinoma. An infiltrating breast carcinoma has been stained with LICR-LON-E[36] and shows cytoplasmic staining of some of the tumor cells. Original magnification, × 200.

both primary and metastatic tumors. In these studies, antibodies to the carcinoembryonic antigen (CEA), alpha-fetoprotein (AFP), and beta-HCG have mostly been employed.[39] Evidence has gathered to suggest that, in some instances, such antibodies may not localize on the tumor cells but in areas of secretion of these moieties within the tumor itself. Accordingly, monoclonal antibodies directed to tumor cell surface components may offer an advantage.

Our own approach to this technique has been to conjugate anti-breast monoclonal antibodies to bifunctional chelating agents and, then, label them with isotopes more suitable for external scanning procedures. We have used the breast-directed monoclonal antibody, LICR-LON-M8, conjugated with DTPA and then labelled with Indium (^{111}In). This reagent yielded superior results in model xenograft systems and has had limited success in delineating bone metastases.[42]

A recent interesting paper has employed an anti-colorectal carcinoma cell surface-directed monoclonal antibody $F(ab^1)_2$ fragment labelled with ^{131}I to detect retroperitoneal lymph node metastases in patients with colonic carcinomas.[35] Antibody scans were positive while other detection methods were within normal limits. This approach could be of value in breast cancer and the search for axillary and internal mammary nodal involvement in view of the current tendency to more conservative surgery. However, the many nonspecific changes axillary nodes can demonstrate may make the interpretation of scanning data difficult.

IMMUNOCYTOCHEMISTRY AND MICROMETASTASES

Current evidence still dictates that radioimmunolocalization detects breast metastases late in their evolution. Most patients at primary presentation do not have overt evidence of metastases as measured by conventional techniques. Nonetheless, 50% will develop metastases within 5 years. Of these, 57% will be found to have bone metastases at first relapse. One approach could be based on the immunocytochemical use of antibreast probes to detect such tumor cells in bone marrow samples at the time of first presentation.[13, 14, 22]

Conventional cytology can detect tumor cells in the marrow of patients without overt bone metastases but in only a minority (~1%) of patients. Using a polyclonal probe to human breast cell membranes (anti-EMA), it was found that immunocytochemical methods applied to such smears could increase the detection rate in patients with recurrent nonskeletal disease.[44] Such tumor cells occurred not only in small clumps but also as single cells (Fig. 9.7). These patients subsequently pursued a worse prognosis with the earlier development of overt bone metastases than those in whom no tumor cells were demonstrable in the marrow.

Accordingly, this study was extended to marrow smears harvested from 200 patients at the time of their initial presentation and in whom there was no evidence of metastases as determined by detailed clinical, biochemical, and radiographic methodologies.[13] The incidence and number of tumor cells, *i.e.*, "micrometastases," detected by immunocytochemistry are shown in Tables 9.2 and 9.3.

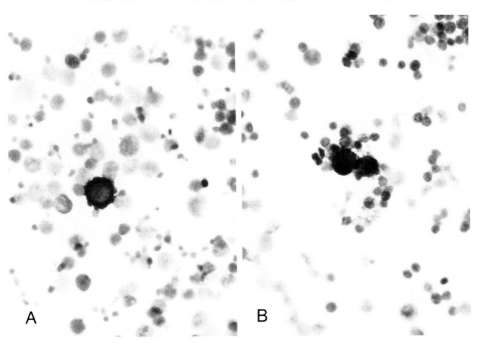

A   B

FIG. 9.7. Human breast carcinoma. Two marrow smears have been stained with LICR-LON-M8 and shown on the *left* are (A) a single cancer cell and on the *right* (B) two such cells. The normal marrow cells are unstained. (A) Original magnification, × 250; (B) original magnification, × 250.

TABLE 9.2. INCIDENCE OF TUMOR CELLS IN THE MARROW AS A FUNCTION OF NODAL STATUS

Axillary Nodal Status	Tumor Cells in the Marrow Detected by Immunocytochemistry		
	Present	Absent	Total
Positive[a]	29(33%)	58	87
Negative	23(20%)	90	113
Total	52(26%)	148	200

[a]One or more nodes involved.

TABLE 9.3. INCIDENCE OF MICROMETASTASES AS A FUNCTION OF SEVERAL PROGNOSTIC INDICES

Prognostic Variables[a]	% Patients with Tumor Cells in the Marrow	
	Present	Absent
VI+, ER−, N+	82	18
VI+, ER−, N−	75	25
VI−, ER+, N+	33	66
VI−, ER+, N−	12	88

[a]VI, intratumoral vascular and/or lymphatic invasion; ER, estrogen receptor status; N, axillary nodal status.

The presence of intratumoral vascular and/or lymphatic permeation has been found to be an important prognostic variable.[5] The incidence of marrow micrometastases appears to correlate well with it and other known prognostic indices (Tables 9.2 and 9.3). Of greatest importance may be the detection of micrometastases in a small subgroup of patients with so-called "good prognosis" disease (*i.e.*, vascular invasion negative (VI-ve), node negative (N-ve), steroid receptor positive (ER + ve) (see Table 9.3). They may benefit from the institution of systemic therapy in the immediate postoperative period.

Present methods are not detecting all the patients who subsequently develop bone marrow metastases. While this may, in part, be a sampling problem, other immune probes, such as to cytoplasmic keratins and/or a cocktail of cell surface-directed monoclonal antibodies,[13] need to be examined for their accuracy of detection.

Appropriate immune probes are also currently available to detect early marrow involvement by other types of tumors such as oat cell, prostatic, thyroid, renal and colonic carcinomas, and neuroblastomas.[39]

PROSPECTS FOR THERAPY

It has long been hoped that antibodies directed towards tumor cell surfaces could be employed as therapeutic agents.[40] This hope had remained elusive until the advent of monoclonal antibodies, when new efforts were made in this direction. Unconjugated monoclonal antibodies have been used to treat patients with leukemias, lymphomas, colonic cancer, and melanomas. In general, remissions were not obtained, although some success was claimed in relation to T cell lymphomas. One outstanding exception has been the use of an anti-idiotypic antibody in a patient with a B cell lymphoma who, several years later, was still in remission.[34]

There are numerous problems with these forms of therapy, including tumor cell antigenic modulation and anti-mouse antibody generation by the patients. With respect to solid tumors, there is also the problem of antibody penetration which may be vascular dependent but could potentially be overcome by repeated doses of antibody if each dose induced some necrosis. In addition, as mentioned before, antigenic heterogeneity to most monoclonals is often apparent so that several monoclonals may be required to be used simultaneously or sequentially. Nonetheless, in model xenograft breast cancer systems, the use of two monoclonal antibodies, both complement dependent, has resulted in tumor cell necrosis, the effects lasting for 4 to 30 days after single doses. Regrowth of the tumors then took place.[11]

More attention has been paid to the use of monoclonal antibodies as homing devices while carrying cytotoxic agents such as ricin, abrin, or pokeweed antiviral protein (PAP) or isotopes.[43, 48]

The problems posed by the detection of bone marrow micrometastases may be amenable in part to the use of "armed" antibreast monoclonal antibodies *in vitro* to assist with bone marrow cleansing. This approach has already had some success in subjects with leukemia and neuroblastoma.[17,41] Bone marrow toxicity represents a limiting feature in most high dose therapeutic regimens. Hence, the possibility of eliminating tumor cells from the marrow, returning it to the patient after high dose therapy and restitution of hematopoeisis, therefore, is of more than academic interest.

With respect to breast and other cancers involving the bone marrow, there is available a monoclonal antibody, LICR-LON-Fib75, which appears to detect an antigen on breast cancer cells but not bone marrow progenitors.[9] The antigen being detected is a 19K cell surface protein, with $\sim 10^6$ copies being expressed per cell.[33] This antibody coupled to the abrin A chain is cytotoxic *in vitro*. Patients' marrows have been harvested, treated with Fib-75-abrin A chain *in vitro*, and returned to them with hematopoiesis being re-established. High dose chemotherapy was also given. The long-term results of this study are awaited.

CONCLUSIONS

Various monoclonal antibodies are now available to probe and understand aspects of the structural and functional differentiation status of the normal and neoplastic human breast. Some of these reagents have a role in the detection of metastases. At first presentation, approximately 30% of patients, with no other evidence of spread, can be found to have tumor cell involvement of the bone marrow. Other monoclonal antibodies are also available which may be used as *in vitro* homing agents to cleanse such marrows of tumor cells as part of a high dose therapeutic regimen. The outcome of patients with micrometastases and their treatment is awaited over the next few years.

REFERENCES

1. Aamdal, S., Børmer, O., Jørgensen, O., Høst, H., Eliassen, G., Kaalhus, O., and Pihl, A. Estrogen receptors and long-term prognosis in breast cancer. *Cancer 53:* 2525–2529, 1984.
2. Amin, A. M., and Ismail, A. A. A. Immunoperoxidase localization of catechol-ø-methyl transferase (COMT) in human breast cancer. *Gegenbaurs Morphol. Jahrb. 129:* 125–128, 1983.
3. Arklie, J., Taylor-Papadimitriou, J., Bodmer, W., Egan, M., and Millis, R. Differentiation antigens expressed by epithelial cells in the lactating breast are also detectable in breast cancers. *Int. J. Cancer 28:* 23–29, 1981.
4. Bailey, A. J., Sloane, J. P., Trickey, B. S., and Ormerod, M. G. An immunocytochemical study of α-lactalbumin in human breast tissue. *J. Pathol. 137:* 13–23, 1982.
5. Bettelheim, R., Mitchell, D., and Gusterson, B. A. Immunocytochemistry in the identification of vascular invasion in breast cancer. *J. Clin. Pathol. 37:* 364–366, 1984.
6. Bjorklund, B. Personal communication, 1984.
7. Brabon, A. C., Williams, J. F., and Cardiff, R. D. A monoclonal antibody to a human breast tumor protein released in response to estrogen. *Cancer Res. 44:* 2704–2710, 1984.
8. Buckman, R., Coombes, R. C., Dearnaley, D. P., Gore, M., Gusterson, B., and Neville, A. Some clinical uses of biological markers. In: *Breast Cancer: Diagnosis and Management*, edited by G. Bonadonna. New York, John Wiley & Sons, 1984, pp. 109–126.
9. Buckman, R., Shepherd, V., Coombes, R. C., McIlhinney, R. A. J., Patel, S., and Neville, A. M. Elimination of carcinoma cells from human bone marrow. *Lancet 2:* 1428–1430, 1982.
10. Bussolati, G. Personal communication, 1984.
11. Capone, P. M., Papsidera, L. D., Croghan, G. A., and Ming Chu, T. Experimental tumoricidal effects of monoclonal antibody against solid breast tumors. *Proc. Natl. Acad. Sci. USA 80:* 7328–7332, 1983.
12. Colcher, D., Hand, P. H., and Nuti, M. A spectrum of monoclonal antibodies reactive with human mammary tumor cells. *Proc. Natl. Acad. Sci. USA 78:* 3199–3203, 1981.
13. Colnaghi, M. I., Canevari, S., Della Torre, G. S., Regazzoni, M., Tagliabue, E., Mariani-Costantini, R., and Rilke, F. Monoclonal antibodies potentially useful in clinical oncology. In:

Monoclonal Antibodies and Cancer, edited by B. D. Boss, R. Langman, I. Trowbridge, and R. Dulbecco. New York, Academic Press, 1983, pp. 207–213.

14. Dearnaley, D. P., Sloane, J. P., Ormerod, M. G., Steele, K., Coombes, R. C., Clink, H. McD., Powles, T. J., Ford, H. T., Gazet, J-C., and Neville, A. M. Increased detection of mammary carcinoma cells in marrow smears using antisera to epithelial membrane antigen. *Br. J. Cancer 44:* 85–90, 1981.

15. Edwards, P. A. W., Brooks, I. M., and Monaghan, P. Expression of epithelial antigens in primary cultures of normal human breast analysed with monoclonal antibodies. *Differentiation 25:* 247–258, 1984.

16. Ekblom, P., Miettinen, M., Forsman, L., and Andersson, L. C. Basement membrane and apocrine epithelial antigens in differential diagnosis between tubular carcinoma and sclerosing adenosis of the breast. *J. Clin. Pathol. 37:* 357–363, 1984.

17. Filipovich, A. H., Youle, R. J., Neville, D. M. Jr., Vallera, D. A., Quinones, R. R., and Kersey, J. H. *Ex-vivo* treatment of donor bone marrow with anti-T-cell immunotoxins for prevention of graft-versus-host disease. *Lancet 1:* 469–471, 1984.

18. Foster, C. S., Dinsdale, E. A., Edwards, P. A. W., and Neville, A. M. Monoclonal antibodies to the human mammary gland. II. Distribution of determinants in breast carcinomas. *Virchows Arch. (Pathol. Anat.) 394:* 295–305, 1982.

19. Foster, C. S., Edwards, P. A. W., Dinsdale, E., and Neville, A. M. Monoclonal antibodies to the human mammary gland. I. Distribution of determinants in non-neoplastic mammary and extra-mammary tissues. *Virchows Arch. (Pathol. Anat.) 394:* 279–293, 1982.

20. Fournier, S., Kuttenn, F., de Cicco, F., Baudot, N., Malet, C., and Mauvais-Jarvis, P. Estradiol 17β-hydroxysteroid dehydrogenase activity in human breast fibroadenomas. *J. Clin. Endocrinol. Metab. 55:* 428–433, 1982.

21. Gatter, K. C., Abdulaziz, Z., Beverley, P., Corvalan, J. R. F., Ford, C., Lane, E. B., Mota, M., Nash, I. R. G., Pulford, K., Stein, H., Taylor-Papadimitriou, J., Woodhouse, C., and Mason, D. Y. Use of monoclonal antibodies for the histopathological diagnosis of human malignancy. *J. Clin. Pathol. 35:* 1253–1267, 1982.

22. Gugliotta, P., Botta, G., and Bussolati, G. Immunocytochemical detection of tumour markers in bone metastases from carcinoma of the breast. *Histochem. J. 13:* 953–959, 1981.

23. Gusterson, B. A., and McIlhinney, R. A. J. Personal communication, 1984.

24. Gusterson, B. A., Warburton, M. J., Mitchell, D., Ellison, M., Neville, A. M., and Rudland, P. S. Distribution of myoepithelial cells and basement membrane proteins in the normal breast and in benign and malignant breast disease. *Cancer Res. 42:* 4763–4770, 1982.

25. Heyderman, E., Steele, K. and Ormerod, M. G. A new antigen on the epithelial membrane: Its immunoperoxidase localization in normal and neoplastic tissue. *J. Clin. Pathol. 32:* 35–39, 1979.

26. Inaba, N., Renk, T., Daume, E., and Bohn, H. Ectopic production of placenta-'specific' tissue proteins (PP$_5$ and PP$_{11}$) by malignant breast tumors. *Arch. Gynecol. 231:* 87–90, 1981.

27. King, W. K., and Greene, G. L. Monoclonal antibodies localize oestrogen receptor in the nuclei of target cells. *Nature 307:* 745–747, 1984.

28. Kohler, G., and Schulman, J. J. Cellular and molecular restrictions of the lymphocyte fusion. *Curr. Top. Microbiol. Immunol. 81:* 143, 1978.

29. Laurence, D. J. R., and Neville, A. M. The detection and evaluation of human tumor metastases. *Cancer Metastasis Rev. 2:* 351–374, 1983.

30. Levy, R., and Miller, R. A. Biological and clinical implications of lymphocyte hybridomas: Tumor therapy with monoclonal antibodies. *Annu. Rev. Med. 34:* 107–116, 1983.

31. Liotta, L. A., Rao, C. N., and Barsky, S. H. Tumor invasion and the extracellular matrix. *Lab. Invest. 49:* 636–649, 1983.

32. Lloyd, K. O. Human tumor antigens: Detection and characterization with monoclonal antibodies. In: *Basic and Clinical Tumor Immunology*, edited by R. B. Herberman. Martinus Nijhoff, 1983, pp. 159–214.

33. McIlhinney, R. A. J., and Patel, S. Purification of a human plasma membrane glycoprotein from human red blood cells by affinity chromatography using a monoclonal antibody. *J. Biol. Chem., 260:* 489–494, 1985.

34. Miller, R. A., Maloney, D. G., Warnke, R., and Levy, R. Treatment of B-cell lymphoma with monoclonal anti-idiotype antibody. *N. Engl. J. Med. 306:* 517–522, 1982.

35. Moldofsky, P. J., Sears, H. F., Mulhern, C. B. Jr., Hammond, N. D., Powe, J., Gatenby, R. A., Steplewski, Z., and Koprowski, H. Detection of metastatic tumor in normal-sized retroperitoneal lymph nodes by monoclonal antibody imaging. *N. Engl. J. Med. 311:* 106–107, 1984.

36. Monaghan, P., Roberts, D., Sappino, P., and Neville, A. M. LICR-LON-E36 in rat pituitary. *J. Histochem. Cytochem., 32:* 1041–1047, 1984.

37. Nathrath, W. B. J., Wilson, P. D., and Trejdosiewicz, L. K. Immunohistochemical localisation of keratin and luminal epithelial antigen in myoepithelial and luminal epithelial cells of human mammary and salivary gland tumours. *Pathol. Res. Pract. 175:* 279–288, 1983.

38. Neville, A. M., Edwards, P. A. W., and O'Hare, M. J. Generating human monoclonal antibodies. *Med. Oncol. Tumor Pharmacother. 1:* 73–76, 1984.

39. Neville, A. M., and Gusterson, B. A. Monoclonal antibodies and human tumours: Pathological and clinical aspects. *Eur. J. Clin. Oncol., 21:* 355–369, 1985.

40. Oldham, R. K., Morgan, A. C., Woodhouse, C. S., Schroff, R. W., Abrams, P. G., and Foon, K. A. Monoclonal antibodies in the treatment of cancer: Preliminary observations and future prospects. *Med. Oncol. Tumor Pharmacother. 1:* 51–62, 1984.

41. Prentice, H. G., Janossy, G., Price-Jones, L., Trejdosiewicz, L. K., Panjwani, D., Graphakos, S., Ivory, K., Blacklock, H. A., Gilmore, M. J. M. L., Tidman, N., Skeggs, D. B. L., Ball, S., Patterson, J., and Hofferand, A. V. Depletion of T lymphocytes in donor marrow prevents significant graft-versus-host disease in matched allogeneic leukaemic marrow transplant recipients. *Lancet 1:* 472–476, 1984.

42. Rainsbury, R. M., Westwood, J. H., Coombes, R. C., Neville, A. M., Ott, R. J., Kalirai, T. S., McCready, V. R., and Gazet, J-C. Location of metastatic breast carcinoma by a monoclonal antibody chelate labeled with Indium-111. *Lancet 2:* 934–938, 1983.

43. Ramakrishnan, S., and Houston, L. L. Comparison of the selective cytotoxic effects of immunotoxins containing ricin A chain or pokeweed antiviral protein and anti-thy 1.1 monoclonal antibodies. *Cancer Res. 44:* 201–208, 1984.

44. Redding, W. H., Monaghan, P., Imrie, S. F., Ormerod, M. G., Gazet, J-C., Coombes, R. C., Clink, H. McD., Dearnaley, D. P., Sloane, J. P., and Powles, T. J. Detection of micrometastases in patients with primary breast cancer. *Lancet 2:* 1271–1274, 1983.

45. Schlom, J., Wunderlich, D., Teramoto, Y. A. Generation of human monoclonal antibodies reactive with human mammary carcinoma cells. *Proc. Natl. Acad. Sci. USA 77:* 6841–6845, 1980.

46. Taylor-Papadimitriou, J., Peterson, J. A., Arklie, J., Burchell, J., Ceriani, R. L., and Bodmer, W. F. Monoclonal antibodies to epithelium-specific components of the human milk fat globule membrane: Production and reaction with cells in culture. *Int. J. Cancer 28:* 17, 1981.

47. Toyoshima, S. Mammary carcinoma with argyrophil cells. *Cancer 52:* 2129–2138, 1983.

48. Vitetta, E. S., Krolick, K. A., and Uhr, J. W. Neoplastic B cells as targets for antibody-ricin A chain immunotoxins. *Immunol. Rev. 62:* 159–183, 1982.

49. Warburton, M. J., Ferns, S. A., and Rudland, P. S. Enhanced synthesis of basement membrane proteins during the differentiation of rat mammary tumor epithelial cells into myoepithelial-like cells *in vitro. Exp. Cell Res. 137:* 373–380, 1982.

50. Warburton, M. J., Ormerod, E. J., Monaghan, P., Ferns, S., and Rudland, P. S. Characterization of a myoepithelial cell line derived from a neonatal rat mammary gland. *J. Cell Biol. 91:* 827–836, 1981.

Chapter 10

Carcinoma of the Breast and of the Ovary as a Model for the Application of Monoclonal Antibodies to Diagnostic Pathology

FRANCO RILKE, MARIA I. COLNAGHI, SYLVIE MÉNARD, ELDA TAGLIABUE, RENATO MARIANI-COSTANTINI, AND GABRIELLA DELLA TORRE

During the last few years major efforts have been made to identify tumor-specific or tumor-associated antigenic markers in humans and animals. In the past, the serologic study of the antigenic phenotype of human tumor cells was predominantly approached by use of conventional absorbed heteroantisera or patient sera that usually showed low affinity or insufficient titer of antibodies for the antigens under investigation. Also, the heterogeneity of the antibodies markedly limited the quality of the results obtained. A variety of marker substances, of a number of human carcinomas, have been utilized to better define, and possibly specifically identify, tumor cells. In carcinoma of the breast, for example, the list of such substances[66] includes carcinoembryonic antigen (CEA) and related glycoproteins, placental markers such as human chorionic gonadotropin (HCG) and pregnancy alpha-2-glycoprotein, milk-associated proteins, mammary epithelial antigens,[15] hormones, enzymes, circulating immune complexes[7, 14, 25, 83] and special markers such as a 52,000 molecular weight mouse mammary tumor virus glycoprotein (GP52).[58, 73] Needless to say, in spite of many interesting results, not a single marker has proven to be breast tumor cell specific.

The recent wide-scale application of hybridoma technology [44] to these types of investigation and the use of murine and human monoclonal antibodies (MoAbs) as probes in the search for cancer antigens have produced a large number of new useful findings. The difficulties of identifying antigens strictly specific for tumor cells are still considerable. However, the lack of tumor specificity of an antibody may be acceptable, particularly when tumor cells are to be differentiated from other cell populations not recognized by the antibody.[20, 21] This applies to detectable tumor cells within lymphoid tissue, bone marrow, and serous effusions. In these instances the absence of cross reactivity wth lymphoid, hematopoietic, reticular, and mesothelial cells respectively is utilized.

In this chapter we will concentrate on the MoAbs generated during the last few years at the Istituto Nazionale Tumori of Milan, with special reference to those that react with normal and neoplastic cells of the human breast[57] and with human epithelial ovarian cancer cells.[75] Applications in diagnostic histopathology and cytopathology will be stressed.

BREAST CANCER

Eighty-eight hybridomas producing antibodies were obtained from the fusion of the murine myeloma P3-X63-Ag8-U1 with spleen cells from a mouse immunized with the human breast cancer cell line, MCF-7.[57] After an initial screen, three MoAbs, MBr1, MBr2, and MBr3, with a specificity for the immunizing cells, were identified and further characterized. The three MoAbs were tested by isotopic antiglobulin assay and immunofluorescence on a panel of normal cells or cell membrane preparations, on cells or cell membrane preparations from fresh surgical specimens of various types of carcinoma, and on various tumor cell lines. MBr1 and MBr2 showed specificity for an antigen that seemed to characterize both normal and neoplastic mammary gland epithelial cells. They showed a superimposable spectrum of reactivity and manifested about 70% reciprocal inhibition in cross-inhibition tests, which suggests an identity of the antigenic molecule or of the epitope target of the two MoAbs.

Immunochemical analysis of the determinant recognized by the IgM fraction of MBr1 showed that the antibody identified a low molecular weight neutral glycolipid antigen and that the carbohydrate portion of the molecule constituted the antigenic determinant.[13] More recently, other MoAbs raised against breast cancer have been produced (MBr4-16), and studies on their characterization are being completed (unpublished data). The reactive profile of MBr1 was tested on a variety of human tumors and nonneoplastic tissues by light microscopic immunohistochemistry. Different patterns of immunoreactivity were present in normal tissues, in tissues with inflammatory changes, and in tumors (Figs. 10.1–10.3), including adenocarcinomas and squamous cell carcinomas of various sites (*e.g.*, stomach, lung, carcinoma *in situ* of the cervix, endometrium, and ovary) (for specific details see Ref. 53). The immunohistologic distribution of the MBr1-defined antigen was analyzed in several histologic types of carcinoma of the breast and their metastases and for comparison in normal mammary epithelium, in nonneoplastic breast lesions (Fig. 10.4), as well as in a few nonepithelial breast tumors (for specific details see Ref. 52).

For this purpose, the antibody stock used was derived from a pool of murine MBr1 ascites, purified and diluted to a final concentration of 3 µg/ml. Murine monoclonal IgM B3, substituted with MBr1 in controls, was reactive with murine lymphomas.[22] Owing to its reported sensitivity,[38] we used a slightly modified avidin-biotin-complex[39] immunoperoxidase technique.[53] Controls consisted of substitution with fetal calf serum or an unrelated murine IgM, at a normalized concentration, for MBr1. The tissues studied were routinely fixed in Bouin's and embedded in paraffin.

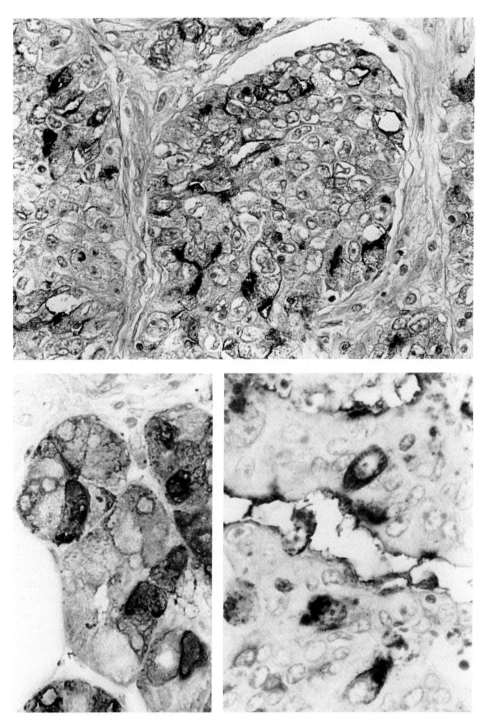

Fig. 10.1. (*Top*) Poorly differentiated adenocarcinoma of the lung stained by monoclonal antibody (MoAb) MBr1. Intraluminal and occasional apical staining and cytoplasmic granular reactivity of tumor cells. Original magnification, × 480.

Fig. 10.2. (*Bottom left*) Diffuse cytoplasmic staining of scattered cells of a paraganglioma by MoAb MBr1. Original magnification, × 835.

Fig. 10.3. (*Bottom right*) Moderately differentiated adenocarcinoma of the endometrium stained by MoAb MBr1. A few cells reveal cytoplasmic staining. Original magnification, × 785.

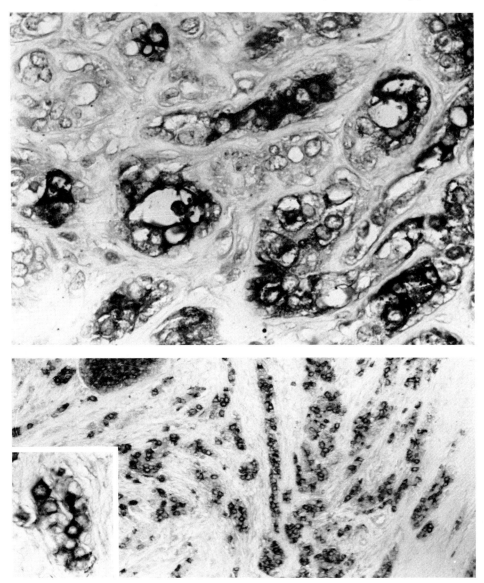

FIG. 10.4. (*Top*) Sclerosing adenosis of the breast stained by MoAb MBr1. Evidence of apical cytoplasmic and intraluminal staining. Original magnification, × 600.

FIG. 10.5. (*Bottom*) Infiltrating lobular carcinoma of the breast in which most of the tumor cells show cytoplasmic staining by MoAb MBr1. Original magnification, × 165. (*Inset*) Focus of infiltrating ductal carcinoma of the same case. Diffuse cytoplasmic staining of most neoplastic cells. Original magnification, × 500.

The main findings were as follows: immunologically detectable antigen was found (with markedly heterogeneous expression as shown by variable staining properties) in infiltrating ductal, lobular (Fig. 10.5), mixed, and tubular carcinomas in 70% of the cases and was never detected on nonepithelial structures. The most common appearance was that of a "patchwork" positivity pattern. Since the staining patterns were classified as apical, intraluminal, diffuse cytoplasmic, focal intracytoplasmic, and marginal, it could be shown that apical luminal staining predominated in well-differentiated ductal carcinomas, whereas marginal and cytoplasmic staining was more commonly encountered in moderately and poorly differentiated ductal carcinomas and in lobular carcinomas. Occasional intracytoplasmic lumens were stained in scattered cells of lobular carcinomas. In medullary carcinomas, focal cytoplasmic staining was present in 20% of the cases; focal apical reactivity was found in 33% of papillary carcinomas. In contrast 50% of colloid carcinomas had marginal labeling of some of the tumor cell nests floating in the mucin. The cells of carcinomas with metaplasia (squamous, spindle cell, or cartilaginous) and carcinoids of the breast were consistently unreactive with MBr1.

In spite of the more common finding of strongly diffusely positive cases and a low incidence of focally reactive cases among well-differentiated ductal carcinomas, differences in immunostaining of ductal carcinomas of various grades were not significant.

The correlation between MBr1 staining and nodal status revealed a high proportion of focally reactive cases and a low proportion of diffusely reactive cases among tumors from patients with more than three positive axillary lymph nodes, but this was without statistical significance. Also, the metastases of well-differentiated ductal carcinomas revealed a trend toward a more diffuse staining.

The age of the patients as well as their menopausal status was unrelated to MBr1 antigen expression. Intraductal carcinoma and lobular neoplasia usually displayed concordant reactivity with the adjacent infiltrating carcinoma. Cribriform areas of intraductal carcinoma often showed luminal staining.

In addition to the classical clinicopathologic parameters,[67] the prognostic significance of the immunohistologic reactivity with MBr1 of primary breast tumors seen from 1973–1980 in a randomized controlled follow-up trial was investigated. This trial compared radical mastectomy with quadrantectomy, axillary dissection, and radiotherapy in T1 N0-N1a patients.[79] Cases with positive axillary lymph nodes were treated with adjuvant radiotherapy (from 1973–1976) or adjuvant chemotherapy according to the CMF regimen (from 1976–1980). All patients were followed in the outpatient clinic, and recurrence-free intervals and overall survival were documented. Actuarial curves revealed no differences in disease-free and overall survival rates related to different treatment modalities.

Primary breast tumors from 243 T1 N0-N1a patients (114 T1 N− and 129 T1 N+) were examined immunohistochemically and were divided into three subsets according to their MBr1 reactivity: unreactive, focally reactive, and reactive. The proportions of these three subsets were comparable in the N− and N+ groups. The incidence of disease relapse, including distant metastases and/or local recurrences, separately considered for the N− and N+ groups, was similar in the MBr1 reactivity subsets. Differences in the incidence of disease relapse, when one considered the unreactive subsets vs. the focally reactive and reactive subsets combined, or the unreactive and focally reactive subsets combined vs. the reactive subset, were also not significant.

The reactivity of metastatic cells in lymph nodes with MBr1 was somewhat lower than that of the corresponding primary tumors. In more than 85% of the cases, the reactivity of the primary and that of the nodal metastases were concordant, whereas discordant cases always had an immunopositive primary. Similar findings were observed in metastatic spread to soft tissues and bone marrow. Sarcomas of the breast (cystoscarcoma phyllodes) and in the breast (malignant lymphomas, malignant fibrous histiocytoma, and angiosarcoma) were negative throughout, except for residual epithelial tissue.

Nonneoplastic mammary epithelium adjacent to breast carcinomas showed an immunoreactivity that correlated with that of the tumor in more than 90% of the cases. There was variable staining of the ducts of the same breast. Usually, the reactivity was both apical and secretory. Lactational breast tissue of pregnant patients with cancer was strongly positive. The epithelial cells of mammary dysplasia, of fibroadenomas, and of gynecomastia were usually reactive, with variations in the apical, secretory, and cytoplasmic staining patterns. A shift from apical labeling in benign epithelial cells to circumferential, intracellular, and cytoplasmic reactivity in neoplastic cells was consistently observed not only in the breast but also in a variety of sites with nonsquamous epithelia. A similar alteration in antigenic reactivity was previously documented with polyclonal sera against human milk fat globule antigens,[40, 71] T antigen,[74] and a variety of lectins that bind carbohydrate moieties.[30, 37, 74]

The distribution of the MBr1 immunohistochemical reactivity in epithelia and carcinomas might reflect functional or evolutionary relationships between molecules in different tissues and tumors but could also be explained by the fortuitous presence of similar or identical epitopes on different molecules in different cell types.[47, 60] Any interpretation must wait for more data on the nature and functional roles of reactive molecules that are recognized in different tissues.

MoAbs reactive with human breast cancer cells have been described by several groups. Some of these antibodies have been reported to be able to discriminate mammary cancer cells from normal breast cells.[19, 69, 76] However, most of the others identify antigenic determinants present on both normal and malignant breast cells.[1]

On the whole, the reactivity of MBr1 revealed similarities to that of MoAbs and polyclonal sera against human milk fat globule membrane (MFGM). Of the four MoAbs reported by Foster *et al.*[28, 29] IgG LICR-LON/M8 appears to be similar to MBr1, in its spectrum of reactivity with ductal, lobular, mucinous, and medullary carcinomas. LICR-LON/M8 also showed some competition to flow cytofluorimetry with a different, recently characterized mouse MoAb, IgM NCRC-11.[26] IgM LICR-LON/M18 differed from MBr1 for its low incidence of reactivity, whereas antibodies LICR-LON/M3 and LICR/LON/M24 could be distinguished from MBr1 in that they reacted with interpithelial cell membranes in nonneoplastic breast epithelium.

Among the two MoAbs described by Thompson *et al.*,[77] only one, the 24.17.2, showed a reactivity reminiscent of MBr1, although differences existed in the reactivity with the respiratory and the genital tracts. The reagent F36/22 described by Papsidero *et al.*,[63] differently from MBr1, reacted with colon carcinoma, whereas the MoAb H59 reported by Yuan *et al.*[82] differed from MBr1 in that it bound to a smaller percentage of malignant breast cancer specimens than MBr1.

An evaluation of the IgM MoAb Ca-1[2] staining on paraffin sections[55] of various breast lesions[18] showed a positive rate of 93% for malignant tumors, whereas fibroadenomas were less commonly and only focally reactive, even though they were more often positive than some of the lesions associated with mammary dysplasia.[70]

The two MoAbs to MFGM reported by Arklie *et al.*[1] appeared very similar immunohistologically to MBr1. In contrast, three MoAbs against an estrogen-induced protein[17] were distinct from MBr1 since they did not react with fibroadenomas, gynecomastia, or lactating breast. Other MoAbs against breast carcinoma-associated antigens[19, 61, 76] clearly differed from MBr1 because they showed limited immunohistochemical binding to nonneoplastic mammary epithelium.

OVARIAN CANCER

The search for immunologic markers of value in detecting ovarian carcinomas in an early phase and in monitoring the course of established disease is essentially related to the ominous prognosis of ovarian cancer due to the usually late diagnosis and rapid dissemination. As for breast tumors, numerous markers have been identified by polyclonal antisera[41] and MoAbs. In this respect, the investigative work performed at this Institution showed that the fusion of the murine myeloma line P3-X63-Ag8-U1 with spleen cells from a mouse immunized with a membrane preparation of a mucinous ovarian cystadenocarcinoma yielded two MoAbs, MOv1 and MOv2.[75] MOv1 and MOv2 are, respectively, an IgG1 and IgM and recognize two different epitopes present on malignant and benign ovarian tumor cells. MOv1 recognizes a high molecular weight glycoprotein secreted by ovarian cells and found to react with all mucinous carcinomas of the ovary tested, whereas MOv2, which also recognizes a high molecular weight glycoprotein, was shown to react with 70% of ovarian carcinomas of various histologic types. Furthermore, MOv2 reacted in frozen sections by indirect immunofluorescence with ovarian and some nonovarian carcinomas. Finally, MOv2 was able to detect the antigen in sera and ascitic fluids from patients with ovarian cystadenocarcinomas but not in control specimens from patients without cancer.[75]

Utilizing the immunoperoxidase technique we investigated a variety of tissues in order to delineate the immunohistochemical profile of MOv2 since the antigen is resistant to Bouin's fixation and paraffin embedding.[50] Immunoperoxidase staining was performed using the avidin-biotin-peroxidase complex method as previously described.[53] Paraffin-embedded tissues, selected from the surgical pathology files, were used for this study. In most cases, paraffin blocks from different areas of the lesion were examined. Partially purified MOv2 syngeneic ascites was used at a protein concentration of 8 μg/ml, and sections of normal colon served as positive controls. The reaction specificity was checked by substituting phosphate-buffered saline with 2% fetal calf serum or the murine monoclonal IgM B3[22] for MOv2 on serial sections.

Evaluation of positive slides took into account the number of immunoreactive cells in relation to the total number of cells of the same type visualized in the tissue section. The cases studied were scored as negative, focally positive (when a few cells in a few high-power fields were stained), or positive (when a substantial percentage of cells was stained). The following patterns of labeling distribution were identified and recorded: intraluminal secretory, apical, interepithelial cell membrane-bound, circumferential, cytoplasmic diffuse, and cytoplasmic focal.

Diffuse immunopositivity was detected in the epithelial cells of most ovarian mucinous cystadeno(fibro)mas, irrespective of their cervical-like or colon-like histologic appearance,[27] and of serous cystadenomas, whose lining resembled that of normal fallopian tubes (Figs. 10.6 and 10.7). The epithelial component of a few benign Brenner's tumors was also immunostained. MOv2 reacted positively with all mucinous and most serous and endometrioid (Fig. 10.8) ovarian carcinomas, whereas the incidence of positive reactions was lower in undifferentiated and clear cell carcinomas. The nonepithelial ovarian neoplasms tested, including benign theca cell and malignant sex cord-stromal, granulosa cell, and endodermal sinus tumors, were immunonegative; the degree of staining heterogeneity was variable in the different types of carcinoma. In most benign and malignant mucinous tumors and, to a lesser extent, in serous tumors, a high percentage of neoplastic cells, uniformly distributed throughout the lesion, reacted with the antibody. In contrast, several endometrioid, undifferentiated, and clear cell types showed only focal reactions. The correlation between the histologic grade of mucinous, serous, and endometrioid carcinomas and their MOv2 immunopositivity revealed that the inci-

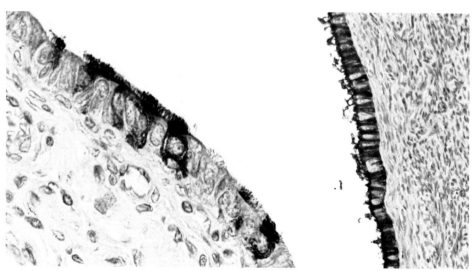

Fɪɢ. 10.6. (*Left*) Epithelium of the fallopian tube. Several ciliated cells reveal strong cytoplasmic staining by MoAb MOv2. Original magnification, × 666.

Fɪɢ. 10.7. (*Right*) Serous cystadenoma of the ovary. Diffuse cytoplasmic staining of the columnar cells by MoAb MOv2. Original magnification, × 165.

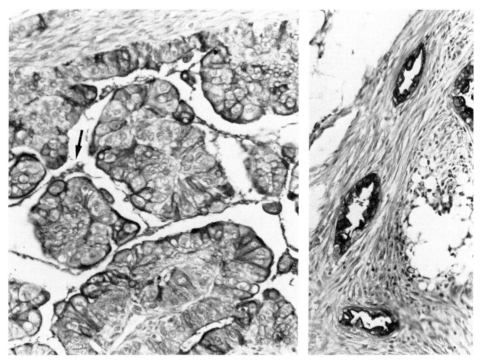

FIG. 10.8. (*Left*) Endometrioid carcinoma of the ovary. Several epithelial cells show circumferential (*arrow*) and apical staining by MoAb MOv2. Original magnification, × 265.

FIG. 10.9. (*Right*) Omental metastasis of a serous carcinoma of the ovary. The cytoplasm of the malignant cells lining the glandular formations is strongly stained by MOv2. Original magnification, × 175.

dence of immunostaining slightly decreased with increasing anaplasia. Mucinous cystadenomas and well-differentiated mucinous carcinomas had strong perinuclear and parabasal labeling, whereas serous cystadenomas and well-differentiated serous carcinomas showed apical staining. Secretion products, mucin and foam cells shed within cystic lumina were generally strongly immunoreactive (For further details see reference 50).

Omental metastases (Fig. 10.9) of ovarian carcinomas were immunostained by MOv2 in most cases and showed focal reactivity only. The immunoreactions of the omental metatases of one mucinous and one serous carcinoma could be compared with those of the primaries (Fig. 10.10), to which they were similar in pattern, intensity, and distribution. Surprisingly, the surface epithelium of eight normal ovaries was immunonegative, whereas normal fallopian tubes showed apical and cytoplasmic epithelial labeling. Also, Walthard's nests were strongly positive. Patches of immunoreactivity were detected in the epithelium of the endometrium and in the columnar epithelium of the endocervix, which showed labeling of apical and interepithelial cell membranes. All of the endometrial and endocervical adenocarcinomas tested exhibited cell membrane and cytoplasmic reactivity. Infiltrating and *in situ* squamous cell carcinomas of the uterine cervix had membrane and cytoplasmic reactivity, which reflected that of intermediate layer keratinocytes of squamous epithelium.

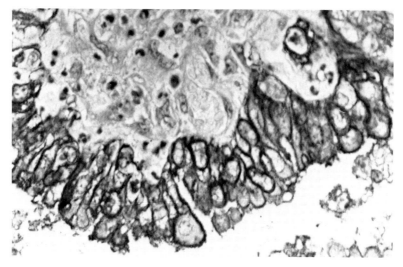

FIG. 10.10. Serous cystadenocarcinoma of the ovary. Localization of the MoAb MOv2 on the plasma membranes of tumor cells. Original magnification, × 625.

Immunoreactivity was also displayed by mammary epithelial cells. Resting epithelia of major ducts and lobular units, as well as mammary alveoli with secretory lactational changes, focally exhibited apical secretion products, cytoplasmic and interepithelial cell membrane-bound positivity.

With regard to breast lesions within the morphologic spectrum of fibrocystic disease, there was well-defined labeling of the attenuated epithelium and secretion products of mammary cysts, of ductal epithelium of sclerosing adenosis and apocrine metaplasia.

Malignant breast lesions frequently reacted with the antibody, although with marked variations in the percentages of positive cells in the specimens tested. Immunohistologic antigen expression was comparable in infiltrating and *in situ* ductal and lobular carcinomas.

As with MBr1, in medullary and mucinous mammary carcinomas, immunostaining was limited to a few cells; the tested papillary carcinomas and carcinoids of the breast were immunonegative. The examination of metastases in axillary lymph nodes of ductal and lobular carcinomas disclosed an incidence of positivity of 60% and a pattern of immunoreactivity similar to that of primary breast carcinomas. One case of pleural, one of omental, and one out of three ovarian metastases from primary breast carcinomas were strongly positive with MOv2.

A variety of normal and malignant epithelial cells of the alimentary system reacted with the antibody. The squamous carcinomas of the oropharynx had strong immunoreactions, whereas columnar cells of gastrointestinal epithelia had a fairly strong cytoplasmic immunostaining, even though the labeling, especially of the colonic epithelium, was consistently stronger and more diffuse than at all other sites. Specimens of fetal small and large intestine had diffuse epithelial immunoreactivity. Adult bile ducts and gallbladder epithelia invariably immunostained. Most of the gastric, pancreatic and colonic adendocarcinomas tested, both noncolloid and colloid types, were diffusely positive with the antibody; their reactive patterns generally paralleled those of adenocarcinomas from other sites.

In the respiratory system, the epithelia of the bronchi, bronchioles, and bronchial glands were strongly immunoreactive, whereas the alveolar respiratory epithelium was immunonegative. Immunostaining was detected in all of the histologic types of malignant tumors of the lung tested; squamous cell carcinoma and adenocarcinoma reacted more consistently and diffusely than the small cell, large cell, bronchioloalveolar and adenocarcinoid varieties.

In the urinary system, the major finding was immunoreactivity of the transitional cell carcinomas tested, which was consistently stronger and more diffuse than that of the normal parent tissue.

In the integumentary system, eccrine and apocrine sweat glands were invariably immunopositive. Positive cells were detected in squamous cell and basal cell carcinomas.

Other reports have also shown that antigenic phenotypes of normal epithelia and of carcinomas of other sites are shared by common epithelial tumors of the ovary. Some of the several glycoprotein antigens reported, such as fetal sulphoglycoprotein antigen,[34] ovarian tumor-specific mucin antigen,[48] colon-specific antigen,[62] colonic mucoprotein antigen,[32] and gastric and intestinal mucus-associated antigens[5, 6] are detected in gastointestinal epithelia and carcinomas as well as in mucinous ovarian tumors only, thus differing from the antigen(s) recognized by MOv2. More similar to the MOv2 antigen are those designated OvC1-2[41] and OCAA-1,[10, 11] even though these antigens were defined by polyclonal sera and characterized by immunodiffusion in gel. CEA was also detected by polyclonal antisera in mucinous carcinomas of the ovary.[16, 24, 33, 35, 49, 78]

Several studies have dealt with MoAbs to ovarian cancer. Two antibodies,[8, 9, 43] designated OC 125 and OC 133, reacted predominantly with serous papillary cystadenocarcinomas, and the same applies to the MoAbs prepared by Bhattacharya *et al.*[12] In contrast, several MoAbs to nonovarian tumors reacted with ovarian carcinomas,[3, 16, 23, 45] including our own MBr1, which failed, however, to react with normal colonic epithelia.

DIAGNOSTIC APPLICATIONS OF MBr1 and MOv2

PAGET'S DISEASE

The special reactive features of MBr1 and MOv2 with reference respectively to carcinoma of the breast and to a large number of adenocarcinomas of the ovary and of other sites prompted comparative immunohistochemical investigations, one of which was carried out on mammary and extramammary Paget's disease. The results were compared with the immunoreactions obtained with an anti-CEA serum and with the data obtained from conventional histochemical methods.[51] Strong immunoreactions with the two antibodies were detected in a high proportion of cases of mammary Paget's disease (60–70%, even though a higher proportion (75%) was immunopositive for CEA. The antisera did not discriminate between mammary and extramammary and extramammary Paget's cells, which was in keeping with the immunostaining of eccrine and aprocrine sweat glands as well as of normal mammary epithelia. In most of the cases of mammary Paget's disease, the antigens recognized by MBr1, MOv2, and anti-CEA were found concordantly on Paget's cells and on the cells of the associated intraductal and/or invasive carcinomas of the breast. The findings support the prevalent theory that Paget's disease is an intra-epidermal adenocarcinoma deriving from cells of adnexal origin.[4, 59, 68] Also supported is the concept that Paget's cells and the cells of the associated carcinomas represent the same neoplastic population.

EFFUSIONS

Another promising application for the diagnostic application of the MoAbs described thus far is the discrimination of malignant breast or ovarian tumor cells in effusions from resting or activated mesothelial cells. This can be done by a direct immunofluorescence assay,[3, 54, 56] since mesothelial cells, poly-morphonuclear leukocytes, and erythrocytes have been shown to be consis-tently negative with MBr1 and MOv2. The difficulties of making this differen-tial diagnosis solely on cytologic criteria have been repeatedly emphasized in the past.[42, 46, 64] Other immunohistochemical approaches to discriminate normal or reactive mesothelial cells from malignant mesothelial cells or carcinomatous cells have used other markers such as CEA, keratin, epithelial membrane antigen (EMA), Ca1 and alpha-1-antichymotrypsin (reviewed by Whitaker and Shilkin [80]). Immunocytochemical staining with a combination of several MoAbs such as HMFG-2, Ca-1[81] and anti-CEA in cytologically negative serous effu-sions from patients with malignancies resulted in an increased diagnostic ac-curacy of 20%.[31]

Our investigation was carried out on 280 pleural fluids and peritoneal effu-sions and peritoneal washings from patients with various neoplastic and non-neoplastic diseases, and the results obtained by immunofluorescence were correlated with those obtained by conventional cytology. Sixty percent of the malignant effusions diagnosed cytologically contained tumor cells reactive with at least one of the two MoAbs tested. However, 16 of 94 effusions cytologically negative for malignant cells were positive by MoAb immu-nofluorescence, which means a retrieval of malignant cells in 17% of the cytologically negative fluids. Interestingly enough, the number of false-nega-tive cases detectable by MoAbs was higher among breast cancer patients than ovarian carcinoma bearers, probably because of the more obvious malignant appearance of ovarian carcinoma cells. The specificity of labeling by the MoAbs was confirmed by immunoelectron microscopy, which demonstrated the positivity of the epithelial cells and the negativity of the mesothelial cells (Figs. 10.11 and 10.12). Preliminary results indicate that the detection rate of carcinoma cells in effusions utilizing the pool of MoAbs raised against different breast and ovarian carcinomas is considerably higher than that obtained by MBr1 or MOv2 (Colnaghi *et al.*, unpublished data.)

BONE MARROW MICROMETASTASES

The prognostic value of MBr1 MoAb is currently under evaluation in another area. It is well known that breast cancer patients with Stage I disease are considered clinically cured if adequately treated, but 20% of them have a recur-

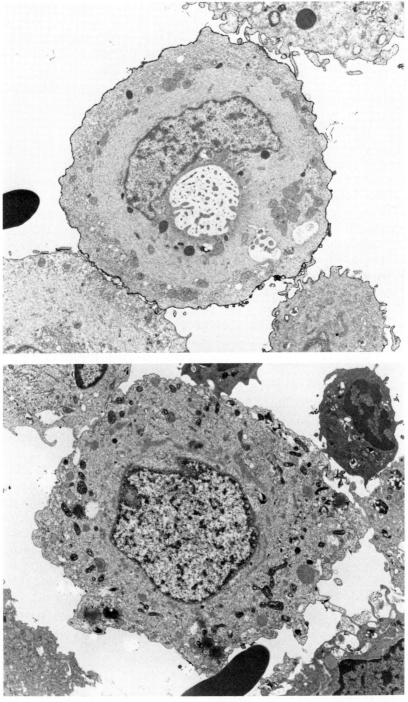

FIG. 10.11. (*Top*) Plasma membrane staining by MoAb MBr1 of a metastatic breast cancer cell in a pleural effusion. Indirect immunoperoxidase technique. Original magnification, × 5600.

FIG. 10.12. (*Bottom*) No evidence of plasma membrane staining by MoAb MBr1 of a mesothelial cell in a pleural effusion. Indirect immunoperoxidase technique. Original magnification, × 6600.

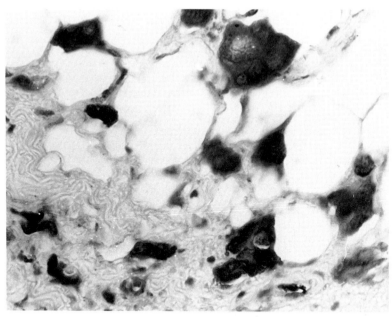

FIG. 10.13. Metastatic infiltrating ductal carcinoma of the breast stained by MoAb MBr1. Diffuse cytoplasmic staining of scattered malignant cells. Original magnification, × 625.

rence within 10 years. At the present time, there are no means of identifying this subpopulation at risk. Since in preliminary studies MoAb MBr1 was proven to be able to detect micrometastases (Fig. 10.13) of breast carcinoma or even single scattered malignant cells in bone marrow biopsy specimens, we are now applying the reagent in a prospective study to verify its capability of selecting patients at high risk for recurrence or metastases. So far, bone marrow samples prepared as cell suspensions from 84 T1-T2 N0 or N1a-b patients have been examined by indirect immunofluorescence. Of the 56 patients pathologically N−, 23% harbored an otherwise undetectable metastatic spread. All patients are being followed to ascertain the significance of this finding, especially in terms of the need for adjuvant chemotherapy and prognostic implications. (See also Chapter 9 by Neville *et al.*)

A detection rate of 24% was reported by Redding *et al.*[65] in patients with breast cancer and negative lymph nodes by applying an anti-EMA[36] antibody on bone marrow cell suspensions with an immunocytochemical method. In contrast, retrospective studies on sections of other sites such as liver and lymph nodes of breast carcinoma-bearing patients revealed that the use of an immunocytochemical technique did not increase the number of positive specimens recognized by conventional stains.[72]

ACKNOWLEDGMENTS

The study was supported in part by Grants 83.00928.96 and 83.00780.96, Controllo della Crescita Neoplastica, Progetto Finalizzato, from the Consiglio Nazionale delle Ricerche, Rome. The authors wish to thank Dr. R. Claren for assistance in the preparation of the manuscript, Ms. B. Johnston for editing it,

Mr. M. Azzini for the photographic art work, and Ms. A. Tosi for secretarial help.

REFERENCES

1. Arklie, J., Taylor-Papadimitriou, J., Bodmer, W., Egan, M., and Millis, R. Differentiation antigens expressed by epithelial cells in the lactating breast are also detectable in breast cancers. *Int. J. Cancer 28:* 23–29, 1981.
2. Ashall, f., Bramwell, M. E., and Harris, H. A new marker for human cancer cells. 1. The Ca antigen and the Ca1 antibody. *Lancet 2:* 1–6, 1982.
3. Atkinson, B. F., Ernst, C. S., Herlyn, M., Steplewski, Z., Sears, H. F., and Koprowski, H. Gastrointestinal cancer-associated antigen in immunoperoxidase assay. *Cancer Res. 42:* 4820–4823, 1982.
4. Azzopardi, J. G. *Problems in Breast Pathology.* London, W. B. Saunders, 1979, pp. 258-261.
5. Bara, J., Loisillier, F., and Burtin, P. Correlation between the presence of gastrointestinal antigens and the histological type of human ovarian mucinous cysts. In *Peptides of Biological Fluids*, edited by H. Peeters. Oxford, Pergamon Press, 1979, pp. 339–342.
6. Bara, J., Malarewics, A., Louisillier, F., and Burtin, P. Antigens common to ovarian mucinous cyst fluid and gastric mucosa. *Br. J. Cancer 36:* 49–56, 1977.
7. Bartorelli, A., Biancardi, C., Ferrara, R., Bailo, M. A., Cavalca, V., and Accinni, R. CEA and/ or CEA-like glycoproteins in breast cancer. In *Markers for Diagnosis and Monitoring of Human Cancer. Proceedings of the Serono Symposia*, edited by M. I. Colnaghi, G. L. Buraggi, and M. Ghine, Vol. 46. London, Academic Press, 1982, pp. 21–33.
8. Bast, R. C., Feeney, M., Lazarus, H., Nadler, L. M., Colvin, R. B., and Knapp, R. C. Reactivity of a monoclonal antibody with human ovarian carcinoma. *J. Clin. Invest. 68:* 1131–1337, 1981.
9. Berkowitz, R., Kabawat, S., Lazarus, H., Colvin, R., Knapp, R., and Bast, R. Comparison of a rabbit heteroantiserum and a murine monoclonal antibody raised against a human epithelial ovarian carcinoma cell line. *Am. J. Obstet. Gynecol. 146:* 607-612, 1983.
10. Bhattacharya, M., and Barlow, J. J. Tumor markers for ovarian cancer. *Int. Adv. Surg. Oncol. 2:* 155-176, 1979.
11. Bhattacharya, M., and Barlow, J. J. Ovarian tumor antigens. *Cancer 42:* 1616-1620, 1978.
12. Bhattacharya, M., Chatterjee, S. K., Barlow, J., and Fuji, H. Monoclonal antibodies recognizing tumor-associated antigen of human ovarian mucinous cystadenocarcinomas. *Cancer Res. 42:* 1650-1654, 1982.
13. Canevari, S., Fossati, G., Balsari, A., Sonnino, S., and Colnaghi, M. E. Immunochemical analysis of the determinant recognized by a monoclonal antibody (MBr1) which specifically binds to human mammary epithelial cells. *Cancer Res. 43:* 1301-1305, 1983.
14. Carpentier, N. A., Egeli, R., Chollet, P., Maurince, P., and Lambert, P. H. Circulating immune complexes as markers for human neoplasia. In *Markers for Diagnosis and Monitoring of Human Cancer, Proceedings of the Serono Symposia*, edited by M. I. Colnaghi, G. L. Buraggi, and M. Ghione, Vol. 46. London, Academic Press, 1982, pp. 9-20.
15. Ceriani, R. L., Thompson, K. E., Peterson, J. A., and Abraham, S. Surface differentiation antigens on human mammary epithelial cells carried on the human milk fat globule. *Proc. Natl. Acad. Sci. U.S.A. 74:* 582–585, 1977.
16. Charpin, C., Bhan, A. K., Zurawski, V. R., and Scully, R. E. Carcinoembryonic antigen (CEA) and carbohydrate determinant 19.9 (Ca 19.9) localization on 121 primary and metastatic ovarian tumors: An immunohistochemical study with the use of monoclonal antibodies. *Int. J. Gynecol. Pathol. 1:* 231-245, 1983.
17. Ciocca, D. R., Adams, D. J., Edwards, D. P., Bjerke, R. J., and McGuire, W. L. Distribution of an estrogen-induced protein with a molecular weight of 24000 in normal and malignant human tissues and cells. *Cancer Res. 43:* 1204-1210, 1983.
18. Clough, D. G. F., Coghill, G. R., and Holley, M. P. Evaluation of the Ca1 antibody in the diagnosis of invasive breast cancer. *J. Clin. Pathol. 37:* 10-13, 1984.
19. Colcher, D., Horan Hand, P., Nuti, J., and Schlom, J. A spectrum of monoclonal antibodies reactive with human mammary tumor cells. *Proc. Natl. Acad. Sci. U.S.A. 78:* 3199-3203, 1981.

20. Colnaghi, M. I., Canevari, S., Della Torre, G., Ménard, S., Miotti, S., Regazzoni, M., and Tagliabue, E. Monoclonal antibodies potentially useful in clinical oncology. In *Monoclonal Antibodies and Cancer*, edited by B. D. Boss, R. Langman, I. Trowbridge, and R. Dulbecco, New York, Academic Press, 1983, pp. 207-213.

21. Colnaghi, M. I., Clemente, C., Della Porta, G., Della Torre, G. Mariani-Costantini, R., Ménard, S., Rilke, R., and Tagliabue, E. Monoclonal antibodies to human breast cancer. In *Monoclonal Antibodies 1982. Progress and Perspectives*, edited by F. Dammacco, G. Doria, and A. Pinchera. Amsterdam, Elsevier, 1983, pp. 79-95.

22. Colnaghi, M. I., Ménard, S. Tagliabue, E., and Della Torre, G. Heterogeneity of the natural humoral anti-tumor immune response in mice as shown by monoclonal antibodies. *J. Immunol. 128:* 2757-2762, 1982.

23. Daasch, V. N., Fernstern, P. D., and Metzgar, R. S. Radioimmune assay studies using a monoclonal antibody to detect an antigen (DU-PAN-2) in the serum and ascites of adenocarcinoma patients (abstr. 1051). In *Proceedings of the American Association for Cancer Research*, Immunology, 1982, p. 266.

24. Donaldson, E. S., Gay, E. C., Sharkey, R. M., Rayburn R., and Goldenberg, D. M. Carcinoembryonic antigen in ovarian epithelial cystadenocarcinomas. The prognostic value of tumor and serial plasma determinations. *Cancer 41:* 2335-2340, 1978.

25. Edgington, T. S., and Nakamura, R. M. Tumor associated and tumor specific markers of human mammary carcinoma. In *Markers for Diagnosis and Monitoring of Human Cancer. Proceedings of the Serono Symposia*, edited by M. I. Colnaghi, G. L. Buraggi, and M. Ghione, Vol. 46. London, Academic Press, 1982, pp. 51-74.

26. Ellis, I. O., Robins, R. A., Elston, C. W., Blamey, R. W., Ferry, B., and Baldwin. R. W. A monoclonal antibody, NCRC-11, raised to human breast carcinoma. 1. Production and immunohistological characterization. *Histopathology 8:* 501-516, 1984.

27. Fenoglio, C. M., Ferenczy, A., and Richart, R. M. Mucinous tumors of the ovary. Ultrastructural studies of mucinous cystadenomas with histogenetic considerations. *Cancer 36:* 1709–1722, 1975.

28. Foster, C. S., Dinsdale, E. A., Edwards, P. A. W., and Neville, A. M. Monoclonal antibodies to the human mammary gland. II. Distribution of determinants in breast carcinomas. *Virchows Arch. (Pathol. Anat.) 394:* 295-305, 1982.

29. Foster, C. S., Edwards, P. A. W., Dinsdale, E. A., and Neville, A. M. Monoclonal antibodies to the human mammary gland. I. Distribution of determinants in non-neoplastic mammary and extra mammary tissues. *Virchows Arch. (Pathol. Anat.) 394:* 279-293, 1982.

30. Franklin, W. A. Tissue binding of lectins in disorders of the breast. *Cancer 51:* 295-300, 1983.

31. Ghosh, A. K., Mason, D. Y., and Spriggs, A. I. Immunocytochemical staining with monoclonal antibodies in cytologically "negative" serous effusions from patients with malignant disease. *J. Clin. Pathol. 36:* 1150-1153, 1983.

32. Gold, D. V. Immunoperoxidase localization of colonic mucoprotein antigen in neoplastic tissues. *Cancer Res. 41:* 767-772, 1981.

33. Goldenberg, D. M., Sharkey, R. M., and Primus, F. J. Immunocytochemical detection of carcinoembryonic antigen in conventional histopathology specimens. *Cancer 42:* 1546-1553, 1978.

34. Häkkinen, I. P. T., and Ilkaa, P. T. FSA. Foetal sulphoglycoprotein associated with gastric cancer. *Transplant. Rev. 20:* 61-76, 1974.

35. Heald, J., Buckley, C. H., and Fox, M. An immunohistochemical study of the distribution of carcinoembryonic antigen in epithelial tumors of the ovary. *J. Clin. Pathol. 32:* 918–926, 1979.

36. Heyderman, E., Steele, K., and Ormerod, M. G. A new antigen on the epithelial membrane: Its immunoperoxidase localisation in normal and neoplastic tissue. *J. Clin. Pathol. 32:* 35-39, 1979.

37. Howard, D. R., and Batsakis, J. G. Cytostructural localization of a tumor associated antigen. *Science 210:* 201-203, 1980.

38. Hsu, S. M., Raine, L., and Fanger, H. A comparative study of the peroxidase-antiperoxidase method and an avidin-biotin complex method for studying polypeptide hormones with radioimmunoassay antibodies. *Am. J. Clin. Pathol. 75:* 734-738, 1981.

39. Hsu, S. M., Raine, L., and Fanger, H. Use of avidin-biotin-peroxidase complex (ABC) in immunoperoxidase techniques. *J. Histochem. Cytochem. 29:* 577-580, 1981.

40. Imam, A., and Tökés, Z. Immunoperoxidase localization of a glycoprotein on plasma membrane of secretory epithelium from human breast. *J. Histochem. Cytochem. 29:* 581-584, 1981.

41. Immamura, N., Takahashi, T., Lloyd, K. O., Lewis, J. L., and Old, L. J. Analysis of human ovarian tumor antigens using heterologous antisera: Detection of a new antigenic system. *Int. J. Cancer 21:* 570-577, 1978.

42. Jarvi, O. H., Kunnas, R. L., Laitio, M. T., and Tyrkko, J. E. S. The accuracy and significance of cytologic cancer diagnosis of pleural effusions (a follow-up study of 338 patients). *Acta Cytol. 16:* 152-158, 1972.

43. Kabawat, S. E., Bast, R. C., Welch, W. R., Knapp, R. C., and Colvin, R. B. Immunopathologic characterization of a monoclonal antibody that recognizes common surface antigens of human ovarian tumors of serous, endometrioid and clear cell types. *Am. J. Clin. Pathol. 79:* 98–104, 1983.

44. Kohler, G., and Milstein, G. Continuous cultures of fused cells secreting antibody of predefined specificity. *Nature (Lond.) 256:* 495-497, 1975.

45. Koprowski, H., Steplewski, Z., Mitchell, K., Herlyn, M., Kerlyn, D., and Fuhrer, P. Colorectal carcinoma antigens detected by hybridoma antibodies. *Somatic Cell Genet. 5:* 957-972, 1979.

46. Koss, L. G. Examination of effusions (pleural, ascitic and pericardial fluids). In *Compendium on Diagnostic Cytology,* 4th ed. edited by G. L. Wied, L. G. Koss, and J. W. Reagan, Chicago, Tutorials of Cytology, 1976.

47. Lane, D., and Koprowski, H. Molecular recognition and the future of monoclonal antibodies. *Nature 296:* 200-202, 1982.

48. Ma, J., Handley , C. J., and de Boer, W. G. R. M. An ovarian tumour specific mucin antigen— immunohistological and biochemical studies. *Pathology 15:* 385-391, 1983.

49. Marchand, A., Fenoglio, C. M., Pascal, R., Richart, R. M., and Bennett, S. Carcinoembryonic antigen in human ovarian neoplasms. *Cancer Res. 35:* 3807-3810, 1975.

50. Mariani-Costantini, R., Agresti, R., Andreola, S., Colnaghi, M. I., Ménard, S., and Rilke, F. Characterization of the specificity by immunohistology of a monoclonal antibody to a novel epithelial antigen of ovarian carcinomas. *Pathol. Res. Pract. 180:* 169–180, 1985.

51. Mariani-Costantini, R., Andreola, S., and Rilke, F. Tumour-associated antigens in mammary and extramammary Paget's disease. *Virchows Arch. (Pathol. Anat.) 405:* 333–340, 1985.

52. Mariani-Costantini, R., Barbanti, P., Colnaghi, M. I., Ménard, S., Clemente, C., and Rilke, F. Reactivity of a monoclonal antibody with tissues and tumors from the human breast. Immunohistochemical localization of a new antigen and clinicopathologic correlations. *Am. J. Pathol. 115:* 47–56, 1984.

53. Mariani-Costantini, R., Colnaghi, M. I., Leoni, F., Ménard, S., Cerasoli, S., and Rilke, F. Immunohistochemical reactivity of a monoclonal antibody prepared against human breast carcinoma. *Virchows Arch. (Pathol. Anat.) 402:* 389-404, 1984.

54. Mariani-Costantini, R., Ménard, S., Clemente, C., Tagliabue, E., Colnaghi, M. I., and Rilke, F. Immunocytochemical identification of breast carcinoma cells in effusions using a monoclonal antibody (letter). *J. Clin. Pathol. 35:* 1037, 1982.

55. McGee, J. O., Woods, J. C., Ashall, F., Bramwell, M. E., and Harris, H. A new marker for human cancer cells. 2. Immunohistochemical detection of the Ca antigen in human tissues with the Ca1 antibody. *Lancet 2:* 7-10, 1982.

56. Ménard, S., Rilke, F., Della Torre, G., Mariani-Costantini, R., Regazzoni, M., Tagliabue, E., Alasio, L., and Colnaghi, M. I. Sensitivity enhancement of the cytologic detection of cancer cells in effusions by monoclonal antibodies. *Am. J. Clin. Pathol. 83:* 571–576, 1985.

57. Ménard, S., Tagliabue, E., Canevari, S., Fossati, G., and Colnaghi, M. I. Generation of monoclonal antibodies reacting with normal and cancer cells of human breast. *Cancer Res. 43:* 1295-1300, 1983.

58. Mesa-Tejada, R., Keydar, I., Ramanarayanan, M., Ohno, T., Fenoglio, C., and Spiegelman, S. Detection in human breast carcinomas of an antigen immunologically related to a group specific antigen of mouse mammary tumor virus. *Proc. Natl. Acad. Sci. U.S.A. 75:* 1529-1533, 1978.

59. Nadji, M., Morales, A. R., Girtanner, R. E., Ziegels-Weissman, J., and Penneys, N. S. Paget's disease of the skin. A unifying concept of histogenesis. *Cancer 50:* 2203-2206, 1981.

60. Nigg, E. A., Walter, G., and Singer, S. J. On the nature of crossreactions observed with antibodies directed to defined epitopes. *Proc. Natl. Acad. Sci. U.S.A. 79:* 5939-5943, 1982.

61. Nuti, M., Teramoto, Y.A., Mariani-Costantini, R., Horan-Hand, P., Colcher, D., and Schlom, J. A monoclonal antibody (B.72.3) defines patterns of distribution of a novel tumor associated antigen in human mammary carcinoma cell populations. *Int. J. Cancer 29:* 539-545, 1982.

62. Pant, K. D., Dahlman, H. L., and Goldenberg, D. M. Further characterization of CSAp: An antigen associated with gastrointestinal and ovarian tumors. *Cancer 42:* 1626-1634, 1978.

63. Papsidero, L. D., Croghan, G. A., O'Connell, M. J., Valenzuela, L. A., Nemoto, T., and Chu, T. M. Monoclonal antibodies (F36/22 and M7/105) to human breast carcinoma. *Cancer Res. 43: 1741-1747, 1983).*

64. Raju, R. N., and Kardinal, C. G. Pleural effusion in breast carcinoma: Analysis of 122 cases. *Cancer 48:* 2524-2527, 1981.

65. Redding, W. H., Coombes, R. C., Monaghan, P., Clink, H. M., Imrif, S. F., Dearnaley, D. P., Ormerod, M. G., Sloane, J. P., Gazet, J. C., Powles, T. J., and Neville, A. M. Detection of micrometastases in patients with primary breast cancer. *Lancet 2:* 1271–1274, 1983.

66. Rilke, F. Influence of pathologic factors on management. In *Cancer Investigation and Management, Breast Cancer: Diagnosis and Management*, edited by G. Bonadonna, Vol. 1. Chichester, Sussex, England, John Wiley & Sons, 1984, pp. 35–62.

67. Rilke, F., Andreola, S., Carbone, A., Clemente, C., and Pilotti, S. The importance of pathology in prognosis and management of breast cancer. *Semin. Oncol. 5:* 360-372, 1978.

68. Roth, L. M., Lee, S. C., and Ehrlich, C. E. Paget's disease of the vulva. A histogenetic study of five cases including ultrastructural observations and review of the literature. *Am. J. Surg. 1:* 193-206, 1977.

69. Schlom, J., Wunderlich, D., and Teramoto, Y. A. Generation of human monoclonal antibodies reactive with human mammary carcinoma cells. *Proc. Natl. Acad. Sci. U.S.A. 77:* 6841-6845, 1980.

70. Simpson, H. W., Candlish, W., Liddle, C., McGregor, M., Mutch, F. and Tinkler, B. A critical investigation of the Oxford tumour marker Ca1 in the histological diagnosis of breast cancer and pre-cancer. *Histopathology 8:* 481-499, 1984.

71. Sloane, J. P., and Ormerod, M. G. Distribution of epithelial membrane antigen in normal and neoplastic tissues and its value in diagnostic tumor pathology. *Cancer 47:* 1786-1795, 1981.

72. Sloane, J. P., Ormerod, M. G., Imrie, S. F., and Coombes, R. C. The use of antisera to epithelial membrane antigen in detecting micrometastases in histological sections. *Br. J. Cancer 42:* 392–398, 1980.

73. Spiegelman, S., Keydar, I., Mesa-Tejada, R., Ohno, T., Ramanarayaran, M., Nayak, R., Bausch, J., and Fenoglio, C. Possible diagnostic implications of a mammary tumor virus-related protein in human breast cancer. *Cancer 46:* 879-892, 1980.

74. Stegner, H. E., Fischer, K., and Poschmann, A. Immunohistochemical localization of Thomsen-Friedenreich antigen in normal and malignant breast tissue using peroxidase-antiperoxidase technique. *Tumor Diagnostik 3:* 127-130, 1981.

75. Tagliabue, E., Ménard, S., Della Torre, G., Barbanti, P., Mariani-Costantini, R., Porro, G., and Colnaghi, M. I. Generation of monoclonal antibodies reacting with human epithelial ovarian cancer. *Cancer Res. 45:* 379–385, 1985.

76. Teramoto, Y. A., Mariani, R., Wunderlich, D., and Schlom, J. The immunohistochemical reactivity of a human monoclonal antibody with tissue sections of human mammary tumors. *Cancer 50:* 241-249, 1982.

77. Thompson, C. H., Jones, S. L., Whitehead, R. H., and McKenzie, I. F. C. A human breast tissue-associated antigen detected by a monoclonal antibody. *J. Natl. Cancer Inst. 70:* 409-419, 1983.

78. van Nagell, J. R., Donaldson, E. S., Gay, E. C., Sharkey, R. M., Rayburn, P., and Goldenberg, D. M. Carcinoembryonic antigen in ovarian epithelial cystadenocarcinomas. *Cancer 41:* 2335-2340, 1978.

79. Veronesi, U., Saccozzi, R., Del Vecchio, M., Banfi, A., Clemente, C., De Lena, M., Gallus, G., Greco, M., Luini, A., Marubini, E., Muscolino, G., Rilke, F., Salvadori, B., Zecchini, A.,

and Zucali, R. Comparing radical mastectomy with quadrantectomy, axillary dissection and radiotherapy in patients with small cancers of the breast. *N. Engl. J. Med. 305:* 6–11, 1981.

80. Whitaker, D., and Shilkin, K. B. Diagnosis of pleural malignant mesothelioma in life—A practical approach. *J. Pathol. 143:* 147-175, 1984.

81. Woods, J. C., Spriggs, A. I., Harris, H., and McGee, J. O. A new marker for human cancer cells. 3. Immunocytochemical detection of malignant cells in serous fluids with the Ca1 antibody. *Lancet 2:* 512-515, 1982.

82. Yuan, D., Hendler, F. J., and Vitetta, E. S. Characterization of a monoclonal antibody reactive with a subset of human breast tumors. *J. Natl. Cancer Inst. 68:* 719-728, 1982.

83. Zangerle, P. F., Collette, J., Hendrich, J. C., Miller, W. B., and Franchimont, P. Milk proteins and breast cancer. In *Markers for Diagnosis and Monitoring of Human Cancer. Proceedings of the Serono Symposia*, edited by M. I. Colnaghi, G. L. Buraggi, and M. Ghione, Vol. 46. London, Academic Press, 1982, pp. 35-49.

Chapter 11

Blood Group Antigens and Ploidy as Prognostic Factors in Urinary Bladder Carcinoma

RONALD S. WEINSTEIN, DANIEL SCHWARTZ, AND
JOHN S. COON

Transitional cell carcinoma arising in human urinary bladder is character-ized, in part, by the variability of its clinical course. Many patients initially present with low grade, low stage disease that is cured by simple resection at cystoscopy. Others present with lesions histologically identical to ones that never recur, but in the ensuing years have recurrences, often repeatedly, with some lesions progressing to invasiveness. Still others present for the first time with deeply invasive tumors but with a brief history of clinical symptoma-tology. The urologist is confronted with difficult decisions in the management of patients in all of these categories. Decisions must be made on the length of follow-up intervals and on the use of topical chemotherapy in patients with superficial lesions, fully recognizing that approximately half of new patients with this clinical presentation are cured by tumor ablation alone, without further intervention. The challenge to the urologist is to identify which half are at risk for recurrent disease. Difficult decisions must also be made for patients with deeply invasive disease since none of the currently available therapeutic options offers acceptable cure rates.

Challenges to the clinical investigator have included, first, identification of molecular markers which can predict tumor recurrences and future invasive-ness in patients presenting with superficial disease and, second, development of methods that can assist in the assessment of drug and/or radiosensivity of deeply invasive tumors. Although neither of these challenges has been fully met, progress has been made in identifying some characteristics of superficial bladder tumors that are potentially useful for discriminating between groups of patients with relatively good or poor prognoses.[40, 64, 65] This chapter will focus attention on several characteristics which fall under an umbrella called tumor markers.

CLASSIFICATION OF TUMOR MARKERS

Tumor markers fall into two broad categories: those that originate in the tumor and those which are produced by normal tissue in response to the

225

presence of the tumor. Examples of the former include oncogenes and tumor cell surface antigens, whereas examples of the later include acute phase proteins, fibrin degradation products, and rheumatoid factor. With respect to research on clinically useful tumor markers in urinary bladder transitional cell carcinoma, one line of promising work involves the characterization of blood group antigen-related substances which are expressed on normal urothelial cells[6] but are often modified on malignant cells from lesions known to have a high potential to become invasive.[7, 11, 34, 37] Also of special interest are studies on tumor cell ploidy and marker chromosomes, which appear to be of diagnostic and prognostic value.[14, 15, 47, 56, 57]

TISSUE BLOOD GROUP ANTIGENS (BGAg)

Many cell surface antigens are altered by malignant transformation, but the BGAg have received the lion's share of the attention in the urology literature to date. Early attention was focused primarily on the ABO(H) antigens,[11, 37, 54] whereas several recent studies have examined the T (Thomsen-Friedenreich) antigen, a relative of MN blood group sustances on erythrocytes.[8, 34] It should be noted at the outset that the term "blood group antigens" is somewhat of a misnomer since these antigens, first detected on red cells near the turn of the century, are present on normal plasma membranes of endothelial and epithelial cells in many organs.[63] With malignant transformation, altered expression of BGAg is manifested two different ways: (1) by the apparent loss of an antigen; and (2) by the emergence of antigens not normally detectable. Either of these alterations in antigen expression could be due to the incomplete synthesis of oligosaccharide chains by neoplastic cells[23] or the action of specific glycosidases or other unmasking enzymes.[34] Changes in the ABH system in transitional cell carcinomas are examples of antigen loss while the expression of the T antigen is an example of antigen emergence.

DETECTION OF BGAg

Several biochemical and immunohistochemical methods are used to measure BGAg expression on tumor cells. Each method has specific advantages and limitations. Immunoperoxidase and immunofluorescence techniques are generally the preferred methods for studying BGAg histologically (Fig. 1) and flow cytometrically[5, 10, 63] whereas other methods have advantages for certain applications. For instance, biochemical analysis of fresh tissue permits quantitation of blood group substances and precise delineation of their molecular structures. Biochemical analysis of glycosyltransferase activities in fresh tissue has also provided insights into the pathogenesis of some BGAg abnormalities.[23-25] The Specific Red Cell Adherence (SRCA) test of Davidsohn[30, 63] is an immunohistological method based on a mixed cell agglutination reaction between erythrocytes and fresh frozen or deparaffinized tissue sections.[30, 63] This is a three-layered mixed-cell agglutination assay, the top layer being homologous indicator red blood cells, the middle layer either antiserum to the A or B antigen or a lectin extracted from the plant *Ulex europaeus* which binds the H antigen, and the bottom layer the BGAg in the tissue. Many early studies on BGAg in transitional cell carcinoma employed the SRCA test, and a

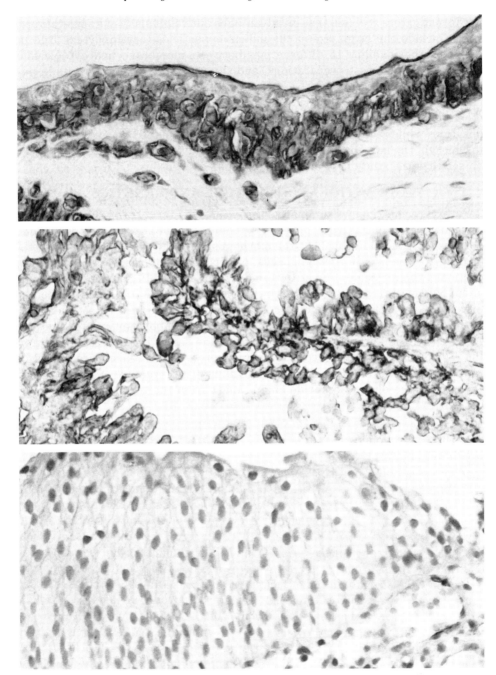

FIG. 11.1. (*Top*) Normal urothelium stained for H antigen by the immunoperoxidase method in a patient with blood group O. In this specimen, basal cells, intermediate cells, and lumenal membrane stain strongly, whereas lateral membranes of superficial cells stain weakly, if at all. Nuclear fast red counterstain. Original magnification, × 500. (*Center*) Immunoperoxidase demonstration of strong H antigen expression in cell membranes of a low-grade human bladder transitional cell carcinoma. Nuclear fast red counterstain. Original magnification, × 500. (*Bottom*) Low grade transitional cell carcinoma of the urinary bladder stained for the T (Thomsen-Friedenreich) antigen by the immunoperoxidase method. Tumor, blood vessels, and stromal elements are T antigen negative. Nuclear fast red counterstain. Original magnification, × 500.

predictive values of positive and negative ABH test results, calculated from data in the literature. The cited studies vary considerably with respect to patient population, length of follow-up, methodology for measuring ABH antigens, tumor grade, and other factors. The results show that ABH testing is highly predictive of a low risk for invasion in patients with a negative ABH test (*i.e.*, ABH antigen is expressed in the tumor) and is somewhat less predictive of subsequent invasion in patients with a positive ABH test.

While these results seem promising, there is a consensus among workers in the field that it is premature to use ABH testing for making therapeutic decisions.[7, 27, 32, 33, 36] Several factors have produced a healthy level of skepticism over the value of ABH testing in the clinical setting. One factor is the heterogeneity of antigen expression in tumors, which complicates the interpretation of test results.[7, 63] Secondly, there are many exceptions to the generalization that antigen expression correlates with future biological aggressiveness (Tables 11.1 and 11.2).[37] A third consideration is the reasonably strong correlation between histologic tumor grade and ABH expression.[32, 37] It remains to be shown in a double-blind prospective study that ABH antigen expression correlates better with tumor invasion than does tumor grade alone.

ABH BLOOD GROUP PRECURSOR SUBSTANCES

Since the blood group-related antigens are synthesized by stepwise elongation of oligosaccharide chains, expression of individual precursor structures

TABLE 11.1 PREDICTIVE VALUES FOR TISSUE ABH TEST

Series	No. of Patients	Predictive Values	
		Negative Test Result (%)	Positive Test Result (%)
DeCenzo *et al.*, 1975	22	100[b]	89[c]
Bergman and Javadpour, 1978	14	100	27
Jakse and Hufstader, 1978	31	100	69
Emmott *et al.*, 1979	26	83	40
Limas *et al.*, 1979	172	85	70
Young *et al.*, 1979	23	89	93
Richie *et al.*, 1980	16	100	71
Johnson and Lamm, 1980	30	100	60
Newman *et al., 1980*	*322*	*96*	*72*
Coon et al., 1982	72	95	38
D'Elia *et al.*, 1982	40	84	73
Limas and Lange, 1982	110	84	63
Wiley *et al.*, 1982	34	100	50
Summers *et al.*, 1983	39	89	52
Total	519 Avg.	93	62

[a]Predictive values, calculated from data reported in the literature. Predictive value is defined as:

$$\text{Predictive value} = \frac{\text{true positives}}{\text{true positives} + \text{false positives}}.$$

[b]Percentage of low stage bladder carcinoma patient with negative ABH test results (*i.e.*, antigen is present) who *did not* develop subsequent invasive carcinoma.

[c]Percentage of low stage bladder carcinoma patients with positive ABH test results (*ie.e.*, antigen is absent) who *did* develop subsequent invasive carcinoma.

TABLE 11.2. RELATIONS OF FOUR MARKERS TO EACH OTHER AND TO CLINICAL COURSE IN PATIENTS WITH BLADDER CANCER[a]

		ABH Ag Present?		TAg Status		
		Yes	No	CrT+	T+	CrT−
Ploidy	< 46	8(0)[b]	4(0)	10(0)	2(0)	0
	46	5(0)	3(0)	5(0)	3(0)	0
	> 46	5(0)	14(11)	5(0)	11(10)	3(3)
Marker	No	9(0)	5(0)	12(0)	2(0)	0
Chromosome	Yes	9(2)	16(11)	8(0)	14(10)	3(3)
ABH Ag	Yes			13(0)	4(1)	1(1)
Present?	No			7(0)	12(9)	2(2)

[a]Adapted from Summers, J. L., et al.[56] and *Cancer Research*.
[b]No. in parentheses refers to no. of patients who developed deep invasion.

may be either increased or decreased in carcinomas, depending upon the point at which oligosaccharide elongation is arrested. We have investigated the prognostic significance of expression of precursor specificities in transitional cell carcinoma of urinary bladder using monoclonal antibodies raised to purified precursor glycolipids by Dr. S.I. Hakomori in Seattle.[38] The immediate precursor of the H antigen, *N*-acetyllactosamine (lactNAc), has been demonstrated in various normal epithelia but is frequently deleted in carcinomas. The prognostic significance of lactNAc expression in transitional cell carcinoma of the urinary bladder was investigated by immunoperoxidase staining of paraffin sections, using a monoclonal antibody to lactNAc. Staining was performed on 38 initial biopsies of Grade I or Grade II, Stage O or Stage A bladder carcinomas with follow-up of over 3 years. All controls expressed lactNAc throughout the entire urothelial width. Twenty-six tumors were lactNAc negative. No patient who had a lactNAc-containing tumor had an invasive recurrence. In the group lacking lactNAc antigen expression, 42% progressed to invasion. Thus, the invasive potential of tumors lacking the immediate precursor of the H antigen appears to be approximately the same as that of tumors that fail to bind *Ulex europeus*, the H antigen specific lectin.

Several other precursor structures to the ABH antigens, including the I and i antigens[18, 20, 42] and other carbohydrate antigens,[39, 48, 67] are of potential value in the evaluation of transitional cell carcinomas.[39, 48, 67]

MN BLOOD GROUP ANTIGEN-RELATED STRUCTURES

Additional BGAg have been examined to determine whether prognostic accuracy might be increased by using batteries of markers.[56, 65] The M, N, T (Thomsen-Friedenreich), and Tn antigens are regarded as a family because they are structurally related[7, 50] These structures and their interrelationships are summarized in Figure 11.3. The T and Tn antigens are cryptic antigens, masked by terminal sugar residues in many normal tissues, including urinary bladder epithelium.[8, 51] Expression of the M and N antigens requires linkage of appropriate oligosaccharide side chains to a specific sequence of *N*-terminal amino acids, as illustrated in Figure 11.3.[2, 46] Neuraminidase treatment of nor-

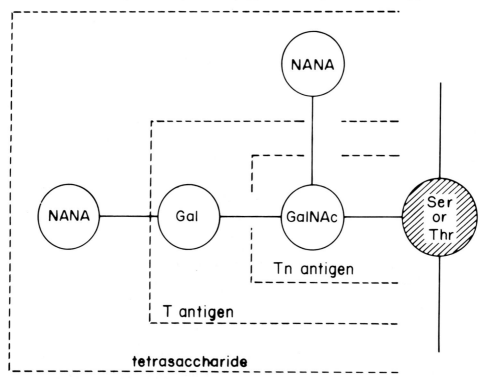

Fɪɢ. 11.3. Diagrammatic representation of probable structures corresponding to different T antigen reactivities of bladder carcinomas. *NANA*, sialic acid; *Gal*, ᴅ-galactose; *GalNAc*, *N*-actyl-ᴅ-galactosamine; *Ser*, serine; *Thr*, threonine.

mal tissue bearing M and N antigens removes terminal sialyl residues, allowing expression of cryptic T antigen. Springer and his co-workers[49-51] developed the concept that the T antigen is expressed on many human carcinoma cells but is masked by sialic acid on homologous normal epithelium.[49-51] Using biochemical methods, Springer [51] found that nearly all breast carcinomas and gastrointestinal carcinomas express the T antigen.

We recently developed immunohistochemical methods that localize T antigen at the cellular level, using a T-specific lectin, peanut (*Arachis hypogaea*) agglutinin (PNA). PNA has a specificity for the disaccharide β-ᴅ-Gal-(1,3)-ᴅ-GalNAc and also reacts with terminal nonreducing ᴅ-Gal but at 1/50th the affinity. The immunoperoxidase methods have been utilized to examine the relationship of T antigen expression to the biological behavior of urinary bladder transitional cell carcinoma.[8] Based on staining with PNA, with or without neuraminidase pretreatment of tissue sections, urinary bladder transitional cell carcinomas have been subclassified into three categories on the basis of differential expression of the T antigen: (1) cryptic T antigen positive (CrT+, Table 11.2), as in normal urothelium; (2) T antigen positive (T+), as in normal urothelium following neuraminidase pretreatment; and (3) T antigen negative both with and without neuraminidase pretreatment, so-called cryptic T antigen negative (CrT −).[8] Clinically useful data has been obtained using immunoperoxidase methods to demonstrate T antigen in bladder tumors.[8,56] In contrast, results obtained thus far with an SRCA test for the T antigen are disappointing.[58]

Several relationships have been established among the features of morphology, T antigen status, and clinical behavior of transitional cell carcinoma. There is a positive correlation in immunoperoxidase studies between tumor grade and T antigen expression. The majority of low grade tumors are CrT + . High grade tumors are generally T + or CrT − , implying defective or incomplete expression of the normal tissue MN-related antigens.[8] T antigen measurements are potentially of greatest value in the evaluation of patients with low stage disease whose tumors are ABH antigen negative. The predictive value of ABH testing in these patients is relatively low compared with the predictive value in patients who express the ABH antigen in their initial lesions (Table 11.1). In an attempt to improve the predictive values, T antigen expression was measured in 32 patients with ABH deletion in their initial lesions. Of those with normal T expression, that is the CrT + phenotype, 17% eventually developed invasive carcinoma. Patients with abnormalities in both ABH and T antigen expression (T + and CrT −) developed invasive carcinoma in 64% of cases.[8]

SURFACE MARKERS IN CARCINOMA *IN SITU*

The relationship of carcinoma *in situ* in urinary bladder to tumorigenesis and prognosis is uncertain but is a topic of great practical importance to urologists (Fig. 11.4).[4,16,17,61,66] Expression of BGAg and related substances by carcinoma *in situ* is of interest for several reasons. First, these markers may help in elucidating the natural history of premalignant bladder lesions.[62] Second, they may aid in identifying the biological equivalent of low grade carcinoma *in situ*, a diagnosis that is difficult to make by conventional histopathology.[62] Third, they may help in identifying early malignancy by cytology. Generally, the characteristic cells of frank carcinoma *in situ* have abnormalities in both ABH and T antigens.[13,40,62] This is expected since tumor cells in Grade III

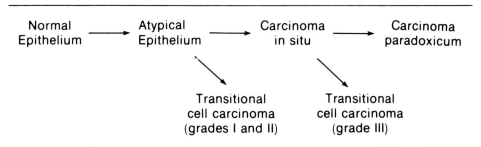

FIG. 11.4. Conceptualization of the origin of low- and high-grade transitional cell carcinoma. It has been proposed that classical carcinoma *in situ* may evolve into either relatively high-grade invasive carcinoma or, in some instances, into a biologically innocuous tumor, for which the term "Carcinoma paradoxicum" has been coined.[66] Lower grade transitional cell carcinomas may arise from so-called atypical epithelium.

transitional cell carcinomas, the morphologically analogous cells to those in classical carcinoma *in situ*, often show abnormal BGAg expression.[8, 37] What is interesting is that areas of atypia and even some areas of normal appearing epithelium in patients with extensive classical carcinoma *in situ* elsewhere in the urinary bladder show ABH[62] and T antigen abnormalities.[3a] Based on these findings, it has been suggested that such areas may represent the elusive precursor lesions of Grade I and Grade II transitional cell carcinoma (Fig. 11.4).[4, 62, 66]

PATHOGENESIS OF ABNORMAL BGAg EXPRESSION

Four theories have been proposed to account for the abnormalities of BGAg expression in tumors:

1. Tumors have abnormalities in specific glycosyltransferases, blocking the incorporation of sugar residues at or near the nonreducing terminus of oligosaccharide chains.[29, 55]
2. Tumors are unable to synthesize certain classes of glycoconjugates because of an inability to form the necessary precursor substances, *e.g.*, glycoproteins and/or glycolipids.[31, 44]
3. Tumors or tumor stroma have highly active glycosidases or proteases acting at the tumor cell surface, causing abnormal degradation of cell surface glyconjugates.[19, 41, 46]
4. Tumors have abnormal terminal glycosylation of oligosaccharide chains, masking normal antigenic determinants.[25, 34]

Data supporting each of these theories have been summarized elsewhere.[7] Suffice it to say that both the disappearance of normal antigens, such as the ABH antigens, and the expression of additional antigens, such as the T and Tn antigens, could be accounted for by the same mechanism.

HETEROGENEITY OF ANTIGEN EXPRESSION IN TUMORS

The concept of heterogeneity of tumor subpopulations is having a major impact on research in basic and clinical oncology. Heterogeneity of BGAg expression is a characteristic of many bladder tumors.[7] The variability in staining patterns that is observed from area to area complicates the interpretation of BGAg test results in many cases and has restricted the clinical usefulness of BGAg measurements. We have observed that in some tumors, BGAg staining is predominantly along the basal cell layer, in some others along the lumenal membrane, whereas in still others the antigen is expressed in all layers, similar to normal urothelium. In some tumors, BGAg are detectable only in sharply circumscribed geographic areas within the tumor or in isolated clusters of tumor cells. It is unknown whether staining heterogeneity is dependent upon clonal diversity within the tumors, cell cycle-dependent fluctuations intensified by variable growth conditions in different areas of the tumor, or other undefined factors.

Since the immunohistological study of solid tumors does not allow dissection of the factors responsible for heterogeneity of BGAg expression, we have studied the expression of these antigens in human urinary bladder carcinoma cell lines by multiparameter flow cytometry and cell sorting. We studied the expression of the A, H, and T antigens in three hyperdiploid bladder transitional cell carcinoma cell lines (647V, Hu456, and HT 1376) using fluoresce-inated blood group antigen-specific lectins (*Dolichos bifloris, Ulex europaeus,* and *Arachis hypogaea*). Cell cycle compartments were quantitated by flow cytometry using propidium iodide staining. Some heterogeneity appeared to be nonheritable and cell cycle-dependent, based upon two-dimensional surface antigen/DNA analysis and the observation of rapid reversion of strongly staining and weakly staining cells in culture to the original phenotype. For example, 90% of Hu 456 cells show strong expression of the H antigen in a Gaussian distribution and have a DNA histogram typical of exponentially growing cells. Surprisingly, the 10% of Hu 456 cells with an intensity of antigen expression at the nonexpression end of the curve (defined as dim) are all in the G_1/G_0 cell cycle compartment. These studies show that H antigen expression is maintained through mitosis. In contrast, expression of the T antigen by 647V cells does not appear to be related to the cell cycle. However, 647V cells sorted by T antigen expression have shown some persistent, heritable antigenic differences after several passages *in vitro*. Resorting the sorted subpopulations after expansion *in vitro* or cloning of sorted dim cells has produced stable subpopulations with antigen expression which is even more different than that of the parental populations. Nevertheless, a substantial portion of the variability of T antigen expression in 647V bladder cancer cells is not heritable, since sorted subpopulations revert toward the parental phenotype after only a few generations in culture, before stabilizing with an intermediate profile after sorting. Since antigen expression by 647V cells does not appear to fluctuate with the cell cycle, the parameters responsible for this nonheritable shift in BGAg expression remain to be defined.[4a]

These findings may help explain some of the observations made in immunohistological studies of BGAg in human bladder carcinomas. The frequent variation of antigen expression among clusters of cells in adjacent areas of the same tumor, and the common staining stratification from basal to superficial cells, could be due to transient variations in antigen expression. Our cytometric data suggest that these transient variations may be only partially attributable to the cell cycle. Empirical immunohistologic observations suggest that focal transient losses of BGAg expression within some tumors are not strongly related to tumor invasion and metastasis in many cases since, generally, it is the tumors with nearly complete antigen loss that have poorer prognoses. It is noteworthy that bladder transitional cell carcinomas with relatively uniformly strong BGAg expression occasionally do behave aggressively. BGAg-negative, aggressive clones which later overgrow other subpopulations or disseminate may dominate the clinical course in such cases. Reversion to normal BGAg expression following dissemination may explain the normal BGAg expression observed in some metastatic lesions. The switching mechanisms for BGAg expression in carcinomas need to be elucidated and could be a fertile area for future investigations.

MARKER CHROMOSOMES AND TUMOR PLOIDY

Cytogenetic studies have demonstrated a strong association between the presence of hyperdiploidy and marker chromosomes in urinary bladder carcinoma cells and a high incidence of tumor recurrences and invasion.[14, 15, 47, 56, 57]

As with other tumor markers, such as the surface antigens, a negative test result (*e.g.*, diploidy, absence of a marker chromosome) is more accurate in predicting which patients will *not* develop subsequent invasion than is a positive test result (*e.g.*, aneuploidy, presence of marker chromosomes) in predicting later invasion. In a comparative study on four markers, ABH antigens, T antigen, marker chromosomes, and ploidy, we found hyperdiploidy to be the best single predictor of recurrences and invasion.[56] The combination of modal chromosome number and T-antigen status was accurate in predicting clinical outcome in 95% of cases for a relatively small series of patients with long-term follow-up (Table 11.2).

Until recently, nuclear DNA content analyses were impractical as routine clinical tests in bladder cancer specimens because of technical difficulties in obtaining suitable karyotypes of many solid tumors and the availability of such testing in a relatively small number of medical centers. Ploidy status and DNA content are of greater significance than specific marker chromosomal abnormalities as prognostic factors[22, 56] and the recent introduction of a method to do flow cytometry on tumor nuclei retrieved from paraffin-embedded tissues[26] should make it feasible to perform nuclear analyses in reference laboratories for purposes of more precisely establishing bladder carcinoma prognosis and for therapeutic monitoring. Furthermore, virtually all tumor specimens are suitable for flow cytometric analysis, whereas conventional cytogenetic analysis has been successful on only a fraction of bladder tumors.[3, 47] Currently, we are routinely obtaining satisfactory DNA histograms from paraffin-embedded bladder carcinoma biopsy specimens (Fig. 11.5) following the method of Hedley *et al.*[26] In brief, 30-μm sections from paraffin blocks are dewaxed, rehydrated, and then mechanically minced with a scissors. The tissue slurry is then digested with 0.5% pepsin in 0.9% NaCl at pH 1.5 for 30 minutes, liberating cell nuclei (Fig. 11.6). The nuclear suspension is then neutralized with buffer, treated with RNAse, and stained with propidium iodide.[59] Stained nuclei are analyzed in a clinical flow cytometer. This method can facilitate the analysis of DNA content in large retrospective series of tumor cases, as well as permit analysis of DNA content in biopsies which are too small to divide for special studies at the time of surgery.

CLINICAL PERSPECTIVES

Until recently, the natural history of urinary bladder carcinoma was pictured as a slow steady progression of carcinoma *in situ* and low grade, low stage tumors to higher grade tumors with deep invasion. This concept was drastically modified several years ago when it was recognized that the majority of patients who will ever have muscle invasion by transitional cell carcinoma present initially with muscle invasion.[9, 28] We suspect that this important cohort of patients has an explosively rapid clinical course. Paradoxically, while superficial urinary bladder carcinoma is the most common form of transitional cell carcinoma in the United States, patients with a history of superficial bladder tumors account for a minority of all deaths from transitional cell carcinoma in this country. It follows that the greatest reduction in overall mortality from transitional cell carcinoma would come from earlier detection of cancer in

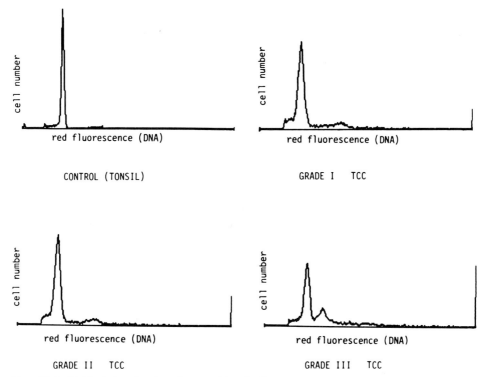

FIG. 11.5. Ploidy determinations for transitional cell carcinomas (*TCC*) and human tonsil made on nuclear suspensions, harvested from paraffin-embedded tissue blocks, by flow cytometry. Tonsil serves as a control and shows a single narrow diploid peak. Grade I and Grade II *TCC*s show a diploid peak, a small tetraploid peak, and a broad distribution of intermediate DNA values compatible with cycling euploid cells. Grade III *TCC* shows a diploid peak plus a second large aneuploid peak (DNA index *1:37*). The diploid peak probably represents stromal or inflammatory cells, whereas the aneuploid peak corresponds to high grade tumor cells.

those patients who currently present with muscle invasion. The markers under consideration in this paper may have little value in this regard unless urinary cytology screening can be made cost effective.

There are several clinical settings in which BGAg and ploidy studies are of potential value although, at the present time, they do not seem to provide clinically useful information in many individual cases beyond that obtainable by more readily available diagnostic procedures, including careful determination of tumor grade and stage, and cytology. In general, patients with solitary low grade transitional cell carcinomas having normal surface antigens and euploidy rarely progress to muscle invasion and can be followed conservatively. Those with abnormal BGAg expression and hyperdiploidy are at a much higher risk to develop invasion and should be followed more energetically. The patients in whom BGAg and ploidy testing are of the greatest potential value are those with Grade II and Grade III, low stage tumors.[21] These are the patients in whom abnormal antigen expression and hyperdiploidy may warrant aggressive monitoring for tumor progression. There are also several clinical settings in which BGAg testing may have little or no practical value. ABH antigen is

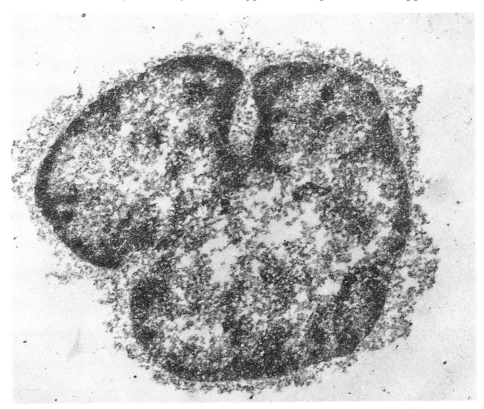

Fɪɢ. 11.6. Thin section electron micrograph of a transitional cell carcinoma cell nucleus re-trieved from a paraffin section by the method of Hedley *et al.*[26] Much of the cytoplasm has been stripped from the nucleus by the procedure, leaving residual polyribosomes which are subse-quently removed by RNAse digestion prior to flow cytometry. Original magnification, × 20,000.

typically expressed by both superficial and deeply invasive squamous cell carci-nomas, with or without concurrent schistosomiasis, negating the usefulness of ABH testing in this particular group of patients.[12, 35] Therapy may also affect BGAg test results and obscure their interpretation[1, 54] but the extent to which this occurs in unclear.[45, 53] BGAg testing is not helpful in evaluating the invasive potential of classical carcinoma *in situ* since BGAg abnormalities are almost invariably present in such lesions, regardless of the occurrence of tumor pro-gression.[13, 62] Ploidy studies on paraffin-embedded carcinoma *in situ* are tech-nically difficult because of the low cell content of these often denuded biopsies. However, there is circumstantial evidence that marker studies may be of value in establishing the diagnosis of low grade carcinoma *in situ*.[13]

ACKNOWLEDGMENTS

Supported in part by NIH-NCI Grants CA-34074 and CA-36641, and by funds from the Otho A. Sprague Memorial Institute.

REFERENCES

1. Alroy, J., Teramura, K., Miller, A. W., III, Pauli, B. U., Gottesman, J. E., Flanagan, M., Davidsohn, I., and Weinstein, R. S. Isoantigens A, B and H in urinary bladder carcinomas following radiotherapy. *Cancer 41:* 1739–1745, 1978.

2. Anstee, D. The blood group MNSs-active sialoglycoproteins. *Semin. Hematol. 18:* 13–31, 1981.

3. Collste, L. G., Darzynkiewicz, Z., Traganos, F., Sharpless, T. K., Sogani, P., Grabstald, H., Whitmore, W. F., Jr., and Melamed, M. R. Flow cytometry in bladder cancer detection and evaluation using acridine orange metachromatic nucleic acid staining of irrigation cytology specimens. *J. Urol. 12:* 478–485, 1980.

3a. Coon, J. S., McCall, A., Miller, A. W., III, Farrow, G. M., and Weinstein, R. S. Expression of blood group-related antigens in carcinoma *in situ* of the urinary bladder. *Cancer 56:* 797–804, 1985.

4. Coon, J. S., Pauli, B. U., and Weinstein, R. S. Precancer of the urinary bladder. *Cancer Surv. 2:* 479–494, 1983.

4a. Coon, J. S., Watkins, J. R., Pauli, B. U., and Weinstein, R. S. Flow cytometric analysis of heterogeneity in blood group-related antigen expression in a human urinary bladder carcinoma cell line, 647V. *Cancer Res. 45:* 3014–3071, 1985.

5. Coon, J. S., and Weinstein, R. S. Detection of ABH tisssue isoantigens by immunoperoxidase methods in normal and neoplastic urothelium. Comparison with the erythrocyte adherence method. *Am. J. Clin. Pathol. 76:* 163–171, 1981.

6. Coon, J. S., and Weinstein, R. S. Variability in the expression of the O(H) antigen in human transitional epithelium. *J. Urol. 125:* 301–306, 1981.

7. Coon, J. S., and Weinstein, R. S. Blood group antigens in tumor cell membranes. In *Biomembranes*, Vol. II., edited by L. Manson and A. Nowotny. New York, Plenum, 1983, pp. 173–205.

8. Coon, J. S., Weinstein, R. S., and Summers, J. Blood group precursor T antigen expression in human urinary bladder carcinoma. *Am. J. Clin. Pathol. 77:* 692–699, 1982.

9. Cutler, S. J., Heney, N. M., and Friedell, G. H. Longitudinal study patients with bladder cancer: Factors associated with disease recurrence and progression. In *Bladder Cancer, AUA Monographs*, edited by W. W. Bonney and G. R. Prout, Jr. Baltimore, Williams & Wilkins, 1982, pp. 35–46.

10. Dabelsteen, E. Quantitative determination of blood group substance A of oral epithelial cells by immunofluorescence and immunoperoxidase methods. *Acta Pathol. Microbiol. Scand. Section (A) 80:* 847–853, 1972.

11. DeCenzo, J. M., Howard, P., and Irish, C. E. Antigenic deletion and prognosis of patients with stage A transitional cell bladder carcinoma. *J. Urol. 114:* 874–878, 1975.

12. El Adl, M. M., Yamase, H. T., Nieh, P. T., Mostofa, A-S., Hinz, C. F., and Walzak, M. P. ABH cell surface isoantigens in invasive bladder carcinoma associated with schistosomiasis. *J. Urol. 131:* 249–251, 1984.

13. Emmott, R. C., Droller, M. J., and Javadpour, N. Studies of A, B or O(H) surface antigen specificity: Carcinoma *in situ* and non-malignant lesions of the bladder. *J. Urol. 125:* 32–35, 1981.

14. Falor, W., and Ward, R. M. DNA banding patterns in carcinoma of the bladder. *J.A.M.A. 226:* 1322–1327, 1973.

15. Falor, W., and Ward, R. M. Prognosis in early carcinoma of the bladder based on chromosomal analysis. *J. Urol. 119:* 44–48, 1978.

16. Farrow, G. M., Utz, D. C., and Rife, C. C. Morphological and clinical observations of patients with early bladder cancer treated with total cystectomy. *Cancer Res. 36:* 2495–2501, 1976.

17. Farrow, G. M., Utz, D. C., Rife, C. C., and Greene, L. F. Clinical observations on sixty-nine cases of *in situ* carcinoma of the urinary bladder. *Cancer Res. 37:* 2784–2798, 1977.

18. Feizi, T., Tuberville, C., and Westwood, J. Blood-group precursors and cancer-related antigens. *Lancet 2:* 391–393, 1975.

19. Fukuda, M. N., Fukuda, M., and Hakomori, S. Cell surface modification by endogalactosidase. Changes of blood group activities and release of oligosaccharides from glycoproteins and glycosphingolipids of human erythrocytes. *J. Biol. Chem. 254:* 5458–5465, 1979.

20. Fukuda, M., Fukuda, M. N., and Hakomori, S. Developmental change and genetic defect in the carbohydrate structure of band 3 glycoprotein of human erythrocyte membrane. *J. Biol. Chem. 254:* 3700–3703, 1979.

21. Giraldo, A. A., Ruby, S. G., and Humes, J. J. Blood group antigens in urothelium in transitional cell carcinoma. *Ann. Clin. Lab. Sci. 13:* 307–314, 1983.

22. Gustafson, H., Tribukait, B., and Esposti, P. L. DNA pattern, histological grade and multiplicity related to recurrence rate in superficial bladder tumours. *Scand J. Urol. Nephrol. 16:* 135–139, 1982.

23. Hakomori, S. Structures and organization of cell surface glycolipids. Dependency on cell growth and malignant transformation. *Biochim. Biophys. Acta 417:* 55–89, 1975.

24. Hakomori, S. Blood group ABH and Ii antigens of human erythrocytes: Chemistry, polymorphism, and their developmental change. *Semin. Hematol. 18:* 39–62, 1981.

25. Hakomori, S. Tumor associated carbohydrate antigens. *Ann. Rev. Immunol. 2:* 102–126, 1984.

26. Hedley, D. W., Friedlander, M. L., Taylor, I. W., Rugg, C. A., and Musgrove, E. A. Method for analysis of cellular DNA content of paraffin-embedded pathological material using flow cytometry. *J. Histochem. Cytochem. 31:* 1333–1335, 1983.

27. Javadpour, N. Tumor markers in urologic cancer. In *Principles and Management of Urologic Cancer,* edited by N. Javadpour. New York, Williams & Wilkins, 1983, p. 32.

28. Kaye, K. W., and Lange, P. H. Mode of presentation of invasive bladder cancer: Reassessment of the problem. *J. Urol. 128:* 31–33, 1982.

29. Kim, Y. S., Isaacs, R., and Perdomo, J. M. Alterations of membrane glycoproteins in human colonic adenocarcinoma. *Proc. Natl. Acad. Sci. USA 71:* 4869–4873, 1974.

30. Kovarik, S., Davidsohn, I., and Stejskal, R. ABO antigens in cancer. Detection with the mixed cell agglutination reaction. *Arch. Pathol. 86:* 12–21, 1968.

31. Krag, S. S. A concanavalin A-resistant Chinese hamster ovary cell line is deficient in the synthesis of (^{3}H) glucosyl oligosaccharide lipid. *J. Biol. Chem. 254:* 9167–9177, 1979.

32. Lange, P. H., and Limas, C. Molecular markers in the diagnosis and prognosis of bladder cancer. *Urology 23*(Suppl.): 46–54, 1984.

33. Limas, C., Coon, J. S., Lange, P., and Weinstein, R. S. ABH antigens in urinary bladder carcinomas: Detection and clinical applications. In *Bladder Cancer, AUA Monograph,* edited by W. Bonney and G. R. Prout. New York, Williams & Wilkins, 1982, pp. 69–79.

34. Limas, C., and Lange, P. Altered reactivity for A, B, and H antigens in transitional cell carcinomas of the urinary bladder: A study of the mechanisms involved. *Cancer 46:* 1366–1373, 1980.

35. Limas, C., and Lange, P. H. Prognostic significance of altered A, B, and H reactivity in transitional cell carcinoma of the urinary bladder. *Dev. Cancer Res. 2:* 133–138, 1980.

36. Limas, C., and Lange, P. H. Tissue blood-group-associated antigens in urothelial neoplasia: Theory and clinical application. *World Urol. Update Ser. 1:* 2–17, 1982.

37. Limas, C., Lange, P., Fraley, E. E., and Vesella, R. L. A, B, and H antigens in transitional cell tumors of the urinary bladder: Correlation with clinical course. *Cancer 44:* 2099–2107, 1979.

38. Luginbuehl, M., Coon, J. S., and Pauli, B. U. H blood group precursor *N*-acetyllactosamine expression in human urinary bladder carcinoma. *Fed. Proc. 43:* 602a, 1984.

39. Nakatsu, H., Kobayashi, I., Onishi, Y., Igawa, M., Ito, H., Tahara, E., and Nihira, H. ABO(H) blood group antigens and carcinoembryonic antigens as indicators of malignant potential in patients with transitional cell carcinoma of the bladder. *J. Urol. 131:* 252–257, 1984.

40. Pauli, B. U., Alroy, J., and Weinstein, R. S. Pathobiology of urinary bladder cancer. In *The Pathology of Bladder Cancer,* Vol. 2, edited by S. Cohen and G. T. Bryan. Boca Raton, FL, CRC Press, 1983, pp. 41–140.

41. Pauli, B., Anderson, S., Memoli, V., and Kuettner, K. Development of an *in vitro* and *in vivo* epithelial tumor model for study of invasion. *Cancer Res. 40:* 4571–4576, 1980.

42. Picard, J., Edward, D., and Feizi, T. Changes in the expression of the blood group A, B, H, Le[a] and Le[b] antigens and the blood group precursor associated I (MA) antigen in glycoprotein-rich extracts of gastric carcinomas. *J. Clin. Lab. Immunol. 1:* 119–128, 1978.

43. Rauvala, H., and Finne, J. Structural similarity of the terminal carbohydrate sequences of glycoproteins and glycolipids. *FEBS Lett. 97:* 1–8, 1979.

44. Reitman, M. L., Trowbridge, I. S., and Kornfeld, S. Mouse lymphoma cell lines resistant to pea lectin are defective in fucose metabolism. *J. Biol. Chem. 255:* 9900–9906, 1980.
45. Richie, J. P., and Yap, W. T. Further observations on the specific red cell adherence test: Effects of radiation therapy. *J. Urol. 125:* 493–495, 1981.
46. Rolih, S. Erythrocyte antigens of the MN system and related structures. In *A Seminar on Antigens on Blood Cells and Body Fluids,* chap. 8, edited by C. Bell, Washington, D.C., American Association of Blood Banks, 1980.
47. Sandberg, A. Chromosomes in bladder cancer. In *Bladder Cancer, AUA Monograph,* edited by W. Bonney and G. Prout. Baltimore, Williams & Wilkins, 1982, pp. 81–94.
48. Simmons, D. A. R., and Perlmann, P. Carcinoembryonic antigen and blood group substances. *Cancer Res. 33:* 313–322, 1973.
49. Springer, G. F., and Desai, P. R. Cross-reacting carcinoma-associated antigens with blood group and precursor specificities. *Transplant. Proc. 9:* 1105–1111, 1977.
50. Springer, G. F., Desai, P. R., Murthy, M. S., Yang, H. J., and Scanlon, E. F. Precursors of the blood group NM antigens as human carcinoma associated antigens. *Transfusion 19:* 233–249, 1979.
51. Springer, G. F., Desai, P. R., Yang, H. J., and Murthy, M. S. Carcinoma-associated blood group MN precursor antigens against which all humans possess antibodies. *Clin. Immunol. Immunopathol. 7:* 426–441, 1977.
52. Srinivas, V., and Kiruluta, H. G. ABO(H) isoantigens in bladder tumors: A new technique of quantitative analysis. *J. Urol. 131:* 245–248, 1984.
53. Stein, B. S., and Kendall, A. R. Blood group antigens and bladder carcinoma: A perspective. *Urology 20:* 229–233, 1982.
54. Stein, B. S., Reyes, J. M., Peterson, R. O., McNellis, D., and Kendall, A. R. Specific red cell adherence: Immunologic evaluation of random mucosal biopsies in carcinoma of the bladder. *J. Urol. 126:* 37–40, 1981.
55. Stellner, K., Hakomori, S., and Warner, G. A. Enzymic conversion of "H_1-glycolipid" to A- or B-glycolipid and deficiency of these enzyme activities in adenocarcinoma. *Biochem. Biophys. Res. Commun. 55:* 439–445, 1973.
56. Summers, J. L., Coon, J. S., Ward, R. M., Falor, W. H., Miller, A. W., III, and Weinstein, R. S. Prognosis in carcinoma of the urinary bladder based upon tissue ABH and T antigen status and karyotype of the initial tumor. *Cancer Res. 43:* 934–939, 1983.
57. Summers, J. L., Falor, W. H., and Ward, R. A 10-year analysis of chromosomes in non-invasive papillary carcinoma of the bladder. *J. Urol. 125:* 177–178, 1981.
58. Vafier, J. A., Javadpour, N., Worsham, G. F., and O'Connell, K. J. Double blind comparison of T-antigen and ABO(H) cell surface antigens in bladder cancer. *Urology 23:* 348–351, 1984.
59. Vindelov, L., Christensen, I., and Nissen, N. A detergent-trypsin method for the preparation of nuclei for flow cytometric DNA analysis. *Cytometry 3:* 323–327, 1983.
60. Watkins, W. M. Genetics and biochemistry of some human blood groups. *Proc. R. Soc. Lond. 202:* 31–53, 1978.
61. Weinstein, R. S. The origin and dissemination of human urinary bladder carcinoma. *Semin. Oncol. 6:* 149–156, 1979.
62. Weinstein, R. S., Alroy, J., Farrow, G. M., Miller, A. W., III, and Davidsohn, I. Blood group isoantigen deletion in carcinoma *in situ* of the urinary bladder. *Cancer 43:* 661–668, 1979.
63. Weinstein, R. S., Coon, J. S., Alroy, J., and Davidsohn, I. Tissue-associated blood group antigens in human tumors. In *Diagnostic Immunohistochemistry,* edited by R. D. DeLellis, New York, Masson, 1981, pp. 239–261.
64. Weinstein, R. S., Coon, J. S., and Pauli, B. U. Characterization of urinary bladder cancer cells. In *Bladder Cancer,* edited by P. H. Smith and G. R. Prout, Jr. Kent, England, Buttersworth, 1984, pp. 12–31.
65. Weinstein, R. S., Miller, A. W., III, and Coon, J. S. Tissue blood group ABH and Thomsen-Friedenreich antigens in human urinary bladder carcinoma. *Prog. Clin. Biol. Res. 153:* 249–260, 1984.
66. Weinstein, R. S., Miller, A. W., III, and Pauli, B. U. Carcinoma *in situ:* Pathobiology of a paradox. *Urol. Clin. North Am. 7:* 525–531, 1980.
67. Wiley, E. L., Mendelsohn, G., Droller, M. J., and Eggleston, J. S. Immunoperoxidase detection of carcinoembryonic antigen and blood group substances in papillary transitional cell carcinoma of the bladder. *J. Urol. 128:* 276–280, 1982.

Chapter 12

Antigenic Markers of Neuroendocrine Tumors:
Their Diagnostic and Prognostic Value

ENRICO SOLCIA, CARLO CAPELLA, ROBERTO BUFFA, PATRIZIA
TENTI, GUIDO RINDI, AND MATTEO CORNAGGIA

The term "neuroendocrine" tumor, in a restricted and more appropriate sense, should be used only to designate tumors like pheochromocytomas and paragangliomas characterized by: (1) known neuroectodermal origin of the tumor cells; and (2) the production of monoamines and/or peptides normally found in nerve cells or endocrine cells or both, thus called neuroendocrine mediators or regulators. However, recently there is a tendency to utilize only the second requisite, and the word neuroendocrine has been used to designate a very wide spectrum of tumors. This includes epithelial endocrine tumors of whatever origin (mostly nonneuroectodermal), neuronal tumors, and related poorly differentiated tumors (i.e., small cell carcinomas, neuroblastomas), if evidence is provided showing the production of (a) neuroendocrine regulatory substances or (b) products (like hormone precursors and carriers) co-secreted with these substances or even (c) related enzymes (as cholinesterases and neuron specific enolase). Both *general markers*, useful for the recognition of the neuroendocrine nature of tumor cells, and *special markers*, useful for the diagnosis of an exact tumor cell type, will be discussed in this chapter.

GENERAL MARKERS OF NEUROENDOCRINE TUMORS

Among possible *enzymatic markers* of neuroendocrine tumors, neuron-specific enolase (NSE) seems to be the only one of practical importance.[56] The immunohistochemical detection of NSE may be especially important for the diagnosis of poorly differentiated tumors as small cell or intermediate cell carcinomas and neuroblastomas, whose scarce content of neurosecretory products may be quite difficult to detect. NSE may also be useful for the recognition of differentiated neuroendocrine tumors whose secretory products remain unknown as, for instance, Merkel cell tumors of the skin.[12]

Tetanus toxin receptor and a related ganglioside antigen A2B5 have been detected on the surface of several neuroendocrine cells and their neoplastic derivatives, including insulinomas, pheochromocytomas, thyroid medullary carcinomas, and neuroblastomas.[21] However, the usefulness of these surface antigens as diagnostic markers of neuroendocrine tumors has not yet been assessed.

The detection of *secretory granules* and *secretory products* remains the more useful way to prove the neuroendocrine nature of a tumor displaying a histologic pattern (solid, trabecular, insular, microlobular, diffuse) suggestive of the diagnoses. Secretory product identification also allows one to distinguish endocrine from nonendocrine tumors showing a similar histological pattern ("solid" carcinomas of the gastrointestinal tract), or to recognize the endocrine nature of tumors lacking a typical neuroendocrine structure (*e.g.*, some gastrinomas and nonargentaffin carcinoids with pseudoglandular structure).

Secretory granules with distinctive ultrastructural features may be identified utilizing electron microscopy. For the histological detection of secretory granules a battery of simple "granule stains" is available. Among these the silver impregnation techniques, especially the Grimelius stain,[31] lead hematoxylin, and "masked (metachromatic) basophilia,[53] are considered the most practical. Although not all neuroendocrine cells and related granules react with Grimelius' silver (Table 12.1), this method is widely used in tumor diagnosis because it is a simple, highly reproducible technique with specificity for endocrine granules (Fig. 12.1). No direct relationship exists between Grimelius reactivity and specific neuroendocrine mediators; a relationship with nonhormonal components of secretory granules, especially with acidic sialoglycoproteins, has been shown.[6, 48] Grimelius-reactive glycoproteins seem to be involved in the intragranular binding of monoamines, either endogenously derived or resulting from the amine precursors uptake and decarboxylation reaction.[48] Recently, chromogranins, a family of acidic sialoglycoproteins,[26] was proposed as the substrate of Grimelius silver.[5, 40]

Chromogranins were first isolated and characterized from adrenal medullary cell granules[47] and sympathetic nerve vesicles.[19] They have been shown to be closely related to the parathyroid secretory protein I or SP-1[13] that is stored in parathyroid secretory granules.[44] Chromogranins are nonhormone components of neuroendocrine granules that probably play a role in hormone storage and release.[13] Polyclonal antibodies directed against bovine chromogranin A and monoclonal antibodies against human chromogranin A have been found to react with secretory granules of a number of endocrine cells and related tumors.[41, 43, 59] Using both polyclonal antibovine chromogranin A antibody (from Prof. H. Winkler[36, 39]) and monoclonal antihuman chromogranin A (from Prof. R. V. Lloyd,[41]) we have confirmed these results and shown a close parallelism between chromogranin A immunoreactivity and a positive Grimelius' silver reaction in normal and neoplastic neuroendocrine cells (Table 12.1 and Figs. 12.2–12.4). Minor discrepancies between the two techniques may be accounted for by their different sensitivity to fixation and embedding procedures. Moreover, the Grimelius reactivity of chromogranins has been directly proven in formaldehyde-fixed model spots.[5] Thus far no chromogranin immunoreactivity has been found in nonneuroendocrine argyrophil cells and related tumors, including most argyrophilic breast carcinomas.

TABLE 12.1. GRIMELIUS STAINING AND CHROMOGRANIN IMMUNOREACTIVITY OF NEUROENDOCRINE TUMORS[a]

Type of Tumor	Grimelius	Chromogranin A[b]
Pheochromocytoma	11/11	3/3
Sympathetic paraganglioma	2/2	2/2
Carotid body paraganglioma	14/14	3/3
Glomus jugulare paraganglioma	12/12	1/1
Thyroid medullary carcinoma	23/23	3/3
Merkel cell tumor	12.19	2/3
Pituitary adenomas		
GH cell	31/88[c]	1/3
PRL cell	14/113[c]	0/3[c]
ACTH cell	3/25[c]	0/5
TSH cell	4/4	2/2
Gonadotrope cell	7/7	2/2
α-chain cell	7/7	2/2
SAG cell	27/27	2/2
Parathyroid adenoma	20/20	3/3
Thymus carcinoid	2/2	1/1
Larynx carcinoid	2/2	1/1
Lung		
Tumorlets	1/1	1/1
Argyrophil carcinoids	35/36	3/3
EC cell carcinoid	1/1	1/1
Neuroendocrine carcinomas		
Moderately differentiated	3/3	1/1
Undifferentiated small and/or intermediate cell	5/20	NT
Pancreatic endocrine tumors		
A cell	5/5	2/2
B cell	4/15	0/2
D cell	1/1[c]	NT
PP cell	2/2	2/2
Gastrinoma	33/36	3/3
Vipoma	13/18	2/2
Gastrointestinal tract		
EC cell carcinoid	22/22	3/3
Gastric ECL cell carcinoid	6/6	3/3
Gastrin cell tumor	12/13	2/2
Rectal L cell carcinoid	10/11	0/3
Non-argentaffin carcinoids, cytologically uncharacterized	4/5	1/1
Liver:PP cell tumor	1/1	1/1
Ovary		
EC cell carcinoid	2/2	1/1
Prostate: endocrine part of mixed carcinoid/carcinoma	2/2	2/2
Breast: argyrophil carcinoma	4/4	0/4

[a] Based on a number of reactive cases/number of cases tested.

[b] LK2H10 monoclonal antibody[41] applied to Grimelius-reactive cases.

[c] Minor cell population.

[d] NT, not tested.

Chromogranin antibodies and, although less conclusive, Grimelius stain are especially useful for the light microscopic diagnosis of neuroendocrine tumors of unknown hormonal product (*e.g.*, gastric argyrophil ECL cell carcinoids, cutaneous Merkel cell tumors, and many nonargentaffin carcinoids from various tissues). These granule-related markers are also useful as a first step in

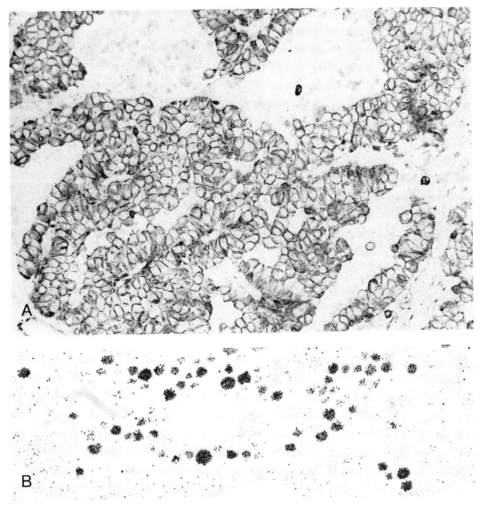

FIG. 12.1. Nonfunctioning pituitary adenoma lacking GH, PRL, ACTH, TSH, beta-FSH, beta-LH, and alpha-chain immunoreactivity, while showing diffuse chromogranin immunoreactivity. (A) Cytoplasmic argyrophilia of tumor cell cords. Paraffin section, Grimelius silver, original magnification, × 120. (B) Electron microscopy of the same tumor showing small (around 120 nm) argyrophil granules (SAG). Aldehyde fixation, Grimelius silver "en block," resin section, original magnification, × 28,000.

the analyses of the neuroendocrine nature of any tumor to be further characterized by specific antihormonal sera and/or ultrastructural investigations.

SPECIFIC NEUROHORMONAL MARKERS

In both normal and neoplastic tissues, neuroendocrine cell typing is based mainly on the identification of specialized hormonal or modulatory substances produced and stored by the cell. This "functional" or, more correctly, "product" characterization of the cells is the most distinctive and reliable criterion for tumor characterization. Besides providing an exact cell identification, it also permits precise correlation with clinical hyperfunctional syndromes and, to some extent, it allows one to predict the natural history of the tumor. However,

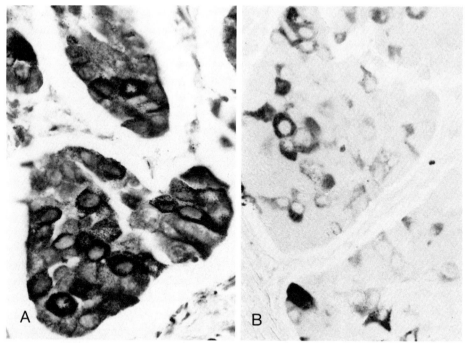

FIG. 12.2. (*A*) Nonfunctioning thymic carcinoid showing argyrophil cells (*A*, Grimelius silver, original magnification, × 400) also reacting with chromogranin A monoclonal antibody LK2H10 (*B*, immunoperoxidase; original magnification, × 400).

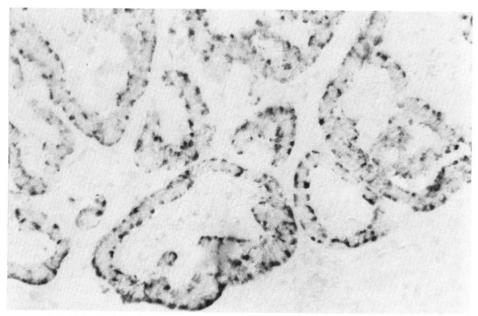

FIG. 12.3. Pyloric endocrine tumor, 10 mm in size, positive with Grimelius silver, lead-hematoxylin, and anti-gastrin (C-terminal) serum (G cell tumor), in a patient also showing gastrin cell hyperplasia in the pyloric mucosa and chronic atrophic gastritis with microcarcinoidosis in the remaining stomach. Tumor cell cords, somewhat mimicking pseudoglandular patterns, react with chromogranin antibody LK2H10. Immunoperoxidase, original magnification, × 200.

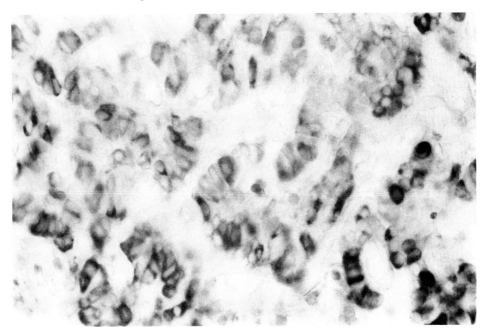

FIG. 12.4. Bronchial nonfunctioning argyrophilic carcinoid showing chromogranin A immunoreactivity. Immunoperoxidase, original magnification, × 400.

it should be noted that in some instances the same substance is produced by entirely different tumors, with different origins, cytology, evolution, and prognosis. This is illustrated by the dual nature of vasoactive intestinal peptide (VIP)-producing tumors, which may be either pancreatic epithelial endocrine tumors or retroperitoneal ganglioneuromas and ganglioneuroblastomas.[9] Thus, parallel histopathologic and ultrastructural investigations are needed to establish correct diagnosis. Ultrastructural immunocytochemistry, by combining the ultrastructural characterization of tumor cells and the immunochemical identification of their neuroendocrine products, may be quite helpful in tumor diagnosis (Fig. 12.5).

The coexistence of multiple endocrine cell types in an endocrine tumor or even of different hormonal products inside the same tumor cell[7, 18, 23, 38] may make it difficult to classify neuroendocrine tumors on purely cytologic grounds. However, most difficulties are overcome when both the cytologic and clinical findings are taken into consideration. This is especially true when one identifies the clinically functional syndrome, even in those patients who have immunocytochemically heterogeneous tumors.[50]

PANCREAS

Four endocrine cell types are universally recognized in the human pancreas: glucagon A, insulin B, somatostatin D, and pancreatic polypeptide PP cells. Cells of unknown function containing very small, round, haloed granules (P cells) and rare 5-hydroxytryptamine-producing enterochromaffin (EC) cells have been also identified.[11, 25] Tumors related to cells comprising the normal

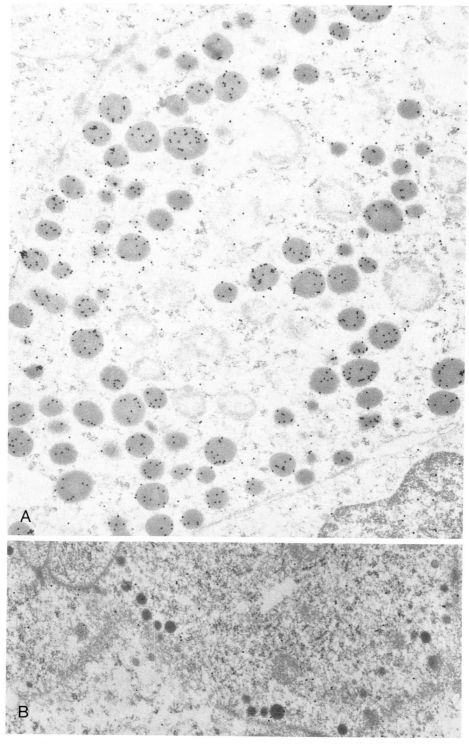

Fig. 12.5. Pituitary tumor associated with acromegaly and increased blood GH levels. Alde-hyde-fixed resin section stained with anti-GH serum followed by gold-labeled protein A. Note immunoreactive, large GH cell granules (A, original magnification, × 28,000) and unreactive small granules in a SAG cell found in the same section of the same tumor (B, original magnification, × 28,000).

endocrine pancreas are called "islet cell tumors," while hormones unrelated to these cells are considered "inappropriate."

The classification of pancreatic endocrine tumors in Table 12.2 is based on extensive immunohistochemical, ultrastructural, and clinicopathologic correlations.[4, 11, 14, 33]

Unexpected, clinically silent islet cell tumors (Table 12.2, Group A1), usually of small size, are found not infrequently in autopsy or surgical material. A, PP, and D cells are often detected in these tumors, most of which are to be interpreted as harmless adenomas.[3, 32, 45] Eighty-five percent of pancreatic endocrine tumors associated with the insulinoma syndrome (insulinomas) have been shown to be benign,[54] and most are now diagnosed when rather small, usually less than 2 cm. Tumors associated with either the glucagonoma or the somatostatinoma syndrome are generally much larger. For 32 patients with glucagonomas reported in the literature, the mean size is 7.4 cm.[45] In these tumors it is likely that a larger tumor mass or a longer history is required for development of the clinically hyperfunctional syndrome. This may artificially select for faster-growing tumors, thus explaining their higher malignancy rate (62%).[45] Similarly, the higher incidence of malignancy (around 50%) among nonfunctioning tumors which produce local symptoms (Table 12.2, Group A5) may be related to their larger size.[33] Tumors with cells producing inappropriate hormones such as gastrin, VIP (Fig. 12.6), ACTH, PTH, or calcitonin are usually malignant if associated with a clinically hyperfunctional syndrome.[49, 50] There is no proof that the detection of inappropriate markers in nonfunctional tumors increases their malignancy rate. However, simple immunohistochemical reactivity for the alpha-chain of human chorionic gonadotropin (α-HCG) and pituitary glycoprotein hormones (Fig. 12.7) might represent a marker of malignancy for all types of pancreatic endocrine tumors.[33]

TABLE 12.2. PANCREATIC ENDOCRINE TUMORS

A)	Islet cell tumors	
	1) Clinically silent A, B, D, PP, EC, and P cell tumors	Mostly adenomas
	2) Insulinoma: B cells with or without other islet cells	
	3) Glucagonoma: A cells with or without other islet cells	
	4) Somatostatinoma: D cells with or without other islet cells	Mainly low grade carcinomas
	Non-functioning A, B, D, EC, and P cell tumors with local symptoms	
B)	Inappropriate tumors	
	1) Gastrinoma: gastrin cells with or without other cells	
	2) Vipoma: VIP cells with or without other cells	Mostly low grade carcinomas
	3) Other functioning tumors with inappropriate (ACTH, ADH, calcitonin, neurotensin, PTH, GRF, *etc.*) syndromes and cells, with or without islet cells.	
C)	Poorly differentiated carcinomas	High malignant

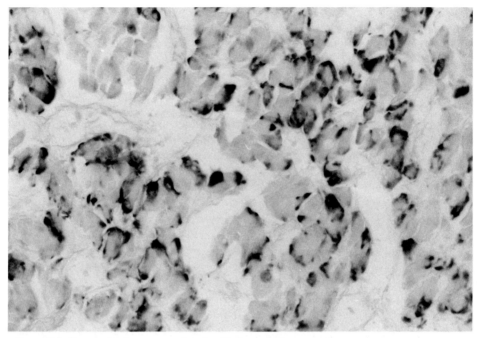

Fig. 12.6. Pancreatic tumor associated with increased serum VIP levels and diarrheogenic syndrome. Many tumor cells react with anti-VIP serum. Immunoperoxidase, original magnification, × 300. Other cells (not shown) also reacted with PP and neurotensin antisera.

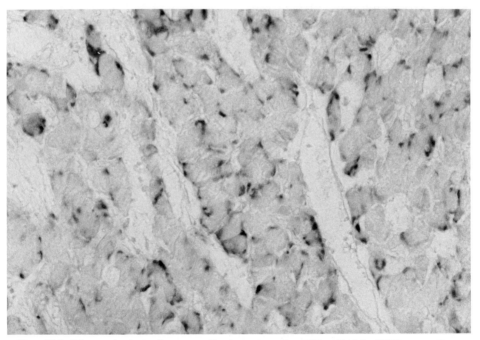

Fig. 12.7. Liver metastasis of a pancreatic vipoma reacting with anti-alpha HCG serum. Immunoperoxidase, original magnification, × 150.

Gastrointestinal Tract

The present status of cytologic studies on gut endocrine tumors is outlined in Table 12.3. Some group A tumors may develop hyperfunctional syndromes, as in the "carcinoid" syndrome associated with EC cells tumors ("argentaffinic carcinoids"), or the gastrinoma syndrome. Like islet cell tumors, gut tumors developing a hyperfunctional syndrome are much more frequently malignant than their nonfunctional counterpart. Practically all argentaffinic carcinoids with the carcinoid syndrome (mostly from distal small bowel) are malignant, while the majority of those lacking the syndrome, including nearly all EC cell tumors from the appendix, are benign.[28] Moreover, clinically silent, apparently benign gastrin cell tumors are not infrequently found in the duodenum,[2] while 38% of duodenal tumors associated with the gastrinoma syndrome are malignant (Fig. 12.8).[35] Nonfunctioning somatostatin cell tumors may also arise in the duodenum.[37] L cells producing enteroglucagon (glicentin) and PP-related sequences occur in rectal endocrine tumors more frequently than any other endocrine cell type, including somatostatin, EC, and enkephalin-containing cells.[1, 24, 42] PP-related antigens of tumor L cells include sequences normally expressed in phylogenetically related pancreatic PP cells rather than in colorectal L cells.[50]

Some ultrastructurally characterized cells with unknown function are present in the gut. These include ECL, D_1, P, and X cells of the gastric mucosa.[51] Tumors related to these cells fit into Group B of Table 12.3 and lack immunohistochemical reactivity for known peptides and amines, although they have Grimelius-positive and chromogranin-reactive granules. Several such tumors have been characterized ultrastructurally and histopathologically.[10, 35]

Unfortunately, large numbers of nonargentaffinic endocrine tumors are still diagnosed by chance in routine material, in the absence of any special immunohistochemical or ultrastructural information. For these Group C tumors the traditional term "nonargentaffinic carcinoid" is retained.

Inappropriate endocrine tumors containing cells immunoreactive for ACTH,[34] parathyroid hormone, calcitonin,[16] VIP,[9] insulin,[1] and alpha-HCG immunoreactive cells[52] occur in the gut much less frequently than in the pan-

---

TABLE 12.3. Gut Neuroendocrine Tumors

A) *Cytologically and functionally defined tumors*
   EC cell carcinoids
   1. 5-HT + substance P
   2. 5-HT
      gastrin cell tumor (gastrinoma)
      D cell tumor (somatostatinoma)
      L cell tumor (enteroglucagonoma)
B) Cytologically defined tumors
   ECL cell tumor (stomach)
   D_1/P cell tumor (stomach, duodenum)
   Paraganglioma (duodenum)
C) Cytologically undefined tumors
   (non-argentaffin carcinoids)
D) Inappropriate tumors (ACTH, insulin, VIP, etc.)
E) Poorly differentiated endocrine carcinomas

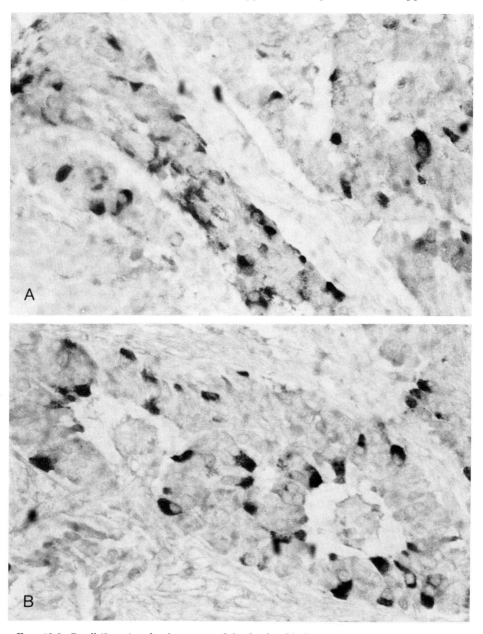

Fig. 12.8. Small (3-mm) endocrine tumor of the duodenal bulb associated with gastric hyperse-cretion and duodenal ulcer. Many tumor cells react with antigastrin serum (A); other cells react with antisomatostatin serum (B). Considering the associated clinicopathologic findings, the diagnosis of gastrinoma was made. Immunoperoxidase, original magnification, × 300.

creas. Unlike the case in pancreatic tumors, alpha-HCG immunoreactivity does not seem to represent a marker for malignancy in gastrointestinal endocrine tumors.[40]

LUNG

A classification of lung endocrine tumors based on cytologic and clinico-pathologic criteria is reported in Table 12.4.

Tumorlets are composed of small, round- to spindle-shaped cells which, ultrastructurally, show very small P-type granules with an argyrophilic core and, histochemically, display diffuse bombesin/gastrin-releasing peptide (BN/GRP) immunoreactivity, variable calcitonin, and scanty 5-HT or ACTH immunoreactivity.[15, 50, 57] Most tumorlets represent unexpected surgical or autopsy findings of no clinical relevance, occurring mainly in elderly patients.

BN/GRP immunoreactive cells have been detected in some bronchial carcinoids.[30, 55, 57] Scattered 5-HT immunoreactive cells have also been observed in some cases.[30, 50] It must be noted that 5-HT or 5-HTP is stored in normal human P cells[58] and that among 5-HT immunoreactive cells of lung carcinoids, 5-HT storing P cells must be distinguished by electron microscopy from EC cells which occur much less frequently in these tumors.[50] Coexistent substance P immunoreactivity may suggest or confirm the presence of EC cells. Of interest is that about half of the bronchial carcinoids associated with the "carcinoid" syndrome are associated with metastases[22] while less than 20% of the tumors unassociated with the syndrome proved to be malignant.[28] Calcitonin, leu-enkephalin, alpha-HCG, somatostatin, ACTH and VIP immunoreactive cells have been also detected in a few cases.[30, 57]

Small cell and intermediate cell *neuroendocrine carcinomas* of high grade malignancy with a scarce and variable content of neuroendocrine substances are known to arise frequently in the lung; their prognosis and behavior do not substantially differ from those of small/intermediate cell carcinomas lacking signs of endocrine differentiation. Poorly differentiated neuroendocrine carcinomas are rarely associated with overt hyperfunctional syndromes. These tu-

TABLE 12.4. NEUROENDOCRINE TUMORS OF THE LUNG

Tumors	Cell Types and Neurohormones	Prognosis
Paraganglioma	Type I cells; enkephalin?	Mostly benign
Tumorlets	P cells with BN/GRP, with/without 5-HT, calcitonin, or ACTH	Benign
Carcinoids	P cells with/without BN/GRP, 5-HT, calcitonin, enkephalin, GRF, *etc.* EC cells with 5-HT ± substance P ACTH cells, somatostatin cells, *etc.*	a) Without syndrome: more than 80% benign b) With syndrome ("carcinoid," Cushing, *etc.*): mainly malignant, low grade
Endocrine carcinomas A) Moderately differentiated B) Poorly differentiated	Mostly P-like cells or granules with/without BN/GRP, ACTH, CRF, ADH, calcitonin, *etc.*	Malignant, intermediate grade Malignant, high grade

mors are distinguishable from moderately differentiated endocrine tumors with less atypia, lower mitotic rates, and better survival.[30] The amount of neuroendocrine products found in the tumor cells or blood, and the frequency of associated endocrine syndromes, although quite variable, are somewhat higher in moderately differentiated carcinomas.

PITUITARY ADENOMAS

Endocrine tumors of the pituitary are characterized by well-differentiated morphologic patterns, lack of inappropriate secretions, and exceptionally low malignancy rate. Cytologic characterization, primarily based on the immuno-histochemical and ultrastructural identification of stored secretory products, is essential for clinicopathologic correlation, including comparison with hyperfunctional syndromes or blood hormone levels and choice of appropriate therapy and postoperative blood hormone monitoring.[23] Table 12.5 shows a hormone-based classification of a series of 307 pituitary tumors we investigated in the last 12 years. Collectively, tumors producing prolactin (PRL), GH (Fig. 12.9), or both hormones (219 cases) accounted for 71% of the tumors, and all were associated with the pertinent endocrine syndrome. Six of the 26 ACTH-secreting tumors were endocrinally nonfunctioning and two developed after bilateral adrenalectomy for Cushing syndrome (Nelson syndrome).

The majority of the remaining tumors were nonfunctioning and, apart from a few cases showing TSH (4), FSH (5), or FSH + LH (2), produced no known

TABLE 12.5. CLASSIFICATION OF 307 CASES OF PITUITARY ENDOCRINE TUMORS

Tumor Type		No. of Cases	%	Mean Age	♂	♀	♂/♀	Main Clinicopathologic Findings
PRL		113	36.8	34.9	29	84	1/2.9	Severe hyperprolactinemia: ♀; amenorrhea ± galactorrhea; impotence; intra or extrasellar
GH		88	28.6	42.9	39	49	1/1.25	Acromegaly, giantism; large intrasellar
GH + PRL		18	5.8	42.5	6	12	1/2	Acromegaly; large intrasellar
ACTH		26	8.4	42.6	3	23	1/7.6	
	a)	18			2	16		Cushing syndrome; microadenomas
	b)	2	(1 malignant)			2		Nelson syndrome; extrasellar
	c)	6			1	5		Nonfunctioning; extrasellar
TSH		4	1.3	51	4	0	4/0	1: Hyperthyroidism; intrasellar
								2: Mild hypothyroidism; extrasellar
								1: Euthyroidism; extrasellar
Gonadotroph		7	2.3	47.7	3	4	1/2.3	Gonadic hypofunction or dysfunction; extrasellar
χ-chain		24	7.8	53.2	13	11	1.1/1	Nonfunctioning; extrasellar
SAG		27	8.8	47.8	17	10	1.7/1	Nonfunctioning; extrasellar

[a]Based on 306 adenomas and 1 carcinoma: 144♂ and 193♀ .

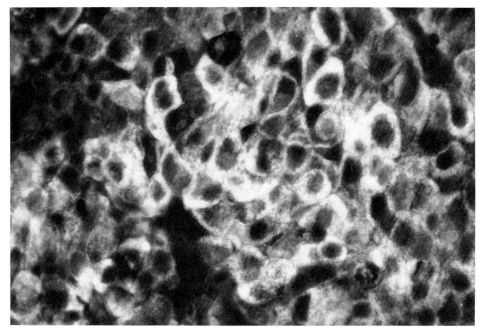

FIG. 12.9. GH immunoreactive cells in a pituitary adenoma associated with acromegaly. Immunofluorescence, original magnification, × 720.

active hormones, although 24 of them (7.8%) reacted with antisera directed against the common, hormonally inactive alpha-chain of pituitary glycoprotein hormones (Figs. 12.10 and 12.11). No reactivity with antisera (National Pituitary Agency) directed against the specific B chain or the whole molecule of the same hormones was demonstrated in these 24 tumors. It seems very likely that alpha-chain cells, like those of human fetal pituitary,[20] represent precursor cells to mature, hormonally active gonadotroph and TSH cells, whose granules are also Grimelius and chromogranin-reactive. Twenty-seven cases (8.8%) lacked any hormone-related immunoreactivity, but showed chromogranin immunoreactive small argyrophil (Grimelius-reactive) granules (SAG), ultrastructurally resembling those of alpha-chain tumors. Most SAG cells should represent precursor cells of the whole glycoprotein hormone cell line, with active (Grimelius-reactive) chromogranin synthesis anticipating that of hormone-related molecules. The close histological, ultrastructural, and clinicopathologic resemblance of SAG and alpha-chain tumors as well as the coexistence of both SAG and alpha-chain cells in alpha-chain tumors support this interpretation.[8] Moreover, pituitary tumors with gonadotroph and TSH cells also showed SAG cells, with or without alpha-chain cells. Together, SAG and alpha-chain tumors represent 17.6% of all pituitary endocrine tumors and compensate for the rarity of mature glycoprotein hormone-producing tumors.

   In general, tumors associated with prominent hyperfunctional syndromes are diagnosed earlier in their natural history while still intrasellar and often small in size, while "nonfunctioning" tumors lacking hyperfunctional syndrome, are diagnosed later, and are more than 1 cm in size (large intrasellar) or

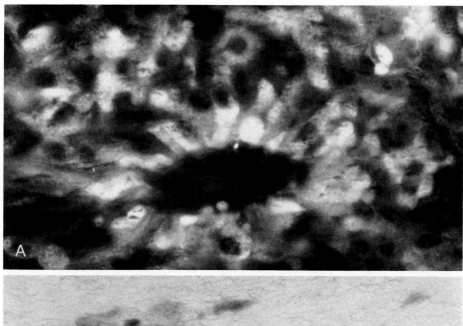

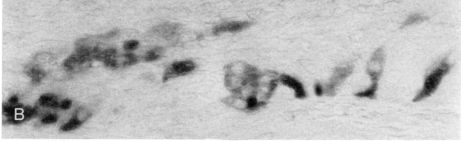

Fig. 12.10. Beta-TSH immunoreactive cells (*A*, immunofluorescence, original magnification, × 720) in an argyrophil, pituitary adenoma also showing chromogranin A immunoreactivity (*B*, immunoperoxidase, original magnification, × 500).

extend into the suprasellar space (extrasellar). In the case of GH and PRL cell tumors, further tumor growth may occur during periods of medical therapy interposed between diagnosis and surgery.

CONCLUSIONS

From the above data it is apparent that a precise identification of tumor cell types and secretory products is essential for the appropriate diagnosis of neuroendocrine tumors. Prognostic evaluation and management require careful comparison of cytologic patterns with blood hormone assays and clinical findings. Generally, well-differentiated tumors characterized by a relative abundance of secretory granules and neuroendocrine products are either benign or of low grade malignancy. Using conventional histologic and cytologic criteria, it is difficult to predict tumor behavior. Mitoses, cellular atypia, and invasive growth are often lacking even in the presence of documented metastases. Evaluating the neuroendocrine differentiation using immunocytochemical analysis may be of help.

In more than 50% of the cases, tumors producing "inappropriate" material

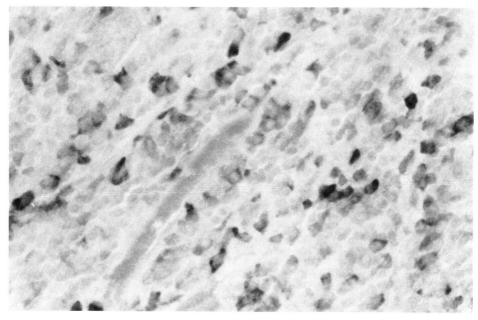

FIG. 12.11. Alpha-HCG-immunoreactive cells in an argyrophil, chromogranin-positive pituitary adenoma lacking beta-HCG, beta-FSH, beta-LH, beta-TSH, ACTH, GH, and PRL immuno-reactivity. Immunoperoxidase, original magnification, × 400.

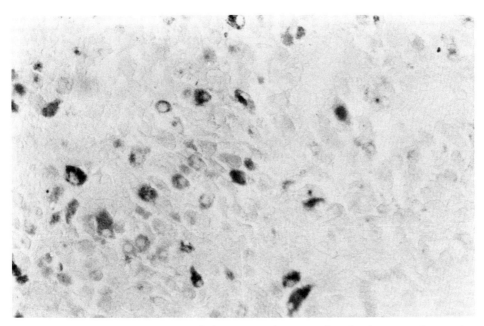

FIG. 12.12. CEA-immunoreactive cells in a metastatic pancreatic endocrine tumor also reacting to Grimelius silver and chromogranin A monoclonal antibody KL2H10. Immunoperoxidase, original magnification, × 300.

proved malignant (*e.g.*, pancreatic gastrinomas and vipomas, extrapituitary tumors producing "ectopic" pituitary hormones, and calcitonin or PTH-producing tumors outside thyroid or parathyroid glands). The malignancy rate is particularly high when neuroendocrine tumors arise in tissues that normally contain no or only scattered neuroendocrine cells (*e.g.*, upper respiratory and digestive tracts, liver, biliary tree, thymus, uterus, bladder, and kidney), and/ or when an overt hyperfunctional syndrome is associated with tumor growth.[50] Inappropriate peptides have also been detected in nontumorous growths (*e.g.*, ACTH in neuroendocrine hyperplasias of the lung[57] or alpha-HCG in hyperplastic gastric mucosa[52]). The oncologic potential of these growths, if any, remains to be determined.

Most well-differentiated tumors producing ectopic hormones behave in a benign fashion, including islet cell tumors, pituitary tumors, parathyroid tumors, pheochromocytomas, paragangliomas, and carcinoids. These tumors are especially benign when nonfunctioning and of small size. Clinically silent, small tumors composed of well-differentiated, appropriate endocrine cells are a relatively frequent finding in autopsy, surgical, or biopsy specimens from the pancreas, gut, or pituitary and, as a rule, are benign. Exceptions to this are thyroid medullary carcinoma and Merkel cell tumors. It must be noted that medullary carcinomas are something more than a simple calcitonin-producing tumor. Somatostatin, 5-HT, substance P, BN/GRP, ACTH, ACTH-releasing factor (CRF), GH-releasing factor (GRF), VIP, neurotensin, alpha-chain of HCG, nerve growth factor (NGF), carcinoembryonic antigen (CEA), histaminase, and kallikrein are all "inappropriate" substances found in these tumors.[7, 17, 18, 39, 46]

Although Merkel cell tumors closely resemble normal human Merkel cells,[27] the exact neuroendocrine substances produced by Merkel cells are still unknown. Thus, we have no possibility of ascertaining the appropriate nature of tumor cell products, although some cases producing inappropriate neuroendocrine substances like calcitonin, somatostatin, or ACTH have been reported.[29]

REFERENCES

1. Alumets, J., Alm, P., Falkmer, S., Håkanson, R., Ljungberg, O., Mårtensson, H., Sundler, F., and Tibblin, S. Immunohistochemical evidence of peptide hormones in endocrine tumours of the rectum. *Cancer 48:* 2409–2415, 1981.
2. Berger, G., Patricot, L. M., Guillaud, M. T., Buerlet, J., Frappart, L., and Vauzelle, J. L. Les gastrinomes silencieux pyloro-duodénaux. A propos de trois observations. *Ann. Anat. Pathol (Paris) 22:* 5–20, 1977.
3. Bordi, C., Ravazzola, M., Baetens, D., Gorden, P., Unger, R. H., and Orci, L. A study of glucagonomas by light and electron microscopy and immunofluorescence. *Diabetes 28:* 925–936, 1979.
4. Bordi, C., and Tardini, A. Electron microscopy of islet cell tumors. In *Progress in Surgical Pathology*, edited by C. M. Fenoglio and M. Wolff. New York, Masson, 1980, pp. 135–155.
5. Buffa, R., Rindi, G., Sessa, F., Tortora, O., and Solcia, E. Chromogranin A, B and C in immunoreactivities of mammalian endocrine cells. Distribution, distinction from costored hormones-prohormones, and relationship with the argyrophil component of secretory granules. *Histochemistry*, in press, 1986.
6. Bussolati, G., Capella, C., Vassallo, G., and Solcia, E. Histochemical and ultrastructural studies on pancreatic A cells. Evidence for glucagon and non-glucagon components of the α granule. *Diabetologia 7:* 181–188, 1971.

7. Capella, C., Bordi, C., Monga, G., Buffa, R., Fontana, P., Bonfanti, S., Bussolati, G., and Solcia, E. Multiple endocrine cell types in thyroid medullary carcinoma. Evidence for calcitonin, somatostatin, ACTH, 5-HT and small granule cells. *Virchows Arch. Pathol. Anat. 377:* 111–128, 1978.

8. Capella, C., Buffa, R., Usellini, L., Frigerio, B., Jehenson, P., Sessa, F., and Solcia, E. Alpha and beta subunits of glycoprotein hormones in argyrophil pituitary tumors with small granule cells. *Ultrastruct. Pathol. 4:* 35–50, 1983.

9. Capella, C., Polak, J. M., Buffa, R., Tapia, F. J., Heitz, P. U., Bloom, S. R., and Solcia, E. Morphological patterns and diagnostic criteria of VIP-producing endocrine tumours. A histological, histochemical, ultrastructural and biochemical study of 32 cases. *Cancer 52:* 1860–1874, 1983.

10. Capella, C., Polak, J. M., Frigerio, B., and Solcia, E. Gastric carcinoids of argyrophil ECL cells. *Ultrastruct. Pathol. 1:* 411–418, 1980.

11. Capella, C., Solcia, E., Frigerio, B., Buffa, R., Usellini, L., and Fontana, P. The endocrine cells of the pancreas and related tumours. Ultrastructural study and classification. *Virchows Arch. A Pathol. Anat. Histol. 373:* 327–352, 1977.

12. Carlei, F., and Polak, J. M. Antibodies to neuron-specific enolase for the delineation of the entire diffuse neuroendocrine system in health and disease. *Semin. Diagn. Pathol. 1:* 59–70, 1984.

13. Cohn, D. V., Zangerle, R., Fischer-Colbrie, R., Chu, L. L. H., Elting, J. J., Hamilton, J. W., and Winkler, H. Similarity of secretory protein I from parathyroid gland to chromogranin A from adrenal medulla. *Proc. Natl. Acad. Sci. USA 79:* 6056–6059, 1982.

14. Creutzfeldt, W. Endocrine tumors of the pancreas. In *The Diabetic Pancreas*, edited by B. W. Volk and K. F. Wellman. New York, Plenum, 1977, pp. 551–590.

15. Cutz, E., Chan, W., Kay, J. M., and Chamberlain, D. W. Immunoperoxidase staining for serotonin, bombesin, calcitonin and Leu-enkephalin in pulmonary tumorlets, bronchial carcinoids and oat cell carcinoma. *Lab. Invest. 46:* 16A, 1982.

16. Deftos, L. J., McMillan, P. J., Sartiano, G. P., Abuid, J., and Robinson, A. G. Simultaneous ectopic production of parathyroid hormone and calcitonin. *Metabolism 25:* 534–550, 1976.

17. De Lellis, R. A., Rule, A. H., Spiler, I., Nathanson, L., Tashjan, A. H., Jr., and Wolfe, H. J. Calcitonin and carcinoembryonic antigen as tumor markers in medullary thyroid carcinoma. *Am. J. Clin. Pathol. 70:* 587–594, 1978.

18. De Lellis, R. A., Tischler, A. S., and Wolfe, H. J. Multidirectional differentiation in neuroendocrine neoplasms. *J. Histochem. Cytochem. 32:* 899–904, 1984.

19. De Potter, W., Smith, A. D., and de Shaepdyver, A. F. Subcellular fractionation of splenic nerve: ATP, chromogranin A, and dopamine-β-hydroxylase in noradrenergic vesicles. *Tissue Cell. 2:* 529–546, 1970.

20. Dubois, P. M., and Begeot, M. Immunocytological localization of LH, FSH, TSH and their subunits in the pituitary of normal and anencephalic human fetuses. *Cell Tissue Res. 191:* 249–265, 1978.

21. Eisenbarth, G. S., Shimizu, K., Bowring, M. A., and Wells, S. Expression of receptors for tetanus toxin and monoclonal antibody A2B5 by pancreatic islet cells. *Proc. Natl. Acad. Sci. USA 79:* 5066–5070, 1982.

22. Even, P., Caubarrère, I., Boutillier, J., Luna, D., and Brouet, G. Biologie des carcinoides des bronches. *Rev. Franc. Malad. Resp. 1:* 239–298, 1973.

23. Ezrin, C., Kovacs, K., and Horvath, E. Pathology of the adenohypophysis. In *Endocrine Pathology*, edited by J. M. B. Bloodworth. Baltimore, Williams & Wilkins, pp. 101–132.

24. Fiocca, R., Capella, C., Buffa, R., Fontana, P., Solcia, E., Hage, E., Chance, R. E. and Moody, A. J. Glucagon-, glicentin-, and pancreatic polypeptide-like immunoreactivities in rectal carcinoids and related colorectal cells. *Am. J. Pathol. 100:* 81–92, 1980.

25. Fiocca, R., Sessa, F., Tenti, P., Usellini, L., Capella, C., O'Have, M. M. T., and Solcia, E. Pancreatic polypeptide (PP) cells in the PP-rich lobe of the human pancreas are identified ultrastructurally and immunocytochemically as F cells. *Histochemistry 77:* 511–523, 1983.

26. Fischer-Colbrie, R., Schachinger, M., Zangerle, R., and Winkler, H. Dopamine β-hydroxylase and other glycoproteins from the soluble content and the membranes of adrenal chromaffin granules: isolation and carbohydrate analysis. *J. Neurochem. 38:* 725–732, 1982.

27. Frigerio, B., Capella, C., Eusebi, V., Tenti, P., and Azzopardi, J. G. Merkel cell carcinoma of the skin: The structure and origin of normal Merkel cells. *Histophathology 7:* 229–249, 1983.

28. Godwin, J. D. Carcinoid tumors. An analysis of 2837 cases. *Cancer 36:* 560–569, 1975.
29. Gould, V. E., Dardi, L. E., and Memoli, V. A. Neuroendocrine carcinomas of the skin: Light microscopic, ultrastructural, and immunohistochemical analysis. *Ultrastruct. Pathol. 1:* 499–509, 1980.
30. Gould, V. E., Linnoila, I., Memoli, V. A., and Warren, W. H. Neuroendocrine components of the bronchopulmonary tract: Hyperplasias, dysplasias, and neoplasms. *Lab. Invest. 49:* 519–537, 1983.
31. Grimelius, L. A silver nitrate stain for α_2 cells in human pancreatic islets. *Acta Soc. Med. Upsal. 73:* 243–270, 1968.
32. Grimelius, L., Hultquist, G. T., and Stenkvist, B. Cytological differentiation of asymptomatic pancreatic islet cell tumours in autopsy material. *Virchows Arch. Pathol. Anat. 365:* 275–288, 1975.
33. Heitz, P. U., Kasper, M., Polak, J. M., and Klöppel, G. Pancreatic endocrine tumors: Immunocytochemical analysis of 125 tumors. *Hum. Pathol. 13:* 263–271, 1982.
34. Hirata, Y., Sakamoto, N., Yamamoto, H., Matsukura, S., Imura H., and Okada S. Gastric carcinoid with ectopic production of ACTH and β-MSH. *Cancer 37:* 377–385, 1976.
35. Hofmann, J. W., Fox, P. S., and Milwaukee, S. D. W. Duodenal wall tumors and the Zollinger-Ellison syndrome. *Arch. Surg. 107:* 334–338, 1973.
36. Hörtnagl, H., Lochs, H., and Winkler, H. Immunological studies on the acidic chromogranins and on dopamine β-hydroxylase (EC 1.14.2.1) of bovine chromaffin granules. *J. Neurochem. 22:* 197–199, 1974.
37. Kaneko, H., Yanaihara, N., Ito, S., Kusumoto, Y., Fujita, T., Ishikawa, S., Sumida, T., and Sekiya, M. Somatostatinoma of the duodenum. *Cancer 44:* 2273–2279, 1979.
38. Larsson, L-I., Grimelius, L., Håkanson, R., Rehfeld, J. F., Stadil, F., Holst, J., Angervall, L., and Sundler, F. Mixed endocrine pancreatic tumors producing several peptide hormones. *Am. J. Pathol. 79:* 271–284, 1975.
39. Lippman, S. M., Mendelsohn, G., Trump, P. L., Wells, S. A., and Bylin, S. B. The prognostic and biological significance of cellular heterogeneity in medullary thyroid carcinoma: A study of calcitonin, L-dopa decarboxylase, and histaminase. *J. Clin. Endocrinol. Metab. 54:* 233–240, 1982.
40. Lloyd, R. V., Mervak T., Schmidt, K., Khazaeli, M. B., and Wilson, B. S. Immunohistochemical detection of chromogranins, neuron-specific enolase, and HCG in gastroenteropancreatic neuroendocrine tumors. *Lab. Invest. 50:* 35A, 1984.
41. Lloyd, R. V., and Wilson, B. S. Specific endocrine tissue marker defined by a monoclonal antibody. *Science 222:* 628–630, 1983.
42. O'Brian, D. S., Dayal, Y., De Lellis, R. A., Tischler, A. S., Bendon, R., and Wolfe, H. J. Rectal carcinoids as tumors of the hindgut endocrine cells. A morphological and immunohistochemical analysis. *Am. J. Surg. Pathol. 6:* 131–142, 1982.
43. O'Connor, D. T., Burton, D., and Deftos, L. J. Chromogranin A: Immunohistology reveals its universal occurrence in normal polypeptide hormone producing endocrine glands. *Life Sci. 33:* 1657–1664, 1983.
44. Ravazzola, M., Orci, L., Habener, J. F., and Potts, J. T. Jr. Parathyroid secretory protein: Immunocytochemical localisation within cells that contain parathyroid hormone. *Lancet 2:* 371–372, 1978.
45. Ruttman, E., Klöppel, G., Bommer, G., Kiehn, M., and Heitz, P. U. Pancreatic glucagonoma with and without syndrome. *Virchows Arch. A Pathol. Anat. Histol. 388:* 51–67, 1980.
46. Shrabanek P., Cannon, D., Dempsey, J., Kirrane, J., Neligan, M., and Powell, D. Substance P in medullary carcinoma of the thyroid. *Experientia 35:* 1259, 1979.
47. Smith, A. D., and Wikler, H. Purification and properties of an acidic protein from chromaffin granules of bovine adrenal medulla. *Biochem. J. 103:* 483–492, 1967.
48. Solcia, E., Capella, C., Buffa, R., and Frigerio B. Histochemical and ultrastructural studies on the argentaffin and argyrophil cells of the gut. In *Chromaffin, Enterochromaffin and Related Cells*, edited by R. E. Coupland and T. Fujita. Amsterdam, Elsevier, 1976, pp. 209–225.
49. Solcia, E., Capella, C., Buffa, R., Frigerio, B., and Fiocca, R. Pathology of the Zollinger-Ellison syndrome. In *Progress in Surgical Pathology*, edited by C. M. Fenoglio. New York, Masson, 1980, pp. 119–133.

50. Solcia E., Capella, C., Buffa, R., Frigerio, B., Usellini, L., Fiocca, R., Tenti, P., Sessa, F., and Rindi, G. Cytology of tumours in the gastroenteropancreatic and diffuse neuroendocrine system. In *Evolution and Tumour Pathology of the Neuroendocrine System*, edited by R. Håkanson, and S. Falkmer. Amsterdam, Elsevier, 1984, pp. 453–480.

51. Solcia, E., Capella, C., Buffa, R., Usellini, L., Frigerio, B., and Fontana, P. Endocrine cells of the gastrointestinal tract and related tumors. *Pathobiol. Annu. 9:* 163–203, 1979.

52. Solcia, E., Capella, C., Frigerio, B., and Fiocca, R. Tumour cytology of the diffuse endocrine system. In *Endocrine Tumours: The Pathobiology of Regulatory Peptide Producing Tumours*, edited by J. M. Polak and S. R. Bloom. Edinburgh, Churchill Livingstone, 1985, pp. 144–161.

53. Solcia, E., Capella, C., and Vassallo, G. Lead-haematoxylin as a stain for endocrine cells. Significance of staining and comparison with other selective methods. *Histochemie 20:* 116–126, 1969.

54. Stefanini, P., Carboni, M., Patrassi, N., and Basoli, A. Beta-islet cell tumors of the pancreas: Results of a study on 1067 cases. *Surgery 75:* 597–609, 1974.

55. Tamai, S., Kameya, T., Hamaguchi, K., Yanai, N., Abe, K., Yanaihara, N., Yamazaka, H., and Kageyama, K. Peripheral lung carcinoid tumor producing predominantly gastrin releasing peptide (GRP). Morphological and hormonal studies. *Cancer 52:* 273–281, 1983.

56. Tapia, F. J., Barbosa, A. J. A., Marangos, P. J., Polak, J. M., Bloom, S. R., Dermody, C., and Pearse, A. G. E. Neuron specific enolase is produced by neuroendocrine tumours. *Lancet 2:* 808–811, 1981.

57. Tsutsumi, Y., Osamura, Y., Watanabe, K., and Yanaihara, N. Immunohistochemical studies on gastrin-releasing peptide- and adrenocorticotropic hormone-containing cells in the human lung. *Lab. Invest. 48:* 623–632, 1983.

58. Wharton, J., Polak, J. M., Cole, G. A., Marangos, P. J., and Pearse, A. G. E. Neuron-specific enolase as an immunocytochemical marker for the diffuse neuroendocrine system in human fetal lung. *J. Histochem. Cytochem. 29:* 1359–1364, 1981.

59. Wilson, B. S., Lloyd, R. V. Detection of chromogranin in neuroendocrine cells with a monoclonal antibody. *Am. J. Pathol. 115:* 458–468, 1984.

Chapter 13

Diagnosing the Anaplastic Tumor

TIMOTHY J. TRICHE

Although tumor diagnosis is necessarily founded in the correlation of clinical, gross, and light microscopic features in a given case, recent developments in the fields of cell biology, immunology, biochemistry, and molecular biology have provided a variety of new tools applicable to the diagnosis of human cancer. These techniques are unnecessary for the vast majority of tumors, but they have specifically provided the means of establishing a precise and clinically relevant diagnosis in a small but significant population of tumors which in the past defied diagnosis. These tumors, which generally lack identifiable gross or light microscopic features which would allow a diagnosis, are frequently generically referred to as primitive, anaplastic, undifferentiated, or small, round-blue tumors. Perhaps the most common form of presentation for this group of lesions is that of metastatic tumor in a lymph node in a patient with an unknown primary. A recent study indicates that the most likely diagnosis in such cases is lymphoma.[30] Conversely, extranodal presentation of lymphoma, often in a cutaneous soft tissue sight or in bone, presents the reverse problem, i.e., an apparent undifferentiated soft tissue malignancy. Large retroperitoneal tumors discovered at surgery, mediastinal masses, lytic bone lesions, or coin lesions of lung discovered during radiologic examination and anemia subsequently discovered to be secondary to diffuse replacement of marrow elements by tumor cells are but a few examples of the manifold ways in which these tumors may present clinically. These neoplasms are frequently morphologically similar to one another, even though they retain ultrastructural features, antigenic determinants, enzymatic content, metabolites, secretory products, or tissue components that allow one to potentially identify the cell or tissue of origin.

For discussion purposes, the most diagonally useful techniques, or those with the greatest potential in the future, can be categorized as follows:

1. Electron microscopy
2. Catecholamine fluorescence
3. Immunocytochemistry
4. Combined electron microscopy and immunocytochemistry
5. Monoclonal antibodies

6. Tissue culture
7. Cytogenetics
8. Oncogene expression

ELECTRON MICROSCOPY

Historically, electron microscopy represents the first significant alternative to routine light microscopic diagnosis. First applied to biological material in the 1950s, electron microscopy had little impact on routine tumor diagnosis until a sufficient body of information concerning the ultrastructural appearance of normal and pathologically altered tissues, especially tumors, was generated in the ensuing decade. By the 1970s, a vast body of literature had been created which delineated in minute detail the expected ultrastructural features of every normal tissue as well as of the majority of tumors. It soon became apparent that many tumors retain at least some features found in their normal tissue counterparts. Thus, ultrastructural features such as microvillus border, junctional complexes, secretory granules, extensive Golgi apparatus, apical basal polarity of cell organelles, and a basal lamina were appreciated as features of adenocarcinoma. Many refinements on this theme have been subsequently described, e.g., the presence of a dense actin filament core within microvilli extending into the cytoplasm as rootlets, with lateral interconnections forming a terminal web, are features both of normal colonic mucosa and colon carcinoma.[33] Thus it became possible to definitively diagnose some cases of metastatic colonic adenocarcinoma. Many other examples of tissue-specific ultrastructural features upon various epithelial or mesenchymal tumors are now documented in the literature. Unfortunately, many exceptions also exist. For example, although pancreatic islet cells contain ultrastructurally specific secretory granules such as insulin-containing beta granules, glucagon-containing alpha granules, or gastrin-containing delta granules, islet cell tumors deriving from this this cell population frequently lack morphologically unique neurosecretory granules, with the possible exception of insulinomas. Commonly, neurosecretory type granules are found in tumors which secrete specific hormones or, in many cases, multiple hormonal products.[10] Thus, a simple correlation with known tissue ultrastructure can be misleading and can lead to an erroneous diagnosis if one fails to appreciate that tumors are not perfect analogs of their normal tissue counterparts.

An additional complication is the frequent atypical appearance of an otherwise normal ultrastructural component. Nowhere is this more diagnostically significant than in the case of melanomas, where the normal maturation of premelanosomes into melanosomes is frequently aberrant, resulting in the appearance of atypical granules not readily recognizable as melanosomes.[12, 13, 46] Abnormal melanogenesis is frequently most evident in precisely those cases representing the greatest diagnostic challenge, that is metasatic amelanotic melanoma presenting in lymph nodes in a patient with no known primary lesion. These abnormal or atypical melanosomes may frequently be admixed with reliably identified melanosomes,[46] but in some cases no normal melanosomes can be identified, and the evidence for melanoma may be circumstantial at best.[13] These granules are frequently isomorphous with lysosomes and phagolysosomes, and this is, in fact, one pathway in the catabolism of normal melanosomes in both melanocytes and normal macrophages ingesting degraded melanoma cells.

Conversely, the appearance of unequivocal melanosomes in tumor cells which otherwise bear no resemblance to a known melanoma has both lead to diagnostic confusion and ultimately to a greater appreciation of the manifold appearances of neural crest-derived melanocytic neoplasia. Nowhere is this more evident than in the case of clear cell sarcoma of tendon sheath, as it was originally known.[27] This lesion, originally thought to be related to synovial sarcoma, is now appreciated as a melanoma of soft tissues and has been renamed recently by the original author.[15] Classic melanosomes have long been appreciated in this neoplasm, and these features in conjunction with subsequent studies employing other techniques has confirmed the neural crest phenotype of this neoplasm. In addition, further ultrastructural studies have generated an appreciation of the close relationship of this tumor to nerve sheath tumors,[6] which thus completes the spectrum at one extreme of melanoma and at the other extreme of malignant nerve sheath tumors, with melanotic malignant schwannomas, clear cell sarcomas, and neutralization of malignant melanomas representing intermediate tumors spanning the spectrum from pure nerve sheath to purely melanocytic differentiation, respectively.

CATECHOLAMINE FLUORESCENCE

Although more sophisticated ultrastructural analysis of tumors based on a broader knowledge of the many ultrastructural forms of common organelles such as melanosomes has become possible, it nonetheless remains true that tumor cells lacking any variant of these structures remain undiagnosable by electron microscopy alone. This has necessitated recourse to nonmorphologic techniques which identify a precise tumor product. Although this approach has been profitably applied to tumor metabolites detected by serum or urine assays, successful morphologic detection within sections of a given tumor were not possible until the application of a technique designed to detect catecholamine fluorescence in the diverse group of so-called amine-precursor uptake and decarboxylation (APUD) tumors first described by A. G. E. Pearse. This technique, first described by neurobiologists,[17] is based on the observation that all catecholamines and catecholamine precursors from dihydroxyphenylalanine onward in the catecholamine metabolic pathway can be detected by their characteristic fluorescence in tissue sections if the tissue is first exposed to the vapor phase of formaldehyde. Thus, imprints or frozen sections which have been rapidly air-dried are exposed in a closed vessel to paraformaldehyde vapor at 80°C for an hour. Under these circumstances, the unstained, unfixed tissue, when subsequently examined in a fluorescence microscope equipped with an appropriate filter pack, will reveal an apple green or yellow fluorescence in those cells which contain any of the catecholamine metabolites. This includes all of the APUD tumors, and the application of this technique has been especially valuable in diagnosing amelanotic melanoma[26] and neuroblastoma,[60] two tumors which not infrequently demonstrate an unusual clinical presentation and sometimes lack ultrastructural evidence of either melanosomes or neurosecretory granules, respectively. Catecholamine fluorescence has thus been a valuable tool for precisely identifying the histogenetic origin of a diverse group of tumors which have been historically difficult to diagnose in as sizeable percent of cases. Nonetheless, the technique is limited to a small group of tumors. Furthermore, a negative result does not necessarily exclude the diagnosis of an APUD tumor due to the inordinate dependence of the technique on precisely controlled technical considerations. These factors have undoubtedly limited the widespread application of this technique, especially because of the requirement for fresh tissue, although a recent report has suggested that even in conventional 4% formalin fixed tissues the technique may occasionally be diagnostic.[34]

IMMUNOCYTOCHEMISTRY

As noted above, ultrastructural examination may be helpful in the diagnosis of specific tumors due to the identification of a specific organelle or intracellular structure, but it imparts no new knowledge regarding the biochemical or immunological character of that structure. Thus in the absence of other specific features, the mere identification of a structure may leave one with an imprecise diagnosis. For example, 10-nm filaments of intermediate filaments are present in a variety of cell types, but the biochemical content of these filaments differs, and elucidation of this biochemical difference using an immunocytochemical technique allows one to divide cells into broad categories (Table 12.1). An appreciation of the histogenetic significance of each of these intermediate filament classes has resulted from extensive biochemical and immunological studies of developing and differentiated embryonic and adult tissues.[40, 57]

The application of immunocytochemistry to paraffin-embedded, fixed pathological material has, in many respects, revolutionized tumor diagnosis. The past 5 years have witnessed the rapid creation of a vast body of literature detailing the reactivity of normal and tumor tissues with a virtually unlimited number of immunologic reagents. In many ways, immunocytochemistry is still in its adolescence, and only now is it becoming apparent that important exceptions to the general rules exist. For example, although keratins have been recognized as components of stratified squamous epithelial and other epithelial tissues, it is now apparent that they enjoy a vast distribution throughout ectodermal and entodermal derivatives of the body, as well as several mesenchymal derivatives.[63] Thus mesothelial cells, a bona fide mesenchymally-derived normal tissue component, contain both epithelial-type keratins, as well as mesenchymal-type vimentin filaments.[20] This unfortunately complicates the diagnosis of samples such as malignant pleural effusions, where both metastatic carcinoma cells and reactive pleural mesothelial cells may contain keratin filaments.[58] This problem is further accentuated by the occurrence of vimentin filaments within the metastatic carcinoma cells, like the mesothelial cells. It is now apparent that in both effusions and their *in vitro* analog, tissue culture, epithelia of diverse type apparently re-express a more embryonal or undifferentiated phenotype, i.e., coexistence of both vimentin and keratin intermediate fliaments.[39] Situations such as these have necessitated a more sophisticated application of immunocytochemistry. In addition, it must be noted that diagnostically relevant antigenic determinants may not be detectable in routinely processed tissue. Thus, a negative result by immunocytochemistry is of little relevance, especially in the absence of appropriate controls. *It cannot be overemphasized that immunocytochemistry in the absence of appropriate controls is of little, if any, diagnostic value.* The combination of false-positive and false-negative results necessitates the routine use of appropriate tissue controls. Preferably, these controls should represent comparable tumors to those under consideration. This problem is particularly evident in the diagnoses of poorly differentiated tumors. The use of a differentiated or keratinizing squamous cell carcinoma as a positive control for antikeratin antibodies when a primitive carcinoma is being evaluated can be tremendously misleading. In this setting, a positive result with the control and a negative result in the tumor tissue is not indicative that tumor is not of epithelial origin and does not contain keratin filaments.

It has become evident that the family of cytokeratins is diverse[51] and appears sequentially from less to more "differentiated" in the normal differentiation of epithelial tissue.[29] Unfortunately, many of the antikeratin antibodies commerically available are against terminally differentiated tissues such as callus, which contains only mature keratins. Likewise, monoclonal antikeratin antibodies can be extremely misleading, since many tumors fail to express a complete array of cytokeratins, or may express keratins indicative of greater or lesser differentiation than those identified by the specific monoclonal antibody employed.[21, 55]

In addition to these technical considerations regarding the detection of tissue-specific antigenic determinants in a given tumor, one must also appreciate that certain tumors exist for which there is no normal tissue counterpart. Synovial sarcoma, for example, shows no verifiable relationship to normal synovia[66] and, in fact does not originate from a joint capsule, despite its frequent close anatomic association. Nonetheless, synovial sarcoma, as its name indicates, is generally regarded as at least a partly mesenchymally derived malignant tumor, i.e., a sarcoma. As one would expect of such a neoplasm, vimentin filaments are routinely identifiable in the spindled cell stromal component.[49] In contrast, the glandular component of biphasic synovial sarcomas is frequently positive for keratin filaments.[18, 47, 49] These are identifiable by electron microscopy as well as by immunocytochemistry. The problem is compounded by the appearance of keratin-type filaments in the stromal component of at least some monophasic synovial sarcomas[18, 50] and by the coexistence of keratin and vimentin filaments within the glandular component in some cases of biphasic synovial sarcoma,[18] analogous to the situation described for mesothelioma and epithelioid sarcoma.[14, 48]

Results such as those described above have made it apparent that the simple distinction of epithelial from mesenchymal tumors by keratin *vs.* vimentin filament content, respectively, is unreliable in the absence of an appreciation of the complexity of the issues involved. Similar complications exist with regard to the expression of other intermediate filament proteins. For example, it has been suggested that desmin is a reliable marker of myogenous differentiation.[1]

Desmin appears to be a less reliable marker than originally thought and, in particular, may be found in tissues not generally thought of as myogenous, *e.g.*, malignant fibrous histiocytoma[47] in which presumably myofibroblastic differentiation has occurred. Thus, although the presence of that filament type may be indicative of a potential function, *e.g.*, contractility, its presence is not reliable evidence of myogenous differentiation, *e.g.*, rhabdomysosarcoma or leiomyosarcoma. In addition, desmin is generally a relatively late appearing intermediate filament in normal myogenesis,[22] so it is not expressed in the more primitive rhabdomysarcomas and leiomyosarcomas.[2] Therefore, antisera to this intermediate filament protein has not achieved widespread diagnostic utility. The final two major classes of intermediate filament proteins, glial fibrillary acidic protein (GFAP) and neurofilament triplet protein, are generally less applicable in routine pathology in that they are generally expressed only in the central nervous system.[75] Although the detection of GFAP by anti-GFAP antisera may be useful in the categorization of a given glial neoplasm, other more conventional histopathological characteristics are frequently of greater value. Neurofilament triple protein, although present in peripheral[41] as well as central neural tissue,[40, 41] has also failed to be of routine diagnostic value in the diagnosis of neural neoplasia. In contrast, other nonfilamentous antibodies have enjoyed wider diagnostic use.

The number of antisera to other antigenic determinants in normal and neoplastic tissues is steadily increasing. Some of these antisera are of significantly greater diagnostic value than others for a variety of reasons, including detectability in routinely processed tissue and the frequency of expression of the antigenic determinant in a given tumor type. Thus, the expression of neuron-specific enolase (NSE) in tumors of neural origin, combined with its general retention in formalin-fixed tissues, has generated a body of literature on the use of this antiserum in the diagnosis of diverse neural crest neoplasia.[23, 24, 70, 76, 83] NSE in fact appears to be a general marker of neural crest derivatives and is expressed in tissues as diverse as all the so-called APUD tumors,[45, 64] as well as uncommon but related tumors, *e.g.* melanotic schwannoma. Like all such antigenic determinants, however, the results of staining with antibodies to NSE must be interpreted with caution. Specifically, the existence of alpha-alpha and beta-beta isomers of enolase, the so-called non-neural enolases, as well as the gamma-gamma, or neuronspecific enolase,[65] allows for at least a theoretical possibility of alpha-gamma or beta-gamma heterodimers. This appears to have been confirmed with alpha-gamma dimers in a variety of CNS tumors where such heterodimers have been isolated.[8, 35] The positive results of staining with anti-NSE antisera on liver and smooth and skeletal muscle[76] suggest that a similar situation exists with regard to the beta isomers in these tissues.

COMBINED ELECTRON MICROSCOPY AND IMMUNOCYTOCHEMISTRY

Complications such as those discussed above have necessitated a reevaluation of the role of immunocytochemistry alone in tumor diagnosis. Other factors, including spurious reactivity of tissue sections with diverse, nonspecific antisera as well as normal rabbit serum controls; detection of unrelated epitopes on other tissue antigenic determinants; and problems with the technique, tissue fixation, tumor expression of a given antigen, retention of the tissue antigen after fixation, denaturation by fixative, and the reliability of the antisera employed to detect these determinants have all served to breed a degree of skepticism and caution on the part of those employing routine diagnostic immunocytochemistry.

It may be that the greatest diagnostic utility of immunocytochemistry will be evident when the technique is employed in conjunction with other techniques, specifically, diagnostic ultrastructure,[28] because the shortcomings of each technique tend to complement those of the other. Specifically, electron microscopy (EM) provides no information about the character of a structure identified, and immunocytochemistry provides no information about the morphologic distribution of an antigenic determinant but does allow identification of its biochemical or immunological characteristics. Furthermore, each technique places a different set of demands on the pathologist. Electron microscopy presupposes a familiarity with, and an appreciation of, the diverse forms known ultrastructural features, in context with the reliability of the observations. Immunocytochemistry, in contrast, presumes a degree of familiarity with normal cell biology and the immunological profile of a given tissue and its tumor type. The first is generally somewhat subjective (*i.e.*, Is that a melanosome or lysosome?), while the second is somewhat more pragmatic and objective but fraught with a diverse array of technique problems alluded to above (*i.e.*, Is the brown reaction product in the tumor cells "browner" than the brown pigments in the background?).

Fortunately, cases which are otherwise nondiagnostic often become diagnostic when both techniques are employed.[5] As in the example cited previously, melanoma which expresses only atypical melanosomes, suspected but not proven of being such by electron microscopy, can also be diagnosed with antisera to a melanoma-antigenic marker such as S100 protein, a protein originally described in the CNS[73] but which is also expressed in a variety of other tissues, including nerve sheath and melanocytic cells,[81] as well as various normal (and perhaps tumor) tissue types, such as cartilage[16] and certain components of skin[54] and lymph node.[80] Despite this, in the context alluded to here, the presence of S100 reactive protein in the tumor cells in conjunction with the suspected but unproven atypical melanosomes detected by EM would provide evidence of the presence of melanocytic tumor. It should be noted that neither electron microscopy nor immunocytochemistry provides information regarding malignancy or benignancy; this of course is a determination solely based on the expertise of the pathologist involved.

Both electron microscopy and immunocytochemistry are intended to define tumor histogenesis, especially where it has relevance regarding prognosis and treatment. In this regard, it should be noted that although the application of diagnostic EM and immunocytochemistry presumes some impact on patient management, the corollary is not necessarily true, *i.e.*, that in cases where no impact on patient management is expected, such studies should not be carried out. On the contrary, these techniques have provided more information about the diverse nature of neoplasia and their histogenetic interrelationships than would ever have been possible to provide by routine techniques alone. On the basis of this, new concepts of management and an appreciation of differing prognoses in otherwise morphologically indistinguishable tumors have emerged. This is true, for example, in the case of peripheral neuroepithelioma of chest wall.[3] This tumor, originally classified as a chest wall Ewing's sarcoma, has only recently been appreciated as a biologically unique and prognostically different neoplasm. As a result, new approaches to the clinical management of these patients are being generated, based on an appreciation of the unique character of this neoplasm. Ancillary diagnostic techniques such as diagnostic EM and immunocytochemistry have a role not only in the diagnosis of a given tumor but, perhaps more importantly, they also serve to generate far more sophisticated knowledge of tumor histogenesis and biology, with important clinical implications.

The preceding techniques are now in everyday use in pathology laboratories throughout the world. Although a great deal remains to be learned, a data base has already been created which allows the ready application of these techniques to everyday diagnosis. A body of emerging techniques now exists which is expected to have a diagnostic impact in the forseeable future. Some of these are discussed below.

MONOCLONAL ANTIBODIES

Despite the fact that monoclonal antibodies are increasingly available commercially and have been employed to some extent in routine diagnosis, and even treatment,[53] the widespread application of these highly specific probes of cell or tissue antigens has been impeded by the inherent lack of reactivity of many of these antibodies with tissues routinely processed for pathologic examination.[11] In general, polyclonal antibodies such as those discussed above have superior affinity and broader reactivity with the antigenic determinants in question, due to the fact that a variety of epitopes on a given antigen are recognized by polyclonal antisera. In contrast, monoclonal antibodies by definition recognize only a single epitope. This epitope may be as small as four sugars in carbohydrate determinants or a short amino acid sequence in protein determinants. This precision becomes counterproductive, in that many different antigenic determinants may also express comparable epitopes. Thus, no monoclonal antibody described to date necessarily recognizes a single cell or tissue type. For this reason, the majority of monoclonal antibodies presently used for diagnostic purposes are employed in batteries which recognize a profile of antigenic determinants. This is true among lymphoid neoplasia, in which monoclonal antibodies have been most widely employed,[53] as well as in neuroblastoma diagnosis, in which monoclonal antibodies are emerging as an important diagnostic and therapeutic tool.[37, 38, 74] It is noteworthy and indicative of the problem alluded to above that many of the monoclonal antibodies currently employed in neuroblastoma evaluation were originally generated against lymphoid determinants and show cross-reactivity with both cell and tissue types.[25] Nonetheless, it has become possible to reliably distinguish general categories of tumor types on the basis of positive or negative reactivity of a given panel of antibodies with a specific tumor in question. Such panels of monclonal antibodies have proven reliable in the distinction of lymphoid, neural, and mesenchymal tumors one from another. They have also provided insight into the proper categorization of ill-understood tumors, such as peripheral neuroepithelioma.[25]

A major problem with the application of monoclonal antibodies to tumor diagnosis is the virtual necessity for fresh tumor tissue for frozen section, imprint, cytospin, or cell sorter analysis. This technical consideration has imposed new demands on clinicians and pathologists dealing with portions of fresh tumor tissue, and separate samples for routine paraffin-embedded study are required. In some ways this situation is no different than the necessity of fixing tissue for EM in glutaraldehyde as opposed to formaldehyde. In other respects these tissue demands add a further burden of timeliness to tissue handling. Tissue must be frozen and stored in an appropriate manner for later sectioning in a cryostat. Freezer temperatures of $-20°C$ are inadequate for long-term storage due to the generation of ice crystal damage within the tissue, and freezer space that provides a temperature of $-70°C$ is not widely available in many hospitals. In addition, frozen sections generated at the time of tumor biopsy are generally nonreactive with monoclonal antibodies after a period of time, even when stored at 4°C.

Other techniques, such as tumor cell suspensions for cell sorter analysis, generate greater demands on the pathologist's time and ability and are, for that reason, not commonly employed, nor is it foreseeable that they will be used in the future unless sufficient diagnostic utility is demonstrated. This may be the case with lymphomas, in which cell sorter analysis of lymphoma cell suspensions is becoming widespread, but alternative and less demanding techniques which give similar results are also becoming popular, specifically, frozen section analysis with the same monoclonal antibodies.[32]

Such techniques after the possibility of generating new information about tumors which has not been previously appreciated. For example, the existence of true histiocytic lymphoma (*i.e.*, a neoplasm not of T or B cell lineage), has long been disputed. Results of testing with panels of monoclonal antibodies that delineate normal T and B cell differentiation in normal and neoplastic lymphoid cells, in conjunction with cytochemical and immunologic assays, has allowed the detection of rare tumors that lack all such determinants and which instead appear to be more closely related to true histiocytes or macrophages.[36,78] These tumors, which histologically may be indistinguishable from T-cell lymphoma, appear to be unique entities. The ultrastructural examination of such neoplasms reveals differences from normal lymphomas which have not been previously recognized, such as the existence of very primitive forms of apparent cell-cell contacts, which are never observed in lymphoma but which have been described in true histiocytic lymphoma.[36]

As monoclonal antibodies for tissue diagnosis are more extensively examined, hopefully, certain monoclonal antibodies will emerge that are reliable in the detection of specific tumor histogenesis (see Chapters by Neville *et al.* and Rilke *et al.*) and that might be applied to routinely processed tissue. The recent description of the so-called anti-T200 antigen antibody[7,56] and related monoclonal antibodies[79] represents one such possibility. These monoclonal antibodies have proven to be of potential diagnostic value in detecting all hematopoietic malignancies, even in paraffin-embedded material.[30, 79] Although far more reliable and reactive in frozen sections or imprints, these monoclonal antibodies, can also detect such neoplasms in paraffin-embedded material. Like all monoclonal antibodies, the reactivity has been somewhat capricious and less intense than with polyclonal antibodies. For this reason, further experience will be necessary for a realistic appraisal of the true diagnostic value of such monoclonals.

TISSUE CULTURE

The developing awareness on the part of pathologists that new diagnostic techniques will require new tissue handling techniques has created the possibility of generating a continuous source of tumor tissue for subsequent analysis. Specifically, once tissue has been obtained in a sterile fresh state for frozen section or cell sorter analysis, it requires little additional preparation to establish such tumor tissue in short-term or potentially long-term culture. Although not a technique to be employed in the vast majority of tumor cases, tissue culture has been valuable in establishing a diagnosis in selected cases.[61] Although most tumors will not grow in long-term tissue culture, virtually all tumors will survive in short-term culture. The availability of such tumor cells or tissue has allowed further analysis if initial studies fail to detect any diagnostically specific information, not infrequently due to the primitive character of certain neoplasms. This is particularly true of tumors of neural crest origin, where the initially primitive and undiagnosable tumor may be induced to undergo tissue-specific differentiation in culture, either spontaneously[31, 61, 62] or with the aid of certain differentiating agents.[31, 71] It is well established that neurite extension detectable by phase contrast microscopy of tissue cultures is a unique property of neural tumors.[52] Less well known is the fact that even in the absence of such gross evidence of differentiation, ultrastructural evidence of differentiation frequently appears. Thus, amelanotic melanoma may become pigmented in culture[19]; neuroblastoma cells originally lacking neurosecretory granules may acquire them[61]; or tissue-specific enzymes or proteins may be secreted into the tissue culture medium[62] for analysis by diverse clinical lab techniques such as radioimmunoassay (RIA), enzymatic assays, or high performance liqiud chromatography (HPLC). Thus, even in the absence of morphologically unique characteristics by light or electron microscopy, certain tumors may acquire unique tumor cell products which might otherwise not be detectable even *in vivo* by serum or urine analysis.

CYTOGENETICS

Although chromosomal abnormalities detected by cytogenetics have long been appreciated in certain human tumors such as chronic myelogenous leukemia, where the so-called Philadelphia chromosome is routinely present, recent developments have implicated a variety of chromosomal abnormalities in specific human tumors which were not previously appreciated (see also Yunis chapter). Chromosome 8:2, 8:22, and 8:14 translocations in Burkitt's lymphoma have been described recently,[44] and chromosome I abnormalities of various types have been described in neuroblastoma.[9] In addition, Ewing's sarcoma has recently been noted to routinely display a chromosome 11:22 reciprocal translocation which appears to be unique to that tumor.[4, 77] Because of the complete absence of a specific marker unique to Ewing's sarcoma by ultrastructural or immunocytochemical or enzymatic analysis, the presence of a unique chromosomal abnormality may prove to be of important diagnostic value. However, such results must be viewed with some caution. For example, in our own studies, we have found that although all 20 cases of Ewing's sarcoma studied to date express an 11:22 reciprocal translocation, as already reported by others, we also find that certain neural tumors, (*i.e.*, peripheral neuroepitheliomas) express an apparently identical chromosomal abnormality in some cases.[82] Furthermore, the single case of soft tissue Ewing's sarcoma available for study has failed to express the 11:22 translocation, an observation which suggests that Ewing's sarcoma of bone and of soft tissue, although morphologically indistinguishable, are nonetheless cytogenetically, if not histogenetically, unrelated. No other childhood tumor which we have examined besides Ewing's sarcoma and peripheral neuroepithelioma displays the characteristic 11:22 translocation.

One of the confusing observations made by cytogenetics has been the lack of a uniform chromosome I abnormality in neuroblastoma. Although other tumors with specific chromosomal abnormalities have shown a uniform break point, the abnormalities noted in neuroblastoma have been heterogeneously scattered along chromosome I.[9] The significance and underlying basis for this has only become apparent recently with the advent of the application of molecular biological techniques to human tumors.

ONCOGENE EXPRESSION

Oncogenes in general and their potential role in tumor cell biology have been discussed in detail previously in this course (see chapter by Tomasi) and will not be discussed in detail here. Certain specific observations bear comment. It now appears that neuroblastoma may be unique among human tumors in that it expresses the specific oncogene *n-myc*,[69] an analog of the ubiquitously distributed *c-myc*, with which it shares limited sequence homology.[4] *In situ* hybridization studies of human chromosomal spreads with probes specific for *n-myc* have ascertained that the normal site of this oncogene is on the short arm of chromosome 2.[69] Unlike other oncogenes characterized to date, *n-myc* is unique in that it displays a propensity for variable translocations to other chromosomes, including chromosome I.[69] It thus becomes apparent that the diverse chromosome I abnormalities in neuroblastoma may be due to the variable insertion of *n-myc* along chromosome I in individual cases of that tumor. It has also become apparent that the homogeneous staining regions within a given identifiable chromosome, as well as the extrachromosomal so-called double minutes are, in fact, a morphological manifestation of the *n-myc* oncogene amplification. These structures show intense hybridization with *n-myc* probes and have strongly implicated *n-myc* in the biologic behavior of neuroblastoma.[69] It is recognized that neuroblastoma is a unique neoplasm which undergoes spontaneous regression as well as differentiation to a normal tissue counterpart in an unpredictable fashion in a significant number of cases. A recent report[12] has shown that *n-myc* expression is minimal in Stage 1 and Stage 2 neuroblastoma, in which tumor progression and patient death are unlikely. In contrast, half of advanced stage, *i.e.*, Stages 3 and 4, neuroblastomas show increased *n-myc* expression (3- to 300-fold). It has also been noted that neuroblastomas which fail to grow in culture tend to correlate with good patient outcome, whereas those tumors which can be established in tissue culture are generally derived from patients who ultimately die.[59] In this connection, it is noteworthy that virtually all neuroblastomas in culture (8/9) express variable but high levels of *n-myc*.[67] These observations have strongly suggested that *n-myc* expression is important in the biology and prognosis of given cases of neuroblastoma. Similar results with *c-myc* have been noted in human small cell carcinoma of lung and related neoplasms.[73] Here, oncogene expression has correlated with an unexpectedly adverse response to treatment and poor survival.

Although conventionally viewed as the domain of molecular biologists, oncogene detection in human tumor material by pathologists using reagents and techniques generated by molecular biologists is clearly desirable, as demonstrated by a recent report.[68] Sections of human neuroblastoma were hybridized with radioactive problems to *n-myc*. Hybridization was detected by light microscopic autoradiography and shown to be specific to tumor cells and, in particular, to those cells which pathologists would regard as undifferentiated and biologically aggressive, *i.e.*, small round and/or pleomorphic tumors cells. It has been noted that differentiating neuroblastoma in the absence of undifferentiated neuroblasts has a good prognosis, whereas composite tumors containing both differentiated and undifferentiated elements display a prognosis which more closely parallels that of undifferentiated neuroblastoma. These results with *in situ* hybridization of *n-myc* to human tumor cells serve to substantiate the suspicion that the biologically aggressive cells in neuroblastoma are, in fact, the same small undifferentiated neuroblasts.

Although the results noted above are unique and preliminary in nature, they nonetheless raise the exciting possibility that, in the future, diagnostic pathology will employ highly specific and sophisticated techniques derived from basic research in tumor cell biology which will provide clinically useful diagnostic and prognostic information. It might become possible, for example, to predict in advance of treatment those patients who are destined to a poor outcome in the absence of aggressive treatment *vs.* those patients with an intrinsically less aggressive tumor, requiring less aggressive or little therapy. It is likely that diagnostic pathology in the future will increasingly employ a diverse array of techniques which will allow the gathering of precise, objective information regarding tumor diagnosis and prognosis.

REFERENCES

1. Altmannsberger, J., Osborn, M., Treuner, J., *et al.* Diagnosis of human childhood rhabdomyosarcoma by antibodies to desmin, the structural protein of muscle specific intermediate filaments. *Virchows Arch (Cell Pathol) 39:* 203–215, 1982.
2. Altmannsberger, M., Osborn, M., Weber, K., and Schauer, A. Expression of intermediate

filaments in different human epithelial and mesenchymal tumors. *Pathol. Res. Pract. 175:* 227–237, 1982.

3. Askin, F. B., Rosai, J., Sibley, R. K., *et al.* Malignant small cell tumor of the thoracopulmonary region in childhood. A distinctive clinicopathologic entity of uncertain histogenesis. *Cancer 43:* 2438–2451, 1979.

4. Aurias, A., Rimbaut, C., Buffe, D., *et al.* Translocation involving chromosome 22 in Ewing's sarcoma. A cytogenetic study of four fresh tumors. *Cancer Genet. Cytogenet. 12:* 21–25, 1984.

5. Azar, H. A., Espinoza, C. G., Richman, A. V., *et al.* "Undifferentiatied" large cell malignancies: An ultrastructural and immunocytochemical study. *Hum. Pathol. 13:* 323–333, 1982.

6. Azumi, N., and Turner R. R. Clear cell sarcoma of tendons and aponeuroses: Electron microscopic findings suggesting Schwann cell differentiation. *Hum. Pathol. 14:* 1084–1089, 1983.

7. Battifora, H., and Trowbridge, I. S. A monoclonal antibody useful for the differential diagnosis between malignant lymphoma and nonhematopoietic neoplasms. *Cancer 51:* 816–821, 1983.

8. Beemer, F. A., Vlug, A. M. C., van Veelen, C. W. M., *et al.* Isozyme pattern of enolase of childhood tumors. *Cancer 54:* 293–296, 1984.

9. Biedler, J. L., Meyers, M. B., and Spengler B. A. Homogeneously staining regions and double minute chromosomes, prevalent cytogenetic abnormalities of human neuroblastoma cells. *Ad. Cell Neurobiol. 4:* 267–307, 1983.

10. Bordi, C., and Tardini, A. Electron microscopy of islet cell tumors. In Fenoglio, C. M., and Wolff, M. (eds): *Progress in Surgical Pathology, Vol. I.* New York, Masson, 1980, pp. 135–155.

11. Borowitz, M. J., and Stein R. B. Diagnostic applications of monoclonal antibodies to human cancer. *Arch. Pathol. Lab. Med. 108:* 101–105, 1984.

12. Broudeur, G. M., Seeger, R. C., Schwab, M., *et al.* Amplification of N-myc in untreated human neuroblastomas correlates with advanced disease stage. *Science 224:* 1121–1124, 1984.

13. Carstens, P. H. B., and Kuhns, J. G. Ultrastructural confirmation of malignant melanoma. *Ultrastruct. Pathol. 2:* 147–149, 1981.

14. Chase, D. R., Weiss, S. W., Enzinger, F. M., and Langloss, J. M. Keratin in epithelioid sarcoma. An immunohistochemical study. *Am. J. Surg. Pathol. 8:* 435–441, 1984.

15. Chung, E. B., and Enzinger, F. M. Malignant melanoma of soft parts. A reassessment of clear cell sarcoma. *Am. J. Surg. Pathol. 7:* 405–413, 1983.

16. Cocchia, D., Lauriola, L., Stolfi, V. M., *et al.* S-100 antigen labels neoplastic cells in liposarcoma and cartilaginous tumours. *Virchows Arch. (Pathol. Anat.) 402:* 139–145, 1983.

17. Corrodi, H., and Jonsson, G. The formaldehyde fluorescence method for the histochemical demonstration of biogenic monoamines. A review on the methodology. *J. Histochem. Cytochem. 15:* 65–78, 1967.

18. Corson, J. M., Weiss, L. M., Banks-Schlegel, S. P., and Pinkus, G. S. Keratin proteins in synovial sarcoma. *Am. J. Surg. Pathol. 7:* 107–109, 1983.

19. Costa, J., Rosai, J., and Philpott, G. W. Pigmentation of "amelanotic" melanoma in culture. *Arch. Pathol. 95:* 371–374, 1983.

20. Deleted in galley proof and renumbered as Ref. 39a.

21. Debus, E., Weber, K., and Osborn, M. Monoclonal cytokeratin antibodies that distinguish simple from stratified squamous epithelia: Characterization on human tissues. *EMBO J 1:* 1641–1647, 1982.

22. Denk, H., Krepler, R., Artleib, U., *et al.* Proteins of intermediate filaments. An immunohistochemical and biochemical approach to the classification of soft tissue tumors. *Am. J. Pathol. 110:* 193–208, 1983.

23. Dhillon, A. P., and Rode J. Patterns of staining for neurone specific enolase in benign and malignant melanocytic lesions of the skin. *Diagn. Histopathol. 5:* 169–174, 1982.

24. Dhillon, A. P., Rode, J., and Leathem, A. Neurone specific enolase: An aid to the diagnosis of melanoma and neuroblastoma. *Histopathology 6:* 81–92, 1982.

25. Donner, L., Triche, T. J., Israel, M. A., *et al.* A panel of monoclonal antibodies which discriminate neuroblastoma from Ewing's sarcoma, rhabdomyosarcoma, neuroepithelioma, and hematopoietic malignancies. In *Advances in Neuroblastoma Research*, edited by A. Evans. New York, Alan R. Liss, 1985.

26. Dunn, D. R., and Barth R. F. Identification of melanoma cells by formaldehyde-induced fluorescence. *Cancer 33:* 701–706, 1974.

27. Enzinger F. M. Clear-cell sarcoma of tendons and aponeuroses. An analysis of 21 cases. *Cancer 18:* 1163–1174, 1965.

28. Erlandson, R. A. Diagnostic immunohistochemistry of human tumors. An interim evaluation. *Am. J. Surg. Pathol. 8:* 615, 1984.

29. Fuchs, E., and Marchuk, D. Type I and type II keratins have evolved from lower eukaryotes to form the epidermal intermediate filaments in mammalian skin. *Proc. Natl. Acad. Sci. USA 80:* 5857–5861, 1983.

30. Gatter, K. C., Alcock, C., Heryet, A., *et al.* The differential diagnosis of routinely processed anaplastic tumors using monoclonal antibodies. *Am. J. Clin. Pathol. 82:* 33–43, 1984.

31. Gerson, J. M., Schlesinger, H. R., Sereni, P., *et al.* Isolation and characterization of a neuroblastoma cell line from peripheral blood in a patient with disseminated disease. *Cancer 39:* 2508–2512, 1977.

32. Harris, N. L., and Data, R. E. The distribution of neoplastic and normal B-lymphoid cells in nodular lymphomas: Use of an immunoperoxidase technique on frozen sections. *Hum. Pathol. 13:* 610–617, 1982.

33. Hickey, W. F., and Seiler, M. W. Ultrastructural markers of colonic adenocarcinoma. *Cancer 47:* 140–145, 1981.

34. Inoshita, T., and Youngberg, G. A. Fluorescence of melanoma cells—A useful diagnostic tool. *Am. J. Clin. Pathol. 78:* 311–315, 1982.

35. Ishiguro, Y., Kato, K., Ito, T., and Nagaya, M. Determination of three enolase isozymes and S-100 protein in various tumors in children. *Cancer Res. 43:* 6080–6084, 1983.

36. Jaffe, E. S. Malignant histiocytosis and true histiocytic lymphomas. In *Surgical Pathology of Lymph Nodes and Related Organs,* edited by E. S. Jaffe. Philadelphia, W. B. Saunders, 1985.

37. Kemshead, J. T., and Coakham, H. B. The use of monoclonal antibodies for the diagnosis of intracranial malignancies and the small round cell tumours of childhood. *J. Pathol. 141:* 249–257, 1983.

38. Kemshead, J. T., Fritschy, J., Garson, J. A., *et al.* Monoclonal antibody UJ 127: 11 detects a 220,000–240,000 kdal. Glycoprotein present on a sub-set of neuroectodermally derived cells. *Int. J. Cancer 31:* 187–195, 1983.

39. Lane, B., and Anderton, B. Focus on filaments: Embryology to pathology. *Nature 298:* 706–707, 1982.

39a. Lazarides, E. Intermediate filaments as mechanical integrators of cellular space. *Nature 283:* 249, 1980.

40. Lazarides E. Intermediate filaments. A chemically heterogeneous, developmentally regulated class of proteins. *Annu. Rev. Biochem. 51:* 219–250, 1982.

41. Lee, V., Wu, H. L., and Schlaepfer, W. W. Monoclonal antibodies recognize individual neurofilament triplet proteins. *Proc. Natl. Acad. Sci. USA 79:* 6089–6092, 1982.

42. Linnoila, R. I., Tsokos, M., Triche, T. J., and Chandra, R. Evidence for neural origin and periodic acid-Schiff-positive variants of the malignant small cell tumor of thoracopulmonary region ("Askin tumor"). *Lab. Invest. 48:* 51A, 1983.

43. Little, C. D., Nau, M. M., Carney, D. N., *et al.* Amplification and expression of the c-myc oncogene in human lung cancer cell lines. *Nature 306:* 194–196, 1983.

44. Magrath, I., Erikson, J., Whang-Peng, J., *et al.* Synthesis of kappa light chains by cell lines containing an 8:22 chromosomal translocation derived from a male homosexual with Burkitt's lymphoma. *Science 222:* 1094–1098, 1983.

45. Marangos, P. J., Polak, J. M., and Pearse, A. G. E. Neuron-specific enolase. A probe for neurons and neuroendocrine cells. *Trends Neurol. Sci. 5:* 193–196, 1982.

46. Mazur, M. T., and Katzenstein, A-L. Metastatic melanoma: The spectrum of ultrastructural morphology. *Ultrastruct. Pathol. 1:* 337–356, 1980.

47. Miettinen, M., Lehto, V-P, Badley, R. A., and Virtanen, I. Expression of intermediate filaments in soft-tissue sarcomas. *Int. J. Cancer 30:* 541–546, 1982.

48. Miettinen, M., Lehto, V-P, Vartio, T., and Virtanen, I. Epithelioid sarcoma. Ultrastructural and immunohistologic features suggesting a synovial origin. *Arch. Pathol. Lab. Med. 106:* 620–623, 1982.

49. Miettinen, M., Lehto, V-P, and Virtanen, I. Keratin in the epithelial-like cells of classical biphasic synovial sarcoma. *Virchows Arch. (Cell Pathol.) 40:* 157–161, 1982.

50. Miettinen, M., Lehto, V-P, and Virtanen, I. Monophasic synovial sarcoma of spindle-cell type. Epithelial differentiation as revealed by ultrastructural features, content of prekeratin and binding of peanut agglutinin. *Virchows Arch. (Cell Pathos.) 44:* 187–199, 1983.

51. Moll, R., Franke, W. W., Schiller, D. L., *et al.* The catalog of human cytokeratins: Patterns of expression in normal epithelia, tumors and cultured cells. *Cell 31:* 11–24, 1982.

52. Murray, M. R., and Stout, A. P. Distinctive characteristics of the sympathicoblastoma cultivated *in vitro. Am. J. Pathol. 23:* 429–441, 1947.

53. Nadler, L. M., Ritz, J., Griffin, J. D., *et al.* Diagnosis and treatment of human leukemias and lymphomas utilizing monoclonal antibodies. *Prog. Hematol. 12:* 187–225, 1981.

54. Nakajima, T., Watanabe, S., Sato, Y., *et al.* An immunoperoxidase study of S-100 protein distribution in normal and neoplastic tissues. *Am. J. Surg. Pathol. 6:* 715–727, 1982.

55. Nelson, W. G., Battifora, H., Santana, H., and Sun, T-T. Specific keratins as molecular markers for neoplasms with a stratified epithelial origin. *Cancer Res. 44:* 1600–1603, 1984.

56. Omary, M. B., Trowbridge, I. S., and Battifora, H. A. Human homologue of murine T200 glycoprotein. *J. Exp. Med. 152:* 842–852, 1980.

57. Osborn, M., and Weber, K. Tumor diagnosis by intermediate filament typing: A novel tool for surgical pathology. *Lab. Invest. 48:* 372, 1983.

58. Ramaekers, F. C. S., Haag, D., Kant, A., *et al.* Coexpression of keratin- and vimentin-type intermediate filaments in human metastatic carcinoma cells. *Proc. Natl. Acad. Sci. USA 80:* 2618–2622, 1983.

59. Reynolds, C. P., Frenkel, E. P., and Smith, R. G. Growth characteristics of neuroblastoma *in vitro* correlate with patient survival. *Trans. Assoc. Am. Phys. 93:* 203–211, 1980.

60. Reynolds, C. P., German, D. C., Weinberg, A. G., and Smith, R. G. Catecholamine fluorescence and tissue culture morphology. Technics in the diagnosis of neuroblastoma. *Am. J. Clin. Pathol. 75:* 275–282, 1981.

61. Reynolds, C. P., Smith, R. G., and Frenkel, E. P. The diagnostic dilemma of the "small round cell neoplasm." Catecholamine fluorescence and tissue culture morphology as markers for neuroblastoma. *Cancer 48:* 2088–2094, 1981.

62. Scheiner, C., Aubert, C., Rorsman, M., *et al.* Neuroblastome. Apport de la biochimie et de la culture cellulaire au diagnostic d'une forme indifferenciee. *Ann. Anat. Pathol. 22:* 349–359, 1977.

63. Schlegel, R., Banks-Schlegel, S., and Pinkus, G. S. Immunohistochemical localization of keratin in normal human tissues. *Lab. Invest. 42:* 91, 1980.

64. Schmechel, D., Marangos, P. J., and Brightman, M. Neurone-specific enolase is a molecular marker for peripheral and central neuroendocrine cells. *Nature 276:* 834–835, 1978.

65. Schmechel, D., Marangos, P. J., Zis, A. P., *et al.* Brain enolases as specific markers of neuronal and glial cells. *Science 199:* 313–315, 1978.

66. Schmidt, D., and Mackay, B. Ultrastructure of human tendon sheath and synovium: Implications for tumor histogenesis. *Ultrastruct. Pathol. 3:* 269–283, 1982.

67. Schwab, M., Alitalo, K., Klempnauer, K-H, *et al.* Amplified DNA with limited homology to myc cellular oncogene is shared by human neuroblastoma cell lines and a neuroblastoma tumour. *Nature 305:* 245–248, 1983.

68. Schwab, M., Ellison, J., Busch, M., *et al.* Enhanced expression of the human gene N-myc consequent to amplification of DNA may contribute to malignant progression of neuroblastoma. *Proc. Natl. Acad. Sci. USA 81:* 4940–4944, 1984.

69. Schwab, M., Varmus, H. E., Bishop, J. M., *et al.* Chromosome localization in normal human cells and neuroblastomas of a gene related to c-myc. *Nature 308:* 288–291, 1984.

70. Sheppard, M. N., Corrin, B., Bennett, M. H., *et al.* Immunocytochemical localization of neuron specific enolase in small cell carcinomas and carcinoid tumours of the lung. *Histopathology 8:* 171–181, 1984.

71. Sidell, N., Altman, A., Haussler, M. R., and Seeger, R. C. Effects of retinoic acid (RA) on the growth and phenotypic expression of several human neuroblastoma cell lines. *Exp. Cell Res. 148:* 21–30, 1983.

72. Sondergaard, K., Henschel, A., and Hou-Jensen, K. Metastatic melanoma with balloon cell changes: An electron microscopic study. *Ultrastruct. Pathol. 1:* 357–360, 1980.

73. Takahashi, K., Isobe, T., Ohtsuki, Y., *et al.* Immunohistochemical study on the distribution of α and β subunits of S-100 protein in human neoplasm and normal tissue. *Virchows Arch (Cell Pathol.) 45:* 385–396, 1984.

74. Trojanowski, J. Q., and Lee, V. M-Y. Monoclonal and polyclonal antibodies against neural antigens: Diagnostic applications for studies of central and peripheral nervous system tumors. *Hum. Pathol. 14:* 281–285, 1983.

75. Trojanowski, J. Q., Lee, V. M-Y., and Schlaepfer, W. W. An immunohistochemical study of human central and peripheral nervous system tumors, using monoclonal antibodies against neurofilaments and glial filaments. *Hum. Pathol. 15:* 248–257, 1984.

76. Tsokos, M., Linnoila, R. I., Chandra, R. S., and Triche, T. J. Neuron-specific enolase in the diagnosis of neuroblastoma and other small, round-cell tumors in children. *Hum. Pathol. 15:* 575–584, 1984.

77. Turc-Carel, C., Philip, I., Berger, M-P., *et al.* Chromosome study of Ewing's sarcoma (ES) cell lines. Consistency of a reciprocal translocation t(11;22)(q24;q12). *Cancer Genet. Cytogenet. 12:* 1–19, 1984.

78. Van der Valk, P., de Velde, J., Jansen, J., *et al.* Malignant lymphoma of true histiocytic origin: Histiocytic sarcoma. A morphological, ultrastructural, immunological, cytochemical and clinical study of 10 cases. *Virchows Arch (Pathol Anat.) 391:* 249–265, 1981.

79. Warnke, R. A., Gatter, K. C., Falini, B., *et al.* Diagnosis of human lymphoma with monoclonal antileukocyte antibodies. *N. Engl. J. Med. 309:* 1275–1281, 1983.

80. Watanabe, S., Nakajima, T., Shimosato, Y., *et al.* Malignant histiocytosis and Letterer-Siwe disease. Neoplasms of T-zone histiocyte with S-100 protein. *Cancer 51:* 1412–1424, 1983.

81. Weiss, S. W., Langloss, J. M., and Enzinger, F. M. Value of S-100 protein in the diagnosis of soft tissue tumors with particular reference to benign and malignant Schwann cell tumors. *Lab. Invest. 49:* 299–308, 1983.

82. Whang-Peng, J., Triche, T. J., Knutsen, T., *et al.* rcp(11;22)(q24;q12) in peripheral neuroepithelioma. *N. Engl. J. Med.*, 1985.

83. Wick, M. R., Scheithauer, B. W., and Kovacs, K. Neuron-specific enolase in neuroendocrine tumors of the thymus, bronchus, and skin. *Am. J. Clin. Pathol. 79:* 703–707, 1983.

Index

Page numbers in italics denote figures; those followed by "t" or "f" denote tables or footnotes, respectively.

Index